Functional Brain Tumor Imaging

Jay J. Pillai
Editor

Functional Brain Tumor Imaging

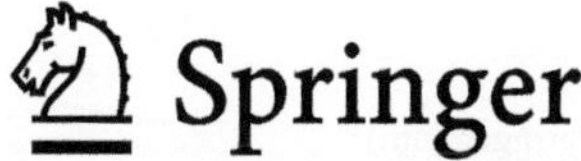

Editor
Jay J. Pillai, MD
Division of Neuroradiology
The Russell H. Morgan Department of Radiology and Radiological Science
Johns Hopkins University School of Medicine and The Johns Hopkins Hospital
Baltimore, MD, USA

ISBN 978-1-4419-5857-0 ISBN 978-1-4419-5858-7 (eBook)
DOI 10.1007/978-1-4419-5858-7
Springer New York Heidelberg Dordrecht London

Library of Congress Control Number: 2013949280

Printed on acid-free paper

Springer is part of Springer Science+Business Media (www.springer.com)

To my parents, brother, wife and two children,
as well as to my many professional mentors over the years.

Preface

The motivation for writing this book was the perceived need on the part of my neuroradiology trainees and colleagues at Johns Hopkins, as well as on the part of some of my neurosurgical and neuro-oncology colleagues, for a comprehensive but concise overview of current state-of-the-art clinical functional/physiologic imaging of brain tumors. Although innumerable research applications have been developed over the last couple of decades in the areas of blood oxygen level-dependent (BOLD) functional magnetic resonance imaging (fMRI), diffusion tensor imaging (DTI), magnetic source imaging/magnetoencephalography (MEG/MSI), MR perfusion imaging and magnetic resonance spectroscopic imaging (MRSI), no single book has been published to date that describes the clinical applications of all of these modalities as they relate specifically to brain tumor imaging. Furthermore, newer more advanced functional imaging techniques, such as sodium imaging at ultra-high field, amide proton transfer (APT) imaging, molecular imaging and high angular resolution diffusion imaging (HARDI), which are generally currently considered to be strictly research level, have found limited clinical application in some settings, and these newer modalities hold much promise for the future of brain tumor imaging. As such, I believe that our colleagues in neuroscience-related fields should be aware of these emerging modalities as well. To date no single book has ever attempted to bring together all of these seemingly disparate imaging modalities to explain how these are currently applied to brain tumor imaging, let alone explain how these may find future application. Thus, although the title of the book suggests an emphasis on BOLD fMRI, I prefer to consider "functional imaging" in its broader context as physiologic imaging. I believe that this book provides a unique conglomeration of descriptions of different techniques that enable physicians in neuro-oncology, neurosurgery, and neuroradiology the opportunity to examine the actual tumor biology and physiology rather than simply rely on current structural MR imaging, which provides very nonspecific information regarding de novo histology, overall prognosis, and therapeutic response. My hope is that understanding of these physiologic imaging modalities and their current applications will serve as a catalyst for future generations of physicians and scientists to build upon what is currently available to improve the overall standard of care for these patients. This book should be useful also to medical students and researchers in the neurosciences who want to quickly learn about what is currently state of the art in physiologic brain tumor imaging as described by those who are recognized leaders in their respective fields, without having to search through countless research papers to build a foundation of knowledge related to these emerging technologies.

The book is divided into three sections. The first deals primarily with the diagnosis and characterization of brain tumors, with three chapters devoted to MR perfusion imaging, DTI, and MRSI, respectively. The second section deals with applications of physiologic/functional imaging to treatment planning and monitoring of therapeutic intervention. This section contains a total of six chapters, including two chapters on BOLD imaging for presurgical mapping (one covering language function and another motor function), one chapter on DTI for presurgical mapping, one on MEG/MSI applications to neurosurgery, one on PET imaging of brain tumors, and one on MRSI of brain tumors. The last section covers future directions in physiologic brain tumor imaging. This last section includes five chapters covering the following topics: APT, HARDI, and other advanced diffusion imaging for surgical planning, ultra-high field MRSI, sodium MRI for the management of human high-grade brain tumors, and future clinical applications of molecular imaging.

The planning and generation of this manuscript required three years of effort to compile contributions from many of the renowned experts in functional imaging, and striking the right balance of descriptions of clinical applications and future potential proved to be challenging. Furthermore, the rapidly evolving nature of these fields made it even more challenging to provide an overview that is truly up-to-date. Much of the current work in genomics and connectomics is extremely preliminary and has not yet found its application in brain tumor imaging, and thus these aspects have been deliberately omitted from this first edition, but as their contributions emerge in the near future, attempts will be made to incorporate them into future editions. It is for this reason that resting state fMRI and diffusion spectrum imaging have been avoided, although these are currently active areas of functional imaging research, both at my institution and across many others in the United States and abroad. However, description of the basics of molecular imaging has been included, because this is one area where clinical translation with respect to brain tumors in the very near future is likely. The authors of the respective chapters and I hope that the readers of this unique volume find the contents to be both enlightening with respect to research applications and clinically useful at the same time. In the end, pragmatic concerns trumped the need to include esoterica, and thus both clinicians and scientists in neuroscience fields will hopefully share my own perspective and find this to be an important contribution to the brain tumor imaging literature that will serve to advance both patient care and research in this rapidly developing field.

Baltimore, MD, USA Jay J. Pillai, MD

Contents

Part I Diagnosis and Characterization of Brain Tumors

1 **MR Perfusion Imaging: ASL, T2*-Weighted DSC, and T1-Weighted DCE Methods** ... 3
Mark S. Shiroishi, Jesse G.A. Jones, Naira Muradyan, Saulo Lacerda, Bihong T. Chen, John L. Go, and Meng Law

2 **Diffusion Tensor Imaging: Introduction and Applications to Brain Tumor Characterization** ... 27
Sumei Wang, Sungheon Kim, and Elias R. Melhem

3 **Diagnosis and Characterization of Brain Tumors: MR Spectroscopic Imaging** ... 39
Peter B. Barker

Part II Physiologic Imaging for Planning and Monitoring of Therapeutic Intervention

4 **BOLD fMRI for Presurgical Planning: Part I** ... 59
Domenico Zacá and Jay J. Pillai

5 **BOLD fMRI for Presurgical Planning: Part II** ... 79
Meredith Gabriel, Nicole P. Brennan, Kyung K. Peck, and Andrei I. Holodny

6 **DTI for Presurgical Mapping** ... 95
Andrew P. Klein, John L. Ulmer, Wade M. Mueller, Flavius D. Raslau, Wolfgang Gaggl, and Mohit Maheshwari

7 **Magnetoencephalographic Imaging for Neurosurgery** ... 111
Phiroz E. Tarapore, Edward F. Chang, Rodney Gabriel, Mitchel S. Berger, and Srikantan S. Nagarajan

8 **Imaging Metabolic and Molecular Functions in Brain Tumors with Positron Emission Tomography (PET)** ... 129
Beril Gok and Richard L. Wahl

9 **Proton Magnetic Resonance Spectroscopy and Spectroscopic Imaging of Primary Brain Tumors** 143
Lester Kwock

Part III Future Directions in Physiologic Brain Tumor Imaging

10 **Role of Amide Proton Transfer (APT)-MRI of Endogenous Proteins and Peptides in Brain Tumor Imaging** 171
Silun Wang, Samson Jarso, Peter C.M. van Zijl, and Jinyuan Zhou

11 **Advanced Diffusion MR Tractography for Surgical Planning** 183
Jeffrey I. Berman

12 **Ultra-High Field MRSI (7T and Beyond)** 195
Peter B. Barker

13 **Sodium Magnetic Resonance Imaging in the Management of Human High-Grade Brain Tumors** 211
Keith R. Thulborn, Ian C. Atkinson, Andrew Shon, Neil A. Das Gupta, John L. Villano, Tamir Y. Hersonskey, and Aiming Lu

14 **Future Clinical Applications of Molecular Imaging: Nanoparticles, Cellular Probes, and Imaging of Gene Expression** 225
Arnav Mehta, Ketan B. Ghaghada, and Srinivasan Mukundan Jr.

Editor's Biography 239

Index 241

Contributors

Ian C. Atkinson, PhD Center for Magnetic Resonance Research, University of Illinois Medical Center, Chicago, IL, USA

Peter B. Barker, DPhil Department of Radiology, Johns Hopkins University School of Medicine, Baltimore, MD, USA

Mitchel S. Berger, MD Department of Neurological Surgery, University of California, San Francisco, CA, USA

Jeffrey I. Berman, PhD Children's Hospital of Philadelphia, and University of Pennsylvania Perelman School of Medicine, Philadelphia, PA, USA

Nicole P. Brennan, BA Department of Radiology, Functional MRI Laboratory, Memorial Sloan-Kettering Cancer Center, New York, NY, USA

Edward F. Chang, MD Department of Neurological Surgery, University of California, San Francisco, CA, USA

Bihong T. Chen, MD Department of Radiology, City of Hope, Duarte, CA, USA

Neil A. Das Gupta, MD Department of Radiation Oncology, Fox Valley Radiation Oncology, Naperville, IL, USA

Meredith Gabriel Department of Radiology, Functional MRI Laboratory, Memorial Sloan-Kettering Cancer Center, New York, NY, USA

Rodney Gabriel, BS Department of Radiology and Biomedical Imaging, University of California, San Francisco, CA, USA

Wolfgang Gaggl, MSE Department of Radiology, Medical College of Wisconsin, Milwaukee, WI, USA

Ketan B. Ghaghada, PhD School of Biomedical Informatics, University of Texas Health Science Center, Houston, TX, USA

John L. Go, MD Departments of Radiology and Otolaryngology, Division of Neuroradiology, Keck School of Medicine, University of Southern California, Los Angeles, CA, USA

Beril Gok, MD Division of Nuclear Medicine, Department of Radiology, Johns Hopkins Hospital, Baltimore, MD, USA

Tamir Y. Hersonskey, MD Provena St. Joseph Medical Center, Joliet, IL, USA

Andrei I. Holodny, MD Department of Radiology, Functional MRI Laboratory, Memorial Sloan-Kettering Cancer Center, Weill Medical College of Cornell University, New York, NY, USA

Samson Jarso Department of Radiology, Johns Hopkins University School of Medicine, Baltimore, MD, USA

F.M. Kirby Research Center for Functional Brain Imaging, Kennedy Krieger Institute, Baltimore, MD, USA

Jesse G.A. Jones, MD Division of Neuroradiology, Department of Radiology, Keck School of Medicine, University of Southern California, Los Angeles, CA, USA

Sungheon Kim, PhD Department of Radiology, Center for Biomedical Imaging, New York University School of Medicine, New York, NY, USA

Andrew P. Klein, MD Department of Radiology, Medical College of Wisconsin, Milwaukee, WI, USA

Lester Kwock, PhD Department of Radiology, University of North Carolina, School of Medicine, Chapel Hill, NC, USA

Saulo Lacerda, MD Department of Radiology, MedImagem-Hospital Beneficencia Portuguesa, São Paulo, SP, Brazil

Meng Law, MD, MBBS, FRACR Department of Radiology, USC Medical Center, Los Angeles, CA, USA

Aiming Lu, PhD Center for Magnetic Resonance Research, University of Illinois Medical Center, Chicago, IL, USA

Mohit Maheshwari, MD Children's Hospital and Health System, Medical College of Wisconsin, Wauwatosa, WI, USA

Arnav Mehta, BS Division of Biology, California Institute of Technology, Pasadena, CA, USA

Elias R. Melhem, MD Department of Diagnostic Radiology and Nuclear Medicine, University of Maryland School of Medicine, Baltimore, MD, USA

Wade M. Mueller, MD Department of Neurosurgery, Medical College of Wisconsin, Milwaukee, WI, USA

Srinivasan Mukundan Jr, MD, PhD Brigham and Women's Hospital, Boston, MA, USA

Naira Muradyan, PhD iCAD, Inc., Nashua, NH, USA

Srikantan S. Nagarajan, PhD Department of Radiology and Biomedical Imaging, University of California, San Francisco, CA, USA

Kyung K. Peck, PhD Department of Radiology, Functional MRI Laboratory, Memorial Sloan-Kettering Cancer Center, New York, NY, USA

Jay J. Pillai, MD Division of Neuroradiology, Russell H. Morgan Department of Radiology and Radiological Science, Johns Hopkins University School of Medicine, Baltimore, MD, USA

Flavius D. Raslau, MD Department of Radiology, Medical College of Wisconsin, Milwaukee, WI, USA

Mark S. Shiroishi Department of Radiology, Keck Medical Center, Keck School of Medicine, University of Southern California, Los Angeles, CA, USA

Andrew Shon Department of Radiology, Physiology and Biophysics, Center for Magnetic Resonance Research, University of Illinois Medical Center, Chicago, IL, USA

Phiroz E. Tarapore, MD Department of Neurological Surgery, University of California, San Francisco, CA, USA

Keith R. Thulborn, MD, PhD Center for Magnetic Resonance Research, University of Illinois Medical Center, Chicago, IL, USA

John L. Ulmer, MD Department of Radiology, Medical College of Wisconsin, Milwaukee, WI, USA

Peter C.M. van Zijl, PhD Department of Radiology, Johns Hopkins University School of Medicine, Baltimore, MD, USA

F.M. Kirby Research Center for Functional Brain Imaging, Kennedy Krieger Institute, Baltimore, MD, USA

John L. Villano, MD Neuro-Oncology Program, University of Illinois, Chicago, IL, USA

Richard L. Wahl, MD Division of Nuclear Medicine, Department of Radiology, Johns Hopkins Hospital, Baltimore, MD, USA

Silun Wang Department of Radiology, Johns Hopkins University School of Medicine, Baltimore, MD, USA

Sumei Wang, MD Division of Neuroradiology, Department of Radiology, Hospital of the University of Pennsylvania, Philadelphia, PA, USA

Domenico Zacá, PhD MR Lab, Center for Mind Brain Sciences, University of Trento, USA

Jinyuan Zhou, PhD Department of Radiology, Johns Hopkins University School of Medicine, Baltimore, MD, USA

F.M. Kirby Research Center for Functional Brain Imaging, Kennedy Krieger Institute, Baltimore, MD, USA

Part I

Diagnosis and Characterization of Brain Tumors

MR Perfusion Imaging: ASL, T2*-Weighted DSC, and T1-Weighted DCE Methods

1

Mark S. Shiroishi, Jesse G.A. Jones, Naira Muradyan, Saulo Lacerda, Bihong T. Chen, John L. Go, and Meng Law

Tumor Biology

Angiogenesis underlies all tumor growth by providing oxygen and nutrients to support increased cellular proliferation and metabolism and to remove waste products. However, tumors cannot create their own blood supply and when malignant tumors are very small, they rely principally on diffusion for survival [3]. If a tumor is to grow beyond a few millimeters in size, angiogenesis will be required [4]. In the central nervous system, gliomas are most studied tumors with regard to MR perfusion imaging and are the primary focus of this discussion.

Glioblastomas produce a number of proangiogenic factors including vascular endothelial growth factor (VEGF), platelet-derived growth factor (PDGF), basic fibroblast growth factor (bFGF), and scatter factor/hepatic growth factor (SF/HGF) [5]. VEGF is the best characterized of these factors [6, 7]. Within the VEGF family are VEGF-A, VEGF-B, VEGF-C, VEGF-D, and placental growth factor (PlGF), but only VEGF-A has been implicated in pathologic angiogenesis [8]. It has also been shown to be a prime vascular permeability factor that contributes to the development of vasogenic edema [9–11]. VEGF acts on the VEGF receptor 2 (VEGFR-2) of endothelial cells via a paracrine loop [12]. VEGF expression varies with tumor type and grade with the greatest seen in glial tumors where expression levels are directly correlated to tumor grade [13–15]. Dedifferentiation of a low-grade into a high-grade glioma involves turning an angiogenic "switch" whereby the balance of vascular inhibitors and promoters is disrupted by overexpression of factors such as VEGF [16]. Astrocytomas initially grow around existing vasculature through a process termed blood vessel co-option. Proliferation 1–2 mm beyond this zone results in hypoxia and necrosis, upregulating hypoxia-inducible factor (HIF) which in turn promotes VEGF expression [17].

M.S. Shiroishi (✉)
Department of Radiology, Keck Medical Center, Keck School of Medicine, University of Southern California, 1520 San Pablo St., Lower Level Imaging L1600, Los Angeles, CA 90033, USA
e-mail: Mark.Shiroishi@med.usc.edu

J.G.A. Jones
Division of Neuroradiology, Department of Radiology, Keck School of Medicine, University of Southern California, Los Angeles, CA, USA

N. Muradyan, Ph.D.
iCAD, Inc., Nashua, NH, USA

S. Lacerda, M.D.
Department of Radiology, MedImagem-Hospital Beneficencia Portuguesa, São Paulo, SP, Brazil

B.T. Chen, M.D.
Department of Radiology, City of Hope, Duarte, CA, USA

John L. Go
Department of Radiology and Otolaryngology, Division of Neuroradiology, Keck School of Medicine, University of Southern California, Los Angeles, CA, USA

M. Law, M.D., M.B.B.S., F.R.A.C.R.
Department of Radiology, USC Medical Center, Los Angeles, CA, USA

J.J. Pillai (ed.), *Functional Brain Tumor Imaging*, DOI 10.1007/978-1-4419-5858-7_1,

T2*-Weighted Dynamic Susceptibility Contrast MR Imaging

Dynamic susceptibility contrast (DSC) perfusion MR imaging, also known as bolus-tracking MRI, represents the most commonly used, clinically validated method of calculating relative cerebral blood volume (rCBV). Absolute values of CBV are typically not obtained because of the technical difficulties encountered with determination of the arterial input function (AIF). Following the bolus intravenous injection of an exogenous, nondiffusible, paramagnetic gadolinium-based contrast agent (GBCA), rapid repeated imaging depicts reduction of signal intensity within the vasculature during the first-pass of bolus administration. For each voxel, a signal intensity–time curve is generated. In the absence of significant contrast agent leakage or recirculation, the transverse relaxivity on spin echo (R2) or gradient echo (R2*) is expressed as

$$\Delta R2^* = \frac{-\ln\left[\frac{SI_t}{SI_0}\right]}{TE}$$

where SI_t is signal intensity at time t, SI_0 is prior to contrast arrival, and TE denotes echo time.

$\Delta R2^*$ is generally assumed to be linearly proportional to contrast agent concentration, although this relationship has been questioned [18–20]. CBV is proportional to the area under the contrast agent concentration–time curve [21–23].

The most commonly used technique in DSC perfusion MRI employs single-shot echo planar imaging (EPI) because it provides very rapid image acquisition. It is usually performed in conjunction with multislice gradient echo (GRE) sequences. Spin echo (SE)-EPI methods have also been used by some. GRE sequences have a higher signal-to-noise ratio (SNR) than SE and therefore allow the use of half the amount of GBCA. GRE also appears to be sensitive to both capillaries and larger vessels while SE is more sensitive to capillaries within a voxel [24]. SE tends to result in fewer susceptibility artifacts compared with GRE sequences and is more sensitive to paramagnetic effects within smaller versus larger vessels. While early studies appeared to demonstrate the utility of SE techniques to grade gliomas, it now appears that GRE demonstrates a better correlation with glioma grade. This is likely due to the fact that the angiogenesis associated with these tumors results in enlarged microvessels that do not resemble capillaries [25–28].

A dose of 0.1 mmol/kg of a GBCA is typically used with a standard GRE-EPI technique. 2D sequences are generally preferred compared to 3D sequences because of their ability to achieve better spatial resolution and shorter TRs and provide a more accurate characterization of bolus passage [29, 30]. In cases where increased spatial coverage is desired, 3D sequences can be substituted. When drawing regions of interest (ROIs), care must be taken to avoid large vessels as GRE sequences are sensitive to macrovessels [26]. Techniques combining SE/GRE methods have been used to determine relative vessel size during antiangiogenic drug treatment [25, 31, 32].

Because traditional T1 dynamic contrast-enhanced (DCE) MRI methods to measure permeability may require minutes (and sometimes hours), there has been some interest in first-pass methods to derive this parameter [27, 33, 34]. Work by Cha et al. recently showed that K^{trans} derived by first-pass DSC methods was well correlated in gliomas compared with steady-state T1 DCE methods, but not so in meningiomas [35]. Other metrics derived from DSC data such as percent signal recovery (PSR) can also give insight into vascular permeability; however, most permeability imaging is currently performed using T1W DCE [36].

Limitations

Contrast agent leakage: Following bolus intravenous injection, the paramagnetic properties of a GBCA induce shortening of T1 and T2/T2* relaxation times of water [37]. Dipole–dipole interactions between tissue water protons and the paramagnetic ions of the GBCA underlie the decrease in T1 relaxation [38]. Because these dipole–dipole interactions are active at only *very short* distances and so the spins to be shortened must be in very close proximity to the gadolinium atom, a marked T1 effect and T1-weighted enhancement will be noted in a region with direct access to a uniform distribution of contrast agent. As a result, intravascular GBCA produces T1 shortening and signal enhancement of the blood pool itself. There is not a significant T2* effect because the uniform distribution of contrast agent does not result in susceptibility-induced gradients.

A different principle underlies the shortening of the T2/T2* relaxation time where susceptibility-induced gradients surround the paramagnetic GBCA and result in spin dephasing. Because the GBCA is compartmentalized within the vascular compartment, there will be a minimal T1 effect and a substantial T2* decrease that extends *beyond* the capillaries [39–41]. This extension of the susceptibility effect into the surrounding tissues results in a more pronounced signal decrease than would be expected relying on only intravascular effects [42].

Preservation of the blood–brain barrier (BBB) allows GBCAs to serve as intravascular tracers during application of the indicator dilution theory in DSC [43]. However, BBB disruption is common in brain tumors as well as other CNS pathologies and this leads to leakage of GBCA into the extravascular extracellular space (EES). This loss of compartmentalization and contrast agent leakage result in competing T1 relaxivity, dipolar T2, and residual T2* effects that interfere with susceptibility signal loss. Without correction algorithms, T1 effects may result in underestimation while T2 and T2* effects may result in overestimation of rCBV [44]. Further complicating matters is that opposing T1 and T2/T2* effects may be present concurrently [45].

There are numerous strategies that have been applied to address leakage correction. These include not correcting for leakage, but mentioning it as a possible confounding variable, only post-processing perfusion data from regions that do not enhance, obtaining dual-echo T2* acquisitions, using low-flip-angle GRE and various mathematical modeling approaches [46–50]. An empirical method that has been proposed involves preloading with GBCA prior to the DSC acquisition in an attempt to saturate the EES tissue T1-weighted signal intensity. This, in theory, should decrease the T1-induced signal intensity increase during the subsequent DSC bolus gadolinium contrast agent administration [44, 45]. A recent preliminary study that combined preload dosing of contrast agent (0.1 mmol/kg) with 6 min of incubation time along with baseline subtraction techniques appeared to improve the diagnostic accuracy of rCBV to differentiate between recurrent glioma and radiation effect [51].

A T1W DCE sequence may be acquired during the preload GBCA administration. At our institution, we administer a 0.05 mmol/kg bolus injection of gadolinium contrast agent during the preload dosing to acquire T1W DCE permeability data. Conventional sequences such as T2-weighted imaging can then be obtained. Then a second 0.05 mmol/kg bolus injection of contrast agent is performed to obtain T2*-w DSC perfusion data.

Alternatives to GBCAs such as macromolecular contrast media (MMCM) or true blood pool agents (molecular weight >50 kDA) are a potential solution to the problem of contrast agent leakage in DSC MRI. These agents remain in the vascular space for a prolonged period of time following injection. However, there are currently no agents that have been approved for routine clinical use. Superparamagnetic iron oxide (SPIO) nanoparticles are a type of MMCM that have been explored as an MRI contrast for brain imaging applications [52]. Recent work involving the use of the iron oxide nanoparticle agent ferumoxytol may provide more accurate estimates of rCBV given its ability to serve as a blood pool agent and not leak out through a damaged BBB in the short term (minutes to hours) [53]. It does appear to slowly leak across a damaged BBB over time, though the mechanism is unclear. Ferumoxytol is unique among iron oxide nanoparticle contrast agents in that it can be safely administered in a rapid bolus fashion and appears to be safe in patients with renal dysfunction where the risk of nephrogenic systemic fibrosis (NSF) is a concern [54].

Other blood pool agents such as albumin, polysaccharide, and polylysine have been explored as alternatives to standard GBCAs; however, they have never reached clinical testing [55–58]. The slow clearance rate of these agents is a potential safety concern [59].

Artifacts: T2*-w DSC imaging is prone to artifact from bone, air, and blood that constitute another source of potential error. Postoperative patients or those harboring tumors at the skull base or postoperative changes may benefit from SE rather than GRE DSC MRI. Reducing slice thickness and applying parallel imaging also limit susceptibility artifact with minimal loss to SNR [24, 60, 61].

T1-Weighted Dynamic Contrast-Enhanced MRI

T1-weighted DCE MR imaging, sometimes referred to as permeability MR imaging, also measures changes in tissue signal intensity over time with administration of a GBCA. However, it typically uses more complex pharmacokinetic models (PKMs) than T2 or T2* DSC perfusion imaging. Resultant analysis of DCE data provides greater tissue detail; however, it incorporates several assumptions that may lead to potential errors. Standard imaging protocols measure T1 relaxation rate before, during, and after the IV administration of a GBCA over several minutes by repeatedly imaging an ROI. A T1-weighted GRE- or spoiled gradient echo (SPGR)-type sequence may be utilized in DCE MRI. The latter is less sensitive to T2 effects that degrade the T1 signal intensity, but with inferior SNR compared to GRE. However, improvement of SNR can be accomplished with the use of 3-dimensional SPGR or equivalent techniques [62]. The techniques used place demands, often conflicting, on high temporal resolution, high spatial resolution, SNR, and anatomical coverage [63].

In general, the acquisition of T1W DCE data involves the use of pre-contrast T1 mapping techniques and dynamic 3D acquisition to create a set of images that give an estimated GBCA concentration at each location and time point. These are then combined with an estimate of the AIF and a PKM to determine metrics such as the volume transfer constant (K^{trans}) and fractional volume of the EES (v_e). PKMs which incorporate the contribution of intravascular tracer to the MR signal will also provide the fractional plasma volume (v_p). *Note that $V_e = v_e \times$ total tissue volume (V_t) and $V_p = v_p \times V_t$ [64].

Signal intensity changes with time must be converted into GBCA concentration–time curves to perform PKM. Unlike computed tomography perfusion, the relationship between MR signal intensity and GBCA concentration is not always linear [65]. Accurate determination of GBCA tissue concentration from T1 mapping can be facilitated by numerous techniques such as the variable flip angle approach, in which baseline pre-contrast T1W images with variable flip angles are acquired just prior to the DCE acquisition. Nevertheless, rapid changes in GBCA tissue concentration (C_t) following the contrast bolus administration impose challenges for measuring T1 quickly over a wide range of values and under conditions of often poor SNR:

$$1/\mathrm{T1} = 1/\mathrm{T1}_0 + R_1 C_t$$

where $\mathrm{T1}_0$ is the relaxation rate before contrast agent injection and R_1 is the relaxivity of the contrast agent [64].

DCE MRI acquisition time plays a major role in brain tumor imaging, where pathologic tissue enhances rapidly. Greater temporal resolution allows for more sophisticated PKM that can determine physiologic markers such as K^{trans} with superior specificity [66]. Iron oxide nanoparticles used as blood pool agents may also improve DCE acquisitions, as less demanding temporal resolution would allow for longer acquisition times to measure permeability [67].

Various PKMs have been developed to fit the contrast agent concentration–time curves of brain tissues to estimate vascular permeability. Arterial flow to the ROI, otherwise known as the AIF, can be determined from DCE data, or, if necessary, estimated from published standards [68]. In most PKMs, it is assumed that the GBCA occupies two tissue compartments: the capillary plasma space (v_p) and the EES (v_e) (Fig. 1.1). The volume transfer constant between the capillary plasma

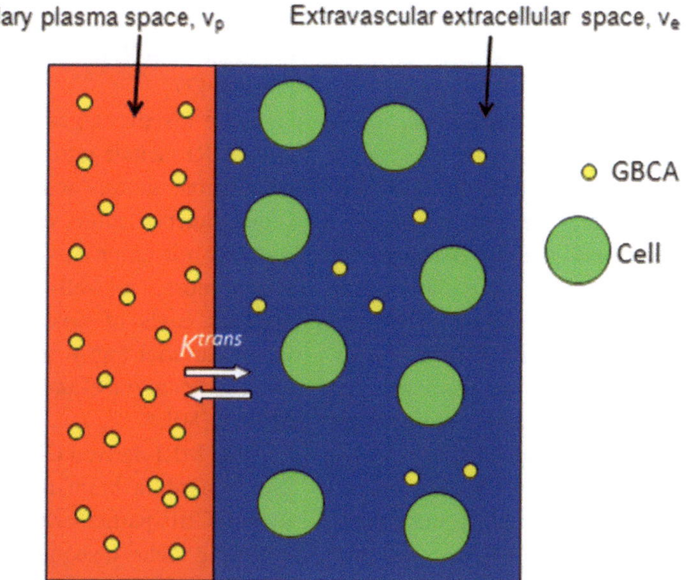

Fig. 1.1 Schematic depicting the two-compartment PKM for contrast agent tracers (GBCA). The GBCA passes from the capillary plasma space (v_p) into the extravascular extracellular space [EES] (v_e). K^{trans} represents the volume transfer constant between the capillary plasma volume and the EES. All GBCAs in clinical use are excluded from the intracellular space

space and EES, K^{trans}, is the most widely utilized vascular permeability metric. It represents a potentially intractable combination of flow, permeability, and surface area [69]. Even with rapid imaging techniques, the temporal resolution may not be able to differentiate the contribution of each factor in the resultant K^{trans} and so the physiologic meaning can differ. Added to this are variations in DCE technique which can make comparison of literature values of K^{trans} problematic [66, 70, 71]. Following IV bolus administration, GBCA initially diffuses within plasma alone, referred to as the vascular or first-pass phase. Regions of BBB disruption then allow GBCA extravasation into v_e. Simpler PKMs ignore the contribution of intravascular GBCA ($v_p = 0$) since the vascular volume in normal brain tissues is small, about 5 %, and the GBCA in the EES is assumed to represent the total GBCA in the tissue of interest [64].

Under conditions of abundant flow and limited permeability, K^{trans} is then equal to the permeability endothelial surface area product (PS) per unit mass of tissue and tissue density (ρ):

$$K^{trans} = PS\rho$$

However, flow-limited tissues such as the necrotic core of a GBM affect K^{trans} differently:

$$K^{trans} = F\rho(1 - \mathrm{Hct})$$

where F denotes blood flow and Hct is hematocrit.

K^{trans} derived from simple PKMs are not as robust as from more complex models incorporating v_p. Highly vascular tumors possess larger intravascular compartments compared with healthy tissues, and require knowledge of the vascular contribution (v_p) into the overall tissue contrast agent concentration. Isolating v_p may also prove useful as a comparison to rCBV derived from DSC, especially in cases where artifacts from bone, air, or blood produce undesirable susceptibility.

More complex modeling such as the adiabatic tissue homogeneity model allows the effects of flow to be differentiated from surface area and capillary permeability [72]. In this model, the intravascular contrast agent concentration is defined in terms of both time and distance within the capillary. However, this complex model requires very high temporal resolution in the range of 1 s [65, 72].

Limitations

Although the prospect of microscopic tissue examination with DCE is enticing, K^{trans}, v_p, and v_e require histopathologic correlation in order to be validated. Animal studies have demonstrated a correlation between these DCE-driven metrics and tissue features such as microvascular density, although the relationship is highly dependent on the spatial resolution [73]. Further studies involving human biopsy and autopsy samples are needed.

Differences in image acquisition methods and PKMs across institutions create challenges when comparing DCE metrics. Quantitation enables description of vascular permeability, but numerical values for metrics such as K^{trans} can vary with scanner model, sequence choice, temporal and spatial resolution, AIF, and PKM used. Standardized imaging protocols attempt to minimize variation, although hardware variations, patient-dependent factors such as cardiac output, and the site of IV injection can confound results. Methodological variation has so far limited comparison of K^{trans} and other metrics, limiting the value of quantification.

Arterial Spin Labeling

Arterial spin labeling (ASL) is an MR perfusion technique capable of estimating absolute CBF without the use of an exogenous contrast agent, instead relying on magnetically labeled water protons as an endogenous tracer [19]. While there are many more perfusion imaging studies that employ exogenous GBCAs, ASL methods do offer some advantages. Because it does not require the injection of a GBCA, it can be considered completely noninvasive, thereby allowing easier repeated measurements, which is particularly notable given the possibility of nephrogenic systemic fibrosis in some patients [74]. Also, because ASL relies on a diffusible tracer (labeled arterial water) it appears to be relatively insensitive to permeability, a major confounder in rCBV [75]. Interestingly, a recent report of a CASL method with a twice-refocused spin-echo diffusion sequence appears to be able to quantify [76]. In addition, there is potential for ASL to be completely operator independent [77].

Some disadvantages of ASL compared with DSC MRI include intrinsically low SNR, longer acquisition times, and a relatively complex acquisition procedure, which may, in part, explain its lower utilization compared with DSC [77–79]. Furthermore, a well-known pitfall of ASL involves cases of severe ischemia where prolonged arterial transit times can result in relaxation of the spin label and produce underestimation of CBF [80].

DSC MRI-derived CBV has been the primary metric used in brain tumor perfusion imaging though CBF, particularly from ASL, has been an emerging focus. It should be noted, however, that CBV and MTT can, in theory, be obtained using ASL following technical modifications but are not yet widely available [81–85].

In an ASL acquisition, a radio-frequency (RF) pulse is used to magnetically "label" arterial blood water. This "label" decays with T1 relaxation, which is on the order of 1-2 [80]. Therefore, only a small amount of arterial spin-labeled water accumulates in the brain. A post-labeling delay is necessary to allow flow of magnetically labeled blood water into the microvasculature and tissue [86]. "Control" images are also obtained where there is no magnetic labeling of arterial blood water but where magnetization transfer effects are accounted for. Pairs of interleaved labeled and control images are produced where the static tissue signals are identical except for where the magnetization of the inflowing blood is different [87]. Labeled acquisitions are subtracted from control experiments without magnetization to determine CBF in ml/100 g/min [80]. The signal difference between inverted and control spins ranges between 0.5 and 1.5 % and experiments must be repeated several times to improve this poor SNR [77].

In practice there are about 30 different techniques of arterial blood labeling schemes and at least 6 different techniques to encode the labeled information during the inflow time and as many readout schemes, potentially leading to a great number of ASL technique variations [77, 78].

There are also multiple methods to quantify ASL-derived CBF without a clear optimal approach [19]. Furthermore, little is known regarding the validation, reproducibility, and sensitivity/specificity of these various methods [79, 88, 89].

While there are a multitude of acronyms in the ASL literature, the two main types of ASL techniques are continuous ASL (CASL) and pulsed ASL (PASL) [90–92]. CASL is the older technique where there is a prolonged RF pulse that continuously labels arterial blood water below the imaging slab until a steady state of tissue magnetization is reached [77]. One consequence of the prolonged RF pulse in CASL is that it leads to magnetization transfer (MT) effects [93]. If the MT effects are present only during the labeling scheme, overestimation of perfusion may result because the saturation effect of the macromolecular pool will result in reduced signal of the free water pool from the tissue of interest [94]. The lack of wide availability of continuous RF transmit hardware and the possibility for large deposition of RF energy into the patient, which can exceed FDA limits for specific absorption rate (SAR), are further issues that have limited the popularity of CASL [79].

While CASL does provide greater perfusion contrast, PASL is comparatively less technically demanding [95, 96]. In PASL, a short RF pulse is used to label a thick slab of arterial blood at a single point in time and imaging is performed following a period of time to allow distribution in the tissue of interest [87]. PASL techniques are divided into two categories depending on whether the labeling is applied in a symmetric or an asymmetric fashion relative to the imaging volume [95]. Compared to CASL, PASL techniques have lower RF power deposition and higher inversion efficiency [79]. A systematic bias in CBF calculation due to PASL's poorly defined distal edge of the labeling plane can be overcome with techniques that employ a saturation pulse following the inversion pulse to sharply define distal edge of the labeling plane [19, 97]. Pseudo-CASL is a relatively newer technique that is a compromise between PASL and CASL that may provide improved balance between labeling efficiency and SNR than conventional ASL methods [98].

Other technical modifications to improve SNR and image quality of ASL include the use of higher field strengths (i.e., 3 T or higher), background suppression of static tissue signal, and the use of a phased array coil as the receiver and introduction of fast 3D sequences as an alternative to traditional EPI approaches [96, 99–102]. Because absolute CBF must be corrected for age- and patient-dependent mean perfusion, relative rather than absolute CBF appears to be sufficient in brain tumor evaluation [103]. However, absolute values can allow comparison of values in a given individual patient throughout the course of treatment.

Clinical Applications of MR Perfusion Imaging

Primary Glial Neoplasms

Diagnosis, Grading, and Outcome: Determination of tumor grade is the most commonly published application of microvascular imaging biomarkers, and while histopathologic diagnosis remains the gold standard and in practice most suspicious tumors are biopsied, these studies can potentially validate these biomarkers [87]. Conventional contrast-enhanced MR imaging is not always accurate in predicting low-grade glioma (LGG) versus high-grade glioma (HGG) because while HGGs more commonly display contrast enhancement, it is not uncommon to be seen in LGG [104].

rCBV has been significantly correlated with histologic features of tumor aggressiveness including vascularity and mitotic activity [105, 106]. rCBV is directly related to elevated microvascular density, a histopathologic marker of malignancy [107]. A strong correlation between glioma grade and rCBV derived from DSC MRI has been well known [104, 108–111] (Figs. 1.2 and 1.3). Peak height, which is calculated as the difference between the pre-contrast T2*-weighted signal intensity and the minimum signal intensity, is an alternative DSC MRI metric that is strongly correlated with rCBV [107].

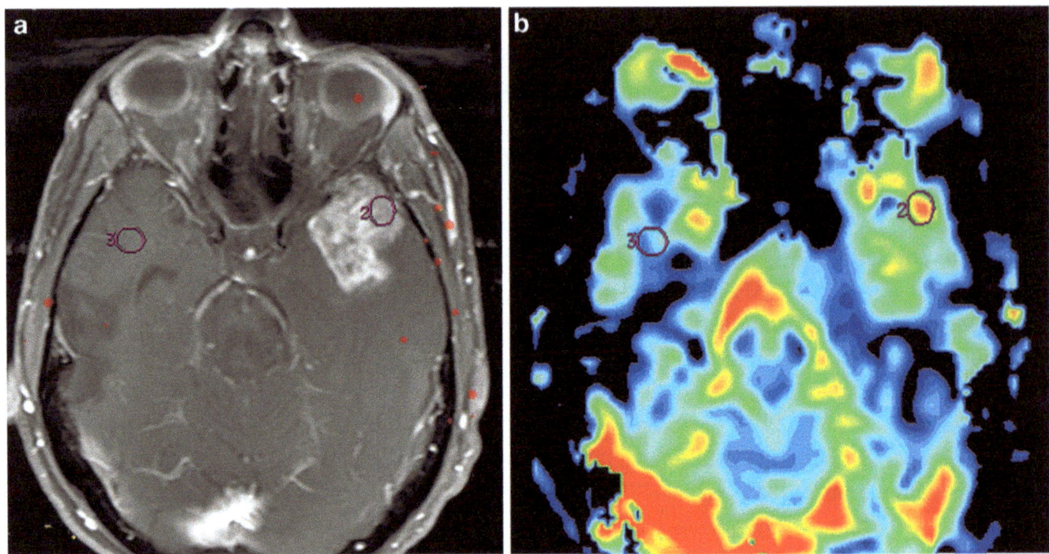

Fig. 1.2 MR perfusion for glioma grading is exemplified by this initial MRI of a 48-year-old man with headaches that revealed an enhancing left temporal lobe mass. Axial T1W post-contrast image (**a**) and accompanying rCBV colormap (**b**) demonstrates increased perfusion within the enhancing mass. A maximum rCBV of 3.04 is consistent with the pathologic diagnosis of GBM

Excluding tumors with oligodendroglial components, an $rCBV_{max} > 4.2$ was predictive of recurrence and $rCBV_{max} \leq 3.8$ was predictive of 1-year survival in astrocytomas [112]. A retrospective study of 189 patients with LGG and HGG demonstrated that an rCBV threshold of 1.75 was able to predict median time to progression independent of histopathological findings [113]. In LGGs undergoing malignant transformation, an increase in rCBV has also been demonstrated up to 12 months prior to the appearance of contrast enhancement on conventional MRI [114].

To address the paucity of multicenter perfusion MRI data in brain tumors, Caseiras et al. sought to examine the value of rCBV to predict clinical outcome in two institutions [115]. Using a standardized imaging and post-processing protocol, their study of 69 patients with LGG found that patients with an adverse event exhibited a significantly higher baseline rCBV than those without. Patients with an rCBV below 1.75 demonstrated a much longer time to progression compared to those above 1.75, implying that LGGs with higher rCBV are more likely to behave like HGGs.

As stated previously, in addition to being the primary agent involved in angiogenesis, VEGF is also a potent promoter of vascular permeability. K^{trans} has also been independently correlated with glioma grade; however the relationship appears to be less strong compared to rCBV [116, 117] (Figs. 1.3 and 1.4). A recent study of 28 patients using individual arterial input functions (iAIFs) and five flip angle T1 mapping at 1.5 T found that K^{trans} was not only able to distinguish LGGs (grade I and II) from HGGs (grade III and IV) but also grade II from grade III [118]. To address the effect of poor estimation of the vascular input function (VIP) on permeability metrics derived from DCE MRI, a recent study by Nguyen et al. employed a phase-derived VIP with the bookend T1 measurement to show that both K^{trans} and V_p derived from DCE MRI could differentiate LGG from HGGs [119]. The use of a phase-derived VIP may be helpful because changes in GBCA contrast agent concentration are known to vary in a *linear* fashion with phase changes in vessels that are more or less parallel to the magnetic field [120, 121]. A study using discriminant functional analysis to distinguish LGGs from HGGs using a combination of immunohistochemical parameters associated with tumor development (VEGF, MMPs, HIF-1α, PRL3 (phosphatase of regenerating liver 3)) and DCE metrics appeared to classify 92.1 %

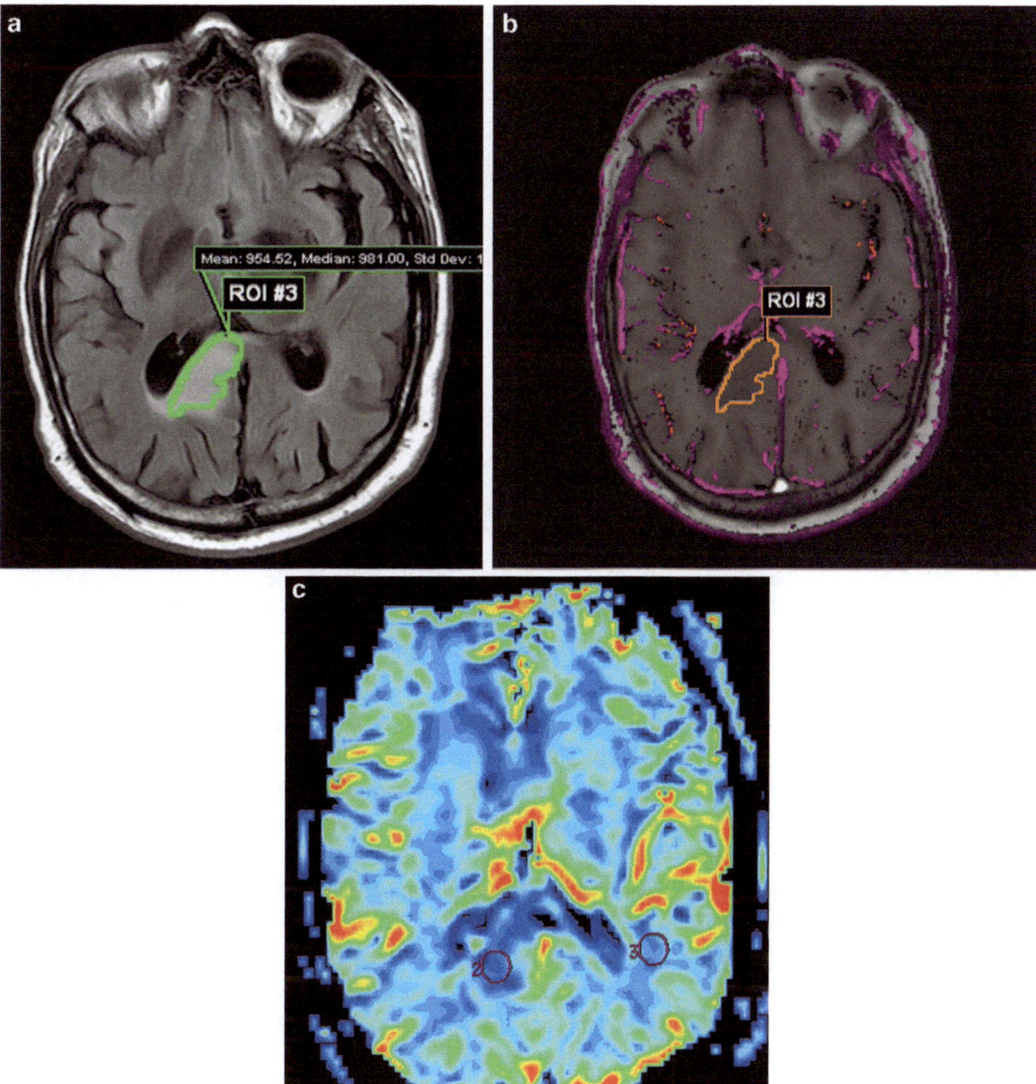

Fig. 1.3 Low-grade glioma in the right corpus callosum/periventricular white matter demonstrates FLAIR hyperintensity (**a**) without contrast enhancement. A volumetric ROI based on the FLAIR abnormality is transferred to K^{trans} colormap (**b**), where only sparse permeability is visualized. DSC MR data also support the diagnosis of LGG; rCBV colormap (**c**) shows low perfusion with a maximum rCBV of 0.5

of cases correctly overall [122]. HIF-1α expression was significantly correlated with rCBV and VEGF expression, rCBV and rCBF correlated with VEGF expression, and MMP-9 expression correlated with k_{ep} (rate constant between EES and plasma).

Most DCE MRI studies of brain tumors have focused on K^{trans} while v_e has been traditionally overlooked. Increased cellularity and grade have been correlated with decreased ADC in gliomas [123–125]. By logical extension, it would seem that since v_e is an estimate of the fractional volume of the EES, both ADC and v_e should be positively correlated. Mills et al. performed the first examination of this hypothesis in glioblastomas and, interestingly, they were not able to demonstrate a correlation between these two measures [126]. This could be a reflection of the current incomplete understanding of these metrics and how they describe the EES; however, the heterogeneous

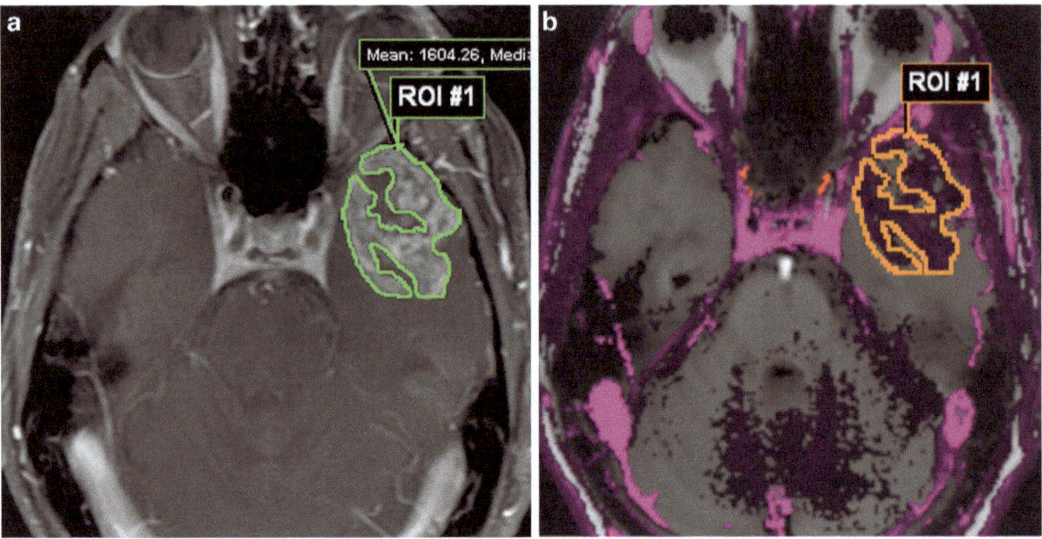

Fig. 1.4 DCE MR of the same patient as in Fig. 1.2. A volumetric ROI through multiple axial T1W post-contrast slices (**a**) with accompanying K^{trans} colormap (**b**) showing regions of high permeability mean $K^{trans} = 0.32\ min^{-1}$

nature of GBMs as well as modeling limitations in the calculation of v_e were also thought to be factors that could have affected the results.

The first report of ASL MR imaging of human brain tumors was in 1996 by Gaa et al. [2]. This study used the PASL technique EPISTAR (echo-planar imaging and signal targeting with alternating radio frequency) in 17 patients with a variety of tumors including LGGs, HGGs, lymphomas, and meningiomas. They found that HGGs demonstrated elevated EPISTAR tumor/white matter contrast with prominent heterogeneity, while LGGs and lymphomas had the lowest EPISTAR tumor/white matter contrast; meningiomas demonstrated the highest values overall. Warmuth et al. reported the first comparison of ASL versus DSC MRI CBF in brain tumors in 2003 [103]. They used PASL (Q2TIPS—quantitative imaging of perfusion by using a single subtraction with addition of thin-section period saturation after inversion and a time delay) in 36 brain tumor patients. This study found that both techniques were able to distinguish between LGGs and HGGs and a good correlation was found between tumor CBF derived by both methods. More recent studies have confirmed that ASL-derived CBF is higher in HGG compared with LGG [75, 127–129]. Recent work using QUASAR (quantitative STAR labeling of arterial regions) ASL at 3 T, a dynamic model-free ASL technique, in 24 glioma patients demonstrated excellent intermodality agreement and reproducibility of tumoral rCBF compared to DSC MRI [130]. In 2011, the first report of an ASL-based CBV (termed arterial blood volume (aBV)) as a marker of CBV in brain tumor patients was reported by van Westen et al. [131]. Using QUASAR ASL at 3 T, they compared aBV and CBV derived from DSC MRI in ten brain tumor patients with HGGs and meningiomas. This study demonstrated good correlation between the two measures; however, further validation is needed and current limitations such as long acquisition times, low SNR, and limited spatial coverage are technical factors that remain to be overcome.

While lower grade neoplasms frequently demonstrate low CBF using ASL, artifactual reasons of why a higher grade lesion may demonstrate artificially low CBF need to be considered such as the presence of calcification, hemorrhage, prominent cystic/necrotic components, or metallic craniotomy clip artifacts [79]. Tumors with elevated ASL-derived CBF are usually thought of as high-grade neoplasms, but low-grade neoplasms such as meningioma and hemangioblastomas characteristically demonstrated elevated CBF as well.

Other Neoplasms

Solitary Metastasis Versus Glioma: MR perfusion characteristics of the peritumoral region may allow one to distinguish between gliomas and solitary metastases, as the former demonstrate elevated rCBV due to infiltration of brain parenchyma whereas the latter do not [127]. Mean peritumoral rCBV has been reported at 1.31 ± 0.97 for gliomas and 0.39 ± 0.19 for metastases [132]. A recent retrospective study reported the first ever examination of the ability of SE DSC to exploit the predominant microvascularity of gliomas compared to metastases, which contain a higher proportion of intermediate-sized vessels. A sensitivity of 88 % and specificity of 72 % were reported using this technique to distinguish a solitary metastasis from a glioma, which appeared to demonstrate significantly higher rCBV [133].

Lymphoma Versus Glioma: Primary central nervous system lymphoma (PCNL) presents another diagnostic dilemma amenable to MR perfusion. PCNL features such as enhancement within deep brain structures including the corpus callosum mimic GBM. rCBV of biopsy-proven PCNL ranges from .42 to 3.41, with mean rCBV significantly below that of glioblastoma yet higher than pyogenic or fungal abscess [24, 134]. Studies of ASL have found similar results [127]. However, given that experience with these disease entities is limited by small subject populations and overlap between rCBV values, MR perfusion should be considered in the context of additional clinical and imaging findings.

Meningioma: While meningiomas are generally benign tumors, their marked vascularity and absence of a BBB can produce much higher rCBVs than intraaxial tumors [24]. Benign meningiomas usually derive their blood supply from dural branches of the external carotid artery. These branches lack a BBB and so there will be little or no return of signal back to baseline on DSC MRI signal intensity–time curves following the first-pass of GBCA [135]. As meningiomas enlarge, pial arteries, which do possess a BBB, may become parasitized. These vessels characteristically show greater return of the baseline signal. Meningiomas with more pial-cortical blood supply appear to be more aggressive and recur is more common. Selective intraarterial GBCA injection of meningiomas before and after embolization can be used to evaluate their perfusion characteristics and blood supply [136]. This method appeared to reveal the blood supply of the meningioma fed by the selected arteries as well as demonstrate the treated and untreated portions of the tumor.

Another study found that rCBV and relative mean time to enhance (rMTE) were significantly elevated in the peritumoral edema of malignant compared to benign meningiomas while there was no significant difference in tumor parenchyma [137]. The elevation of rCBV in malignant meningiomas was thought to be secondary to angiogenesis and tumor invasion of the adjacent brain tissue [138]. Increase of rMTE was thought to be the result of the combined effects of tumor size, microvascular permeability, vessel tortuosity, and vascular compression [139]. Yang et al. found that atypical meningiomas demonstrated higher rCBV and K^{trans} than benign meningiomas, although only the K^{trans} difference was statistically significant [140]. The amount of micronecrosis associated with atypical meningiomas was postulated to be a mechanism of increased permeability.

Biopsy Guidance: The biopsy of brain tumors has traditionally relied on contrast-enhanced CT or MRI [141, 142]. However, up to 25 % of tumors are undergraded because the most malignant portion of a tumor may not necessarily enhance [1, 143]. Targeting of the most malignant portions of a tumor with the aid of rCBV parametric maps is utilized in some centers to better grade tumors [24]. The potential of metrics such as rCBV to predict clinical outcome supports the notion of its use as an adjunct to histopathology as the gold standard to grade gliomas [115].

Monitoring Treatment Response

The Macdonald Criteria are currently the most widely used method to assess therapeutic response in HGGs. These take into consideration two-dimensional measurements of contrast enhancement on MRI along with clinical status and corticosteroid dosage [144]. However, reliance on contrast enhancement has long been known to be problematic because it is a nonspecific reflection of BBB disruption that can be caused by many etiologies including progression of tumor, treatment-related effects, postoperative changes, and ischemia [145–148].

Both delayed radiation necrosis (DRN) and progression of glioblastoma appear as contrast-enhancing masses with surrounding edema and are difficult to differentiate on conventional MRI [146, 149]. In progression of tumor, rCBV appears to be elevated likely due to increased vascular proliferation. However, in DRN there is lower rCBV because it is composed of extensive fibrinoid necrosis, vascular dilation, and endothelial injury [107, 150–153]. Recently, other DSC MRI-derived metrics such as increased PH as well as lower relative PSR have been reported in progression of glioblastoma compared to DRN [107]. The use of DCE MRI to diagnose DRN is much more limited compared to DSC MRI but studies do indicate that there is also lower permeability of DRN compared with recurrent tumor [61, 154]. Recent work by Bisdas et al. appeared to support this in 18 patients with HGG where a K^{trans} threshold of greater than 0.19 produced 100 % sensitivity and 83 % specificity for detecting progression of glioma versus DRN [112]. Narang et al. demonstrated the utility of a nonmodel-based semiquantitative DCE MRI technique to differentiate recurrent/progressive brain tumor from treatment-induced necrosis [155]. Using analysis of signal intensity–time curves, they found that recurrent/progressive tumor demonstrated greater maximum slope of enhancement in the initial vascular phase. Their results indicated that, while semiquantitative metrics are less physiologically specific, they are simple to derive and robust to differentiate the two entities.

In patients with metastatic brain tumors following stereotactic radiosurgery, Weber et al. performed a study employing both DSC and ASL perfusion MRI. They found that rCBF measurements at 6 weeks following treatment were predictive of treatment outcome where an increase in rCBF was indicative of tumor progression while a decrease in rCBF predicted tumor response [128]. In glioma patients following surgery and radiation therapy, Ozsunar et al. examined 30 patients and concluded that ASL may be more accurate than DSC MRI to distinguish recurrent HGG from radiation necrosis, particularly in areas of mixed radiation necrosis, where leakage effects could result in underestimation of DSC MRI-derived rCBV [156].

Pseudoprogression(PsP): Current standard of care for newly diagnosed HGGs involves maximal safe resection, radiation therapy, and temozolamide chemotherapy [157, 158]. These tumors are inherently diffuse neoplasms associated with residual tumor burden despite microscopic surgical removal and absence of contrast enhancement on postoperative MR imaging. Tumor almost inevitably progresses, prompting enrollment of patients into clinical trials. However, this process has become complicated by the recent recognition of PsP. PsP refers to increased enhancement on MRI within the first 3–6 months of chemoradiation, earlier than following radiation therapy alone, that is due to treatment-related changes rather than true early progression (TEP) [159, 160]. While it is estimated that PsP is seen in about 20–30 % of cases following chemoradiation, the exact incidence of PsP is difficult to determine given differences in study design and definitions. In fact, Clarke and Chang estimate that about half of patients with glioblastoma will develop concerning findings on conventional contrast-enhanced MRI following chemoradiation and that many of these patients will be found to have PsP rather than TEP if treatment is not changed [159]. Methylation of the DNA repair gene MGMT promoter region is associated with sensitivity to temozolamide and prolonged survival [161–163]. The cell death associated with MGMT methylation also appears to predispose patients to PsP. Increased permeability associated with BBB disruption is responsible for edema and contrast enhancement in PsP and it can be extremely difficult to differentiate it from TEP on conventional contrast-enhanced MRI [164].

The inability to distinguish PsP versus TEP complicates patient management decisions and clinical trial design. Patients with TEP should change to an alternative therapy, typically a clinical trial [159]. Because the enhancing lesions of PsP typically improve or stabilize over time, there is the possibility of false attribution of efficacy if the patient is switched to a different treatment regimen. Also, a patient who is experiencing PsP and has their treatment changed will be sacrificing an effective therapy. Currently, no advanced imaging methods have been validated to adequately diagnose PsP and follow-up conventional contrast-enhanced MRI remains the standard method to monitor these patients. Some recent reports showing lower rCBV in PsP compared to TEP appear to show the promise of DSC MRI in this context [165, 166]. The use of the iron oxide nanoparticle blood pool agent ferumoxytol may better differentiate PsP from TEP compared to GBCAs using DSC MRI-derived rCBV because of uncertainties raised due to contrast agent leakage [53]. Tissues affected by radiation necrosis demonstrate lower permeability than recurrent brain tumors and the use of DCE MRI may potentially be helpful to distinguish PsP from TEP [155, 167] (Figs. 1.5 and 1.7).

Because of the recognition of PsP, the recent RANO Working Group recommendations state that within 12 weeks of the completion of chemoradiation, the designation of progression of disease can be made only if there is new enhancement outside of the radiation field or if there is unequivocal evidence of tumor on histopathology [168]. There is some concern, however, that these recommendations would exclude the most malignant tumors that progress quickly and that because these patients were not excluded from many prior drug trials, a new element of bias may be introduced when the efficacy of a new drug is compared with historical controls [169].

Radiation Effects: Vascular injury is considered a primary factor in radiation-induced injury to

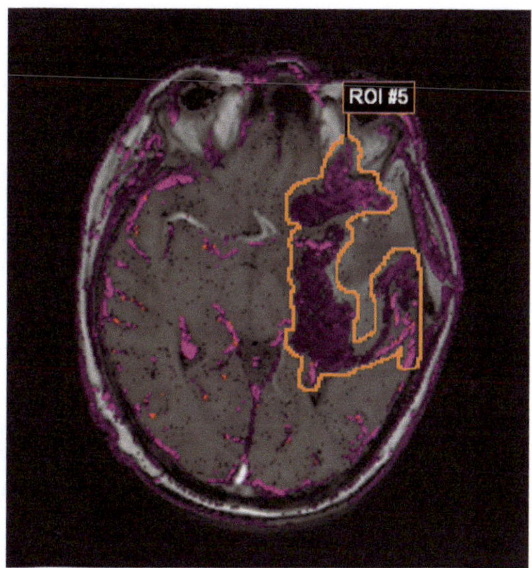

Fig. 1.5 True progression, same patient as Fig. 1.6. Axial slice from a volumetric ROI overlaid onto K^{trans} colormap shows a large area of increased mean K^{trans} of 0.25 min^{-1}. Repeat MRI 2 months later demonstrated interval progression of disease

cerebral tissues [170–173]. In the first year after radiation therapy, a decrease in rCBV is seen with a larger decrease noted in areas receiving higher radiation doses [46, 174]. Using DSC MRI and examining both the first-pass and recirculation phases, Lee et al. found a possible dose-dependent decrease in vascular density and increase in microvascular permeability and/or tortuosity in irradiated normal-appearing brain tissue 2 months after radiation therapy [175]. Recent preliminary results in ten patients who underwent partial brain radiation therapy and DCE MRI appear to demonstrate the potential of v_p and K^{trans} to predict neurocognitive function after radiation therapy [176].

Antiangiogenic Therapy: Therapeutic agents directed against VEGF, such as bevacizumab, dramatically reduce BBB permeability and promote vascular normalization. A rapid decrease in the amount of contrast enhancement can be noted with therapy, raising the possibility that changes in vascular permeability rather than true antitumoral response were underlying these effects [32, 177]. An impressive decrease in the amount of contrast enhancement (often reversible), high response

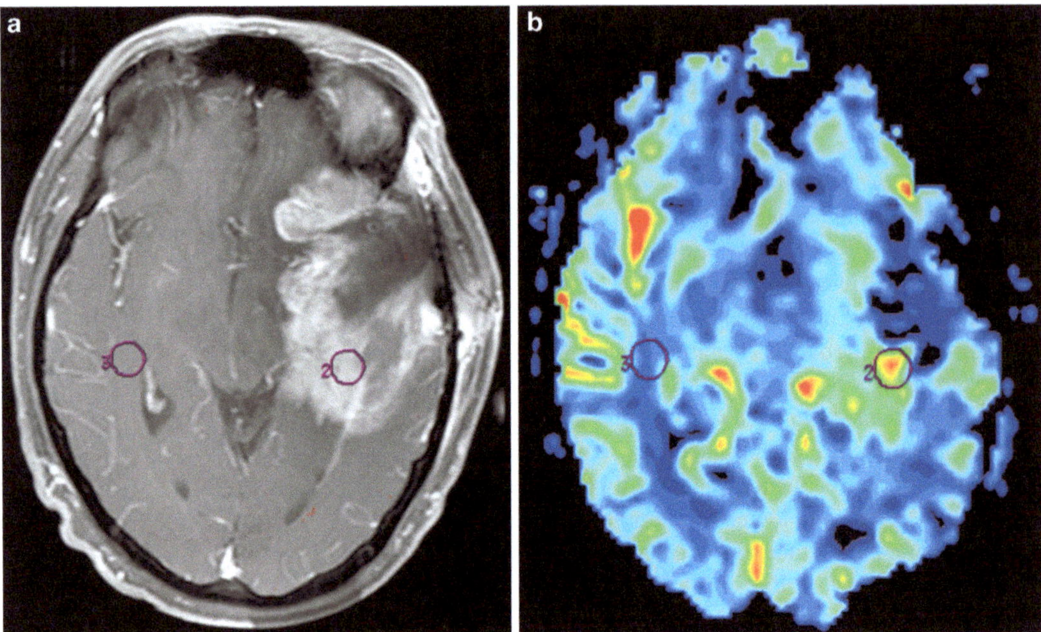

Fig. 1.6 True progression of a 34-year-old man with GBM 2 months following surgery and chemoradiation. Axial T1W post-contrast image demonstrates a large enhancing mass (**a**) with an rCBV colormap (**b**) that demonstrates a maximum rCBV of 4.3

rate, and 6-month progression-free survival but with modest effect on overall survival appear to support this conclusion [32]. Therefore, reliance on a decrease in the amount of contrast enhancement on conventional MRI may not be reliable to determine antitumoral effect. Imaging characteristics of this so-called pseudoresponse, such as increased diffusion restriction and FLAIR signal, have been recently reported [178–180]. A recent report combined changes of K^{trans}, rCBV, and circulating collagen IV into a "vascular normalization index" and found that it was closely associated with both progression-free and overall survival [181]. Regardless of whether a true antitumoral response or pseudoresponse is seen, vascular normalization and its consequent reduction in vasogenic edema can result in decreased steroid usage and decreased morbidity [32, 182].

The recent RANO Working Group now recommends that for patients on antiangiogenic therapy, progression of disease can be considered if there is a significant increase in the amount of non-enhancing T2/FLAIR signal while the patient is on stable/increasing corticosteroid dosage compared with the baseline scan or best response after the start of therapy [168]. However, the exact definition of a "significant" increase in T2/FLAIR signal nor what constitutes a significant change in corticosteroid dosing was not given, raising the prospect of ambiguity [169].

Standardization and the Future of MR Perfusion

Quantitative metrics derived from MR perfusion have enhanced quantitative imaging evaluation of brain tumors. However, there is variability that can be attributable to differences in image acquisition, post-processing, and interpretation. Most methods of data analysis rely on the placement of user-defined ROIs encompassing a portion or the entire lesion [87]. However, no standardization exists. Wetzel et al. demonstrated that the placement of multiple ROIs to determine the highest rCBV provided clinically acceptable

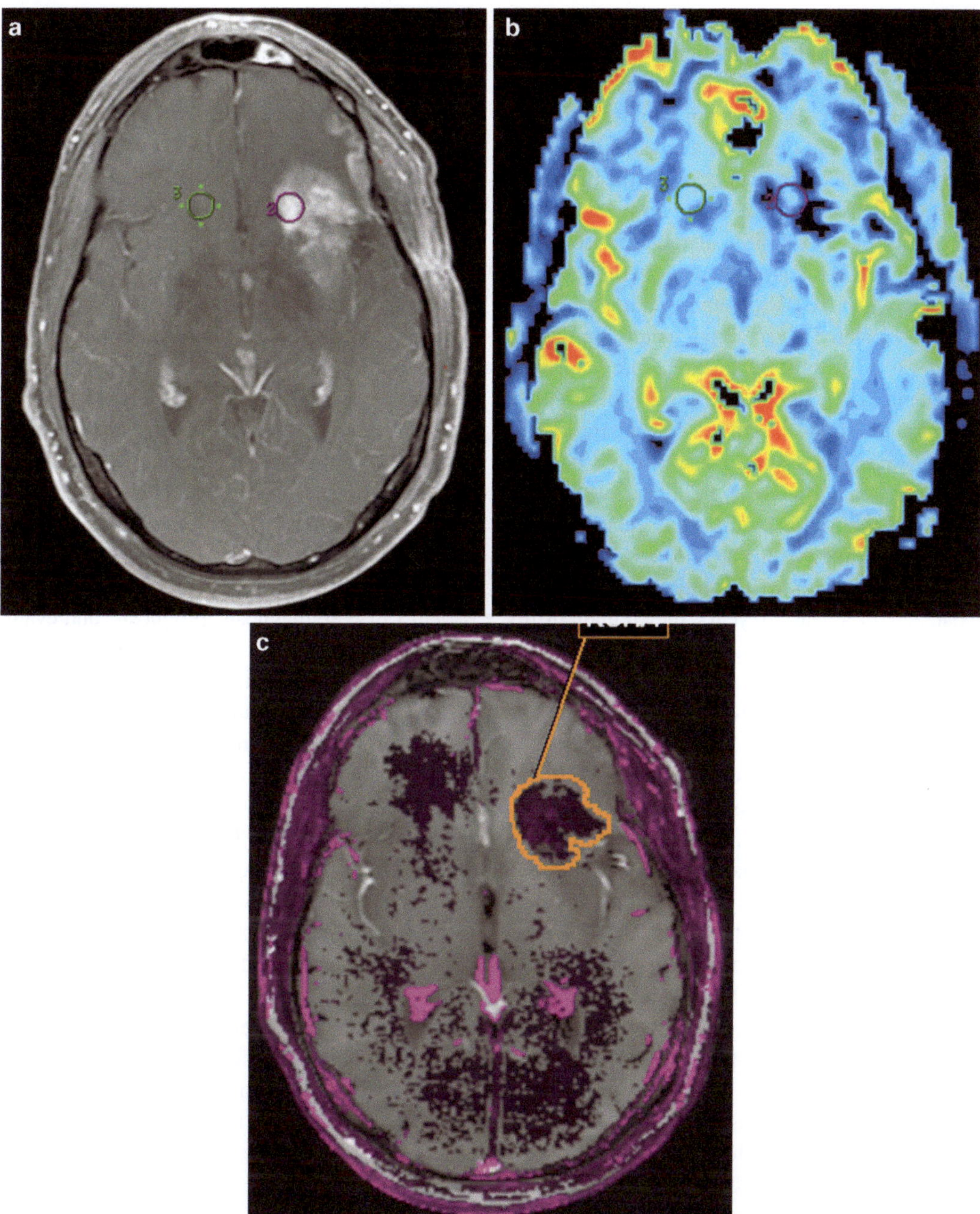

Fig. 1.7 Pseudoprogression, MR perfusion of a 42-year-old man with GBM 3-month status post resection and chemoradiation. (**a**) Axial post-contrast T1-weighted image demonstrates an enhancing mass in the low left frontal region/basal ganglia region. (**b**) rCBV colormap shows max rCBV to be low, 0.8. K^{trans} colormap of the lesion (**c**) demonstrates mean K^{trans} of 0.13 min^{-1}. Follow-up MRI 2 months later was stable to slightly improved. The patient continues on his current treatment regimen

reproducibility amongst multiple neuroradiologists [183]. Analytic approaches such as this have the advantage that it is easy to perform; however, it can result in an excessive level of data reduction [87]. Glioblastomas and treatment effects typically appear heterogeneous and these lesions can be problematic as high and low values in an ROI can cancel each other out. Therefore, other analysis techniques such as histogram-based and voxel-wise analyses have been proposed as alternatives to conventional ROI analysis [184–187]. The use of histograms can describe the heterogeneity of the tissue of interest; however, spatial specificity is lost [188]. Parametric response mapping (PRM) is an advanced method of data analysis where rCBV or other parametric maps are co-registered over serial exams and compared on a voxel-wise basis before and after treatment [186, 187, 189]. While this method appears to show promise, co-registration of image voxels can present a challenge because neoplasms may move in nonlinear ways over time or if the tumor size is small relative to the resolution of the voxel size [190].

While perfusion MRI techniques have been in existence for at least 20 years, they remain firmly within the realm of academia/clinical research and are not yet part of routine standard of care for brain tumor patients. Sorensen points out several reasons behind this [191]. First, there is no specific reimbursement for perfusion MRI. Secondly, no GBCA has been approved specifically for perfusion MRI of the brain. And most importantly, there is a little high-quality data that show an actual clinical impact of these techniques in brain tumor patients. A recent single-center prospective study of glioma patients was reported to address this issue [192]. In this study, 59 consecutive patients with gliomas were examined by three neuroradiologists, first using conventional MRI and then afterward with inclusion of qualitative evaluation of perfusion imaging (both DSC as well as ASL MRI techniques). These imaging data were then evaluated in a multidisciplinary fashion with a clinical neuro-oncology team and hypothetical treatment plans were created for each patient prospectively first using conventional MRI and then using conventional MRI combined with perfusion MRI. The addition of perfusion imaging appeared to have a significant effect on neuroradiologists' and clinicians' confidence in tumor status as well as clinical management decisions. Larger multicenter validation studies are desperately needed.

The application of ASL to brain tumors is still in relative infancy compared with DSC and DCE MRI. ASL's ability to provide absolute CBF values as well as its lack of a need for GBCAs are clearly desirable. In addition, the determination of an ASL-derived blood volume measurement may become fully realized in the future. There exist a multitude of ASL technical variants that will need validation regarding their clinical value. Current technical limitations related to low SNR, long acquisition times, and complex methodology are some hurdles that will need to be overcome. Recent efforts such as "the ASL Network" (http://www.asl-network.org) have been established to improve communication among stakeholders such as physicists, engineers, and physicians.

The development of quantitative imaging biomarkers may help guide and improve efficiency of clinical trials and provide better evaluation of a patient's disease diagnosis, prognosis, and evaluation of therapeutic efficacy beyond those obtained from conventional MRI [191, 193]. A lack of technical standardization and lack of high-quality data demonstrating the clinical benefit of perfusion MRI remain unresolved issues. Organized efforts such as the National Cancer Institute's Quantitative Imaging Network (QIN) and the Quantitative Imaging Biomarkers Alliance (QIBA) are in place with a goal to optimize, validate, and standardize image acquisition and post-processing methods [194, 195]. Standardization of perfusion MRI image acquisition, post-processing, and data interpretation will greatly aid in carrying out well-designed multicenter studies to definitively demonstrate its ability to have a major impact in patient management.

Conclusion

Conventional contrast-enhanced MR imaging is limited in its ability to demonstrate underlying tumor biology. MR perfusion imaging can provide useful information to determine tumor grade, prognosis, and therapeutic efficacy. Variations in acquisition and processing techniques require some degree of expertise and a lack of technical standardization may make widespread clinical adoption of these techniques difficult. Efforts dedicated towards technical standardization and high-quality data demonstrating definite clinical benefit of MR perfusion in neurooncology patients are needed to promote widespread use of imaging biomarkers in routine clinical use.

References

1. Ft E, Kelly PJ, Scheithauer BW, et al. Cerebral astrocytomas: histopathologic correlation of MR and CT contrast enhancement with stereotactic biopsy. Radiology. 1988;166:823–7.
2. Gaa J, Warach S, Wen P, Thangaraj V, Wielopolski P, Edelman RR. Noninvasive perfusion imaging of human brain tumors with EPISTAR. Eur Radiol. 1996;6:518–22.
3. Folkman J, Ingber D. Inhibition of angiogenesis. Semin Cancer Biol. 1992;3:89–96.
4. Knopp MV, Giesel FL, Marcos H, von Tengg-Kobligk H, Choyke P. Dynamic contrast-enhanced magnetic resonance imaging in oncology. Top Magn Reson Imaging. 2001;12:301–8.
5. Quant EC, Wen PY. Novel medical therapeutics in glioblastomas, including targeted molecular therapies, current and future clinical trials. Neuroimaging Clin N Am. 2010;20:425–48.
6. Chaudhry IH, O'Donovan DG, Brenchley PE, Reid H, Roberts IS. Vascular endothelial growth factor expression correlates with tumour grade and vascularity in gliomas. Histopathology. 2001;39:409–15.
7. Varlet P, Guillamo JS, Nataf F, Koziak M, Beuvon F, Daumas-Duport C. Vascular endothelial growth factor expression in oligodendrogliomas: a correlative study with Sainte-Anne malignancy grade, growth fraction and patient survival. Neuropathol Appl Neurobiol. 2000;26:379–89.
8. Norden AD, Drappatz J, Wen PY. Novel anti-angiogenic therapies for malignant gliomas. Lancet Neurol. 2008;7:1152–60.
9. Dvorak HF, Brown LF, Detmar M, Dvorak AM. Vascular permeability factor/vascular endothelial growth factor, microvascular hyperpermeability, and angiogenesis. Am J Pathol. 1995;146:1029–39.
10. Nagy JA, Masse EM, Herzberg KT, et al. Pathogenesis of ascites tumor growth: vascular permeability factor, vascular hyperpermeability, and ascites fluid accumulation. Cancer Res. 1995;55:360–8.
11. Jain RK, di Tomaso E, Duda DG, Loeffler JS, Sorensen AG, Batchelor TT. Angiogenesis in brain tumours. Nat Rev Neurosci. 2007;8:610–22.
12. Millauer B, Shawver LK, Plate KH, Risaui W, Ullrich A. Glioblastoma growth inhibited in vivo by a dominant-negative Flk-1 mutant. Nature. 1994; 367:576–9.
13. Plate KH, Risau W. Angiogenesis in malignant gliomas. Glia. 1995;15:339–47.
14. Amoroso A, Del Porto F, Di Monaco C, Manfredini P, Afeltra A. Vascular endothelial growth factor: a key mediator of neoangiogenesis. A review. Eur Rev Med Pharmacol Sci. 1997;1:17–25.
15. Pietsch T, Valter MM, Wolf HK, et al. Expression and distribution of vascular endothelial growth factor protein in human brain tumors. Acta Neuropathol. 1997;93:109–17.
16. Bergers G, Hanahan D. Modes of resistance to anti-angiogenic therapy. Nat Rev Cancer. 2008;8:592–603.
17. Argyriou AA, Giannopoulou E, Kalofonos HP. Angiogenesis and anti-angiogenic molecularly targeted therapies in malignant gliomas. Oncology. 2009;77:1–11.
18. Kiselev VG. On the theoretical basis of perfusion measurements by dynamic susceptibility contrast MRI. Magn Reson Med. 2001;46:1113–22.
19. Wintermark M, Sesay M, Barbier E, et al. Comparative overview of brain perfusion imaging techniques. Stroke. 2005;36:e83–99.
20. Knutsson L, van Westen D, Petersen ET, et al. Absolute quantification of cerebral blood flow: correlation between dynamic susceptibility contrast MRI and model-free arterial spin labeling. Magn Reson Imaging. 2010;28:1–7.
21. Rosen BR, Belliveau JW, Buchbinder BR, et al. Contrast agents and cerebral hemodynamics. Magn Reson Med. 1991;19:285–92.
22. Rosen BR, Belliveau JW, Vevea JM, Brady TJ. Perfusion imaging with NMR contrast agents. Magn Reson Med. 1990;14:249–65.
23. Rempp KA, Brix G, Wenz F, Becker CR, Guckel F, Lorenz WJ. Quantification of regional cerebral blood flow and volume with dynamic susceptibility contrast-enhanced MR imaging. Radiology. 1994;193:637–41.
24. Cha S, Knopp EA, Johnson G, Wetzel SG, Litt AW, Zagzag D. Intracranial mass lesions: dynamic contrast-enhanced susceptibility-weighted echo-planar perfusion MR imaging. Radiology. 2002;223: 11–29.
25. Schmainda KM, Rand SD, Joseph AM, et al. Characterization of a first-pass gradient-echo spin-echo method to predict brain tumor grade and angiogenesis. AJNR Am J Neuroradiol. 2004;25: 1524–32.
26. Boxerman JL, Schmainda KM, Weisskoff RM. Relative cerebral blood volume maps corrected for contrast agent extravasation significantly correlate with glioma tumor grade, whereas uncorrected maps do not. AJNR Am J Neuroradiol. 2006;27:859–67.
27. Donahue KM, Krouwer HG, Rand SD, et al. Utility of simultaneously acquired gradient-echo and spin-echo cerebral blood volume and morphology maps in brain tumor patients. Magn Reson Med. 2000;43:845–53.
28. Zama A, Tamura M, Inoue HK. Three-dimensional observations on microvascular growth in rat glioma

using a vascular casting method. J Cancer Res Clin Oncol. 1991;117:396–402.
29. van Gelderen P, Grandin C, Petrella JR, Moonen CT. Rapid three-dimensional MR imaging method for tracking a bolus of contrast agent through the brain. Radiology. 2000;216:603–8.
30. Kassner A, Annesley DJ, Zhu XP, et al. Abnormalities of the contrast re-circulation phase in cerebral tumors demonstrated using dynamic susceptibility contrast-enhanced imaging: a possible marker of vascular tortuosity. J Magn Reson Imaging. 2000;11:103–13.
31. Dennie J, Mandeville JB, Boxerman JL, Packard SD, Rosen BR, Weisskoff RM. NMR imaging of changes in vascular morphology due to tumor angiogenesis. Magn Reson Med. 1998;40:793–9.
32. Batchelor TT, Sorensen AG, di Tomaso E, et al. AZD2171, a pan-VEGF receptor tyrosine kinase inhibitor, normalizes tumor vasculature and alleviates edema in glioblastoma patients. Cancer Cell. 2007;11:83–95.
33. Weisskoff R, Boxerman J, Sorensen A, Kulke S, Campbell T, Rosen B. Simultaneous blood volume and permeability mapping using a single Gd-based contrast injection. In: Society of Magnetic Resonance. San Francisco, 1994
34. Johnson G, Wetzel SG, Cha S, Babb J, Tofts PS. Measuring blood volume and vascular transfer constant from dynamic, T(2)*-weighted contrast-enhanced MRI. Magn Reson Med. 2004;51:961–8.
35. Cha S, Yang L, Johnson G, et al. Comparison of microvascular permeability measurements, K(trans), determined with conventional steady-state T1-weighted and first-pass T2*-weighted MR imaging methods in gliomas and meningiomas. AJNR Am J Neuroradiol. 2006;27:409–17.
36. Lupo JM, Cha S, Chang SM, Nelson SJ. Dynamic susceptibility-weighted perfusion imaging of high-grade gliomas: characterization of spatial heterogeneity. AJNR Am J Neuroradiol. 2005;26:1446–54.
37. Calamante F, Thomas DL, Pell GS, Wiersma J, Turner R. Measuring cerebral blood flow using magnetic resonance imaging techniques. J Cereb Blood Flow Metab. 1999;19:701–35.
38. Farrar TC, Becker ED. Pulsed and fourier transform NMR. Introduction to theory and methods. New York: Academic; 1971.
39. Villringer A, Rosen BR, Belliveau JW, et al. Dynamic imaging with lanthanide chelates in normal brain: contrast due to magnetic susceptibility effects. Magn Reson Med. 1988;6:164–74.
40. Fisel CR, Ackerman JL, Buxton RB, et al. MR contrast due to microscopically heterogeneous magnetic susceptibility: numerical simulations and applications to cerebral physiology. Magn Reson Med. 1991;17:336–47.
41. Majumdar S, Zoghbi SS, Gore JC. Regional differences in rat brain displayed by fast MRI with superparamagnetic contrast agents. Magn Reson Imaging. 1988;6:611–5.
42. Roberts TP, Mikulis D. Neuro MR: principles. J Magn Reson Imaging. 2007;26:823–37.
43. Meier P, Zierler KL. On the theory of the indicator-dilution method for measurement of blood flow and volume. J Appl Physiol. 1954;6:731–44.
44. Paulson ES, Schmainda KM. Comparison of dynamic susceptibility-weighted contrast-enhanced MR methods: recommendations for measuring relative cerebral blood volume in brain tumors. Radiology. 2008;249:601–13.
45. Provenzale JM, Schmainda KM. Perfusion imaging for brain tumor characterization and assessment of treatment response. In: Jolesz FA, Newton HB, editors. Handbook of neuro-oncology neuroimaging. New York: Elsevier Ltd.; 2008. p. 265–77.
46. Fuss M, Wenz F, Scholdei R, et al. Radiation-induced regional cerebral blood volume (rCBV) changes in normal brain and low-grade astrocytomas: quantification and time and dose-dependent occurrence. Int J Radiat Oncol Biol Phys. 2000;48:53–8.
47. Hobbs SK, Shi G, Homer R, Harsh G, Atlas SW, Bednarski MD. Magnetic resonance image-guided proteomics of human glioblastoma multiforme. J Magn Reson Imaging. 2003;18:530–6.
48. Giese A, Bjerkvig R, Berens ME, Westphal M. Cost of migration: invasion of malignant gliomas and implications for treatment. J Clin Oncol. 2003;21:1624–36.
49. Uematsu H, Maeda M, Sadato N, et al. Blood volume of gliomas determined by double-echo dynamic perfusion-weighted MR imaging: a preliminary study. AJNR Am J Neuroradiol. 2001;22:1915–9.
50. Babu R, Huang PP, Epstein F, Budzilovich GN. Late radiation necrosis of the brain: case report. J Neurooncol. 1993;17:37–42.
51. Hu LS, Baxter LC, Pinnaduwage DS, et al. Optimized preload leakage-correction methods to improve the diagnostic accuracy of dynamic susceptibility-weighted contrast-enhanced perfusion MR imaging in posttreatment gliomas. AJNR Am J Neuroradiol. 2010;31:40–8.
52. Weinstein JS, Varallyay CG, Dosa E, et al. Superparamagnetic iron oxide nanoparticles: diagnostic magnetic resonance imaging and potential therapeutic applications in neurooncology and central nervous system inflammatory pathologies, a review. J Cereb Blood Flow Metab. 2010;30:15–35.
53. Gahramanov S, Raslan AM, Muldoon LL, et al. Potential for differentiation of pseudoprogression from true tumor progression with dynamic susceptibility-weighted contrast-enhanced magnetic resonance imaging using ferumoxytol vs. gadoteridol: a pilot study. Int J Radiat Oncol Biol Phys. 2011;79:514–23.
54. Neuwelt EA, Varallyay CG, Manninger S, et al. The potential of ferumoxytol nanoparticle magnetic resonance imaging, perfusion, and angiography in central nervous system malignancy: a pilot study. Neurosurgery. 2007;60:601–11. discussion 611-602.
55. Bock JC, Kaufmann F, Felix R. Comparison of gadolinium-DTPA and macromolecular gadolinium-DTPA-polylysine for contrast-enhanced pulmonary time-of-flight magnetic resonance angiography. Invest Radiol. 1996;31:652–7.

56. Boschi F, Marzola P, Sandri M, et al. Tumor microvasculature observed using different contrast agents: a comparison between Gd-DTPA-Albumin and B-22956/1 in an experimental model of mammary carcinoma. Magma. 2008;21:169–76.
57. Sirlin CB, Vera DR, Corbeil JA, Caballero MB, Buxton RB, Mattrey RF. Gadolinium-DTPA-dextran: a macromolecular MR blood pool contrast agent. Acad Radiol. 2004;11:1361–9.
58. Lebduskova P, Kotek J, Hermann P, et al. A gadolinium(III) complex of a carboxylic-phosphorus acid derivative of diethylenetriamine covalently bound to inulin, a potential macromolecular MRI contrast agent. Bioconjug Chem. 2004;15:881–9.
59. Tian M, Wen X, Jackson EF, et al. Pharmacokinetics and magnetic resonance imaging of biodegradable macromolecular blood-pool contrast agent PG-Gd in non-human primates: a pilot study. Contrast Media Mol Imaging. 2011;6:289–97.
60. Young IR, Cox IJ, Coutts GA, Bydder GM. Some consideration concerning susceptibility, longitudinal relaxation time constants and motion artifact in vivo human spectroscopy. NMR Biomed. 1989;2:329–39.
61. Lacerda S, Law M. Magnetic resonance perfusion and permeability imaging in brain tumors. Neuroimaging Clin N Am. 2009;19:527–57.
62. Cercignani M, Symms MR, Schmierer K, et al. Three-dimensional quantitative magnetisation transfer imaging of the human brain. NeuroImage. 2005; 27:436–41.
63. Parker GJ, Padhani AR. T1-W DCE-MRI: T1-weighted dynamic contrast-enhanced MRI. In: Tofts PS, editor. Quantitative MRI of the brain. Chichester, England: John Wiley & Sons; 2003. p. 341–64.
64. Tofts PS, Brix G, Buckley DL, et al. Estimating kinetic parameters from dynamic contrast-enhanced T(1)-weighted MRI of a diffusable tracer: standardized quantities and symbols. J Magn Reson Imaging. 1999;10:223–32.
65. Evelhoch JL. Key factors in the acquisition of contrast kinetic data for oncology. J Magn Reson Imaging. 1999;10:254–9.
66. Paldino MJ, Barboriak DP. Fundamentals of quantitative dynamic contrast-enhanced MR imaging. Magn Reson Imaging Clin N Am. 2009;17:277–89.
67. Turetschek K, Floyd E, Helbich T, et al. MRI assessment of microvascular characteristics in experimental breast tumors using a new blood pool contrast agent (MS-325) with correlations to histopathology. J Magn Reson Imaging. 2001;14:237–42.
68. Tofts PS, Kermode AG. Measurement of the blood-brain barrier permeability and leakage space using dynamic MR imaging. 1. Fundamental concepts. Magn Reson Med. 1991;17:357–67.
69. Parker GJ, Tofts PS. Pharmacokinetic analysis of neoplasms using contrast-enhanced dynamic magnetic resonance imaging. Top Magn Reson Imaging. 1999;10:130–42.
70. O'Connor JP, Jackson A, Asselin MC, Buckley DL, Parker GJ, Jayson GC. Quantitative imaging biomarkers in the clinical development of targeted therapeutics: current and future perspectives. Lancet Oncol. 2008;9:766–76.
71. O'Connor JP, Jackson A, Parker GJ, Jayson GC. DCE-MRI biomarkers in the clinical evaluation of antiangiogenic and vascular disrupting agents. Br J Cancer. 2007;96:189–95.
72. St Lawrence KS, Lee TY. An adiabatic approximation to the tissue homogeneity model for water exchange in the brain: I. Theoretical derivation. J Cereb Blood Flow Metab. 1998;18:1365–77.
73. Aref M, Chaudhari AR, Bailey KL, Aref S, Wiener EC. Comparison of tumor histology to dynamic contrast enhanced magnetic resonance imaging-based physiological estimates. Magn Reson Imaging. 2008;26:1279–93.
74. Grobner T. Gadolinium: a specific trigger for the development of nephrogenic fibrosing dermopathy and nephrogenic systemic fibrosis? Nephrol Dial Transplant. 2006;21:1104–8.
75. Wolf RL, Wang J, Wang S, et al. Grading of CNS neoplasms using continuous arterial spin labeled perfusion MR imaging at 3 Tesla. J Magn Reson Imaging. 2005;22:475–82.
76. Wang J, Fernandez-Seara MA, Wang S, St Lawrence KS. When perfusion meets diffusion: in vivo measurement of water permeability in human brain. J Cereb Blood Flow Metab. 2007;27:839–49.
77. Petersen ET, Zimine I, Ho YC, Golay X. Non-invasive measurement of perfusion: a critical review of arterial spin labelling techniques. Br J Radiol. 2006;79:688–701.
78. Golay X, Guenther M. Arterial spin labelling: final steps to make it a clinical reality. Magma. 2012;25: 79–82.
79. Pollock JM, Tan H, Kraft RA, Whitlow CT, Burdette JH, Maldjian JA. Arterial spin-labeled MR perfusion imaging: clinical applications. Magn Reson Imaging Clin N Am. 2009;17:315–38.
80. Wolf RL, Detre JA. Clinical neuroimaging using arterial spin-labeled perfusion magnetic resonance imaging. Neurotherapeutics. 2007;4:346–59.
81. Wang J, Alsop DC, Song HK, et al. Arterial transit time imaging with flow encoding arterial spin tagging (FEAST). Magn Reson Med. 2003;50:599–607.
82. Petersen ET, Lim T, Golay X. Model-free arterial spin labelling quantification approach for perfusion MRI. Magn Reson Med. 2006;55:219–32.
83. Thomas DL, Lythgoe MF, Calamante F, Gadian DG, Ordidge RJ. Simultaneous noninvasive measurement of CBF and CBV using double-echo FAIR (DEFAIR). Magn Reson Med. 2001;45:853–63.
84. Kim T, Kim SG. Quantification of cerebral arterial blood volume and cerebral blood flow using MRI with modulation of tissue and vessel (MOTIVE) signals. Magn Reson Med. 2005;54:333–42.
85. Kim T, Kim SG. Quantitative MRI of cerebral arterial blood volume. Open Neuroimag J. 2011;5: 136–45.
86. Alsop DC, Detre JA. Reduced transit-time sensitivity in noninvasive magnetic resonance imaging of

human cerebral blood flow. J Cereb Blood Flow Metab. 1996;16:1236–49.
87. Thompson G, Mills SJ, Stivaros SM, Jackson A. Imaging of brain tumors: perfusion/permeability. Neuroimaging Clin N Am. 2010;20:337–53.
88. Petersen ET, Mouridsen K, Golay X. The QUASAR reproducibility study, Part II: Results from a multicenter Arterial Spin Labeling test-retest study. NeuroImage. 2010;49:104–13.
89. Gevers S, van Osch MJ, Bokkers RP, et al. Intra- and multicenter reproducibility of pulsed, continuous and pseudo-continuous arterial spin labeling methods for measuring cerebral perfusion. J Cereb Blood Flow Metab. 2011;31:1706–15.
90. Edelman RR, Siewert B, Adamis M, Gaa J, Laub G, Wielopolski P. Signal targeting with alternating radiofrequency (STAR) sequences: application to MR angiography. Magn Reson Med. 1994;31:233–8.
91. Kwong KK, Chesler DA, Weisskoff RM, et al. MR perfusion studies with T1-weighted echo planar imaging. Magn Reson Med. 1995;34:878–87.
92. Kim HS, Kim SY. A prospective study on the added value of pulsed arterial spin-labeling and apparent diffusion coefficients in the grading of gliomas. AJNR Am J Neuroradiol. 2007;28:1693–9.
93. Wolff SD, Balaban RS. Magnetization transfer contrast (MTC) and tissue water proton relaxation in vivo. Magn Reson Med. 1989;10:135–44.
94. Henkelman RM, Huang X, Xiang QS, Stanisz GJ, Swanson SD, Bronskill MJ. Quantitative interpretation of magnetization transfer. Magn Reson Med. 1993;29:759–66.
95. Golay X, Hendrikse J, Lim TC. Perfusion imaging using arterial spin labeling. Top Magn Reson Imaging. 2004;15:10–27.
96. Wang J, Alsop DC, Li L, et al. Comparison of quantitative perfusion imaging using arterial spin labeling at 1.5 and 4.0 Tesla. Magn Reson Med. 2002;48: 242–54.
97. Yongbi MN, Yang Y, Frank JA, Duyn JH. Multislice perfusion imaging in human brain using the C-FOCI inversion pulse: comparison with hyperbolic secant. Magn Reson Med. 1999;42:1098–105.
98. Wu WC, Jiang SF, Yang SC, Lien SH. Pseudocontinuous arterial spin labeling perfusion magnetic resonance imaging: a normative study of reproducibility in the human brain. NeuroImage. 2011;56:1244–50.
99. Yongbi MN, Fera F, Yang Y, Frank JA, Duyn JH. Pulsed arterial spin labeling: comparison of multisection baseline and functional MR imaging perfusion signal at 1.5 and 3.0 T: initial results in six subjects. Radiology. 2002;222:569–75.
100. Wang Z, Wang J, Detre JA. Improved data reconstruction method for GRAPPA. Magn Reson Med. 2005;54:738–42.
101. Fernandez-Seara MA, Wang Z, Wang J, et al. Continuous arterial spin labeling perfusion measurements using single shot 3D GRASE at 3 T. Magn Reson Med. 2005;54:1241–7.
102. Fernandez-Seara MA, Wang J, Wang Z, et al. Imaging mesial temporal lobe activation during scene encoding: comparison of fMRI using BOLD and arterial spin labeling. Hum Brain Mapp. 2007;28:1391–400.
103. Warmuth C, Gunther M, Zimmer C. Quantification of blood flow in brain tumors: comparison of arterial spin labeling and dynamic susceptibility-weighted contrast-enhanced MR imaging. Radiology. 2003;228:523–32.
104. Law M, Yang S, Wang H, et al. Glioma grading: sensitivity, specificity, and predictive values of perfusion MR imaging and proton MR spectroscopic imaging compared with conventional MR imaging. AJNR Am J Neuroradiol. 2003;24:1989–98.
105. Sugahara T, Korogi Y, Kochi M, et al. Correlation of MR imaging-determined cerebral blood volume maps with histologic and angiographic determination of vascularity of gliomas. AJR Am J Roentgenol. 1998;171:1479–86.
106. Aronen HJ, Glass J, Pardo FS, et al. Echo-planar MR cerebral blood volume mapping of gliomas. Clinical utility. Acta Radiol. 1995;36:520–8.
107. Barajas Jr RF, Chang JS, Segal MR, et al. Differentiation of recurrent glioblastoma multiforme from radiation necrosis after external beam radiation therapy with dynamic susceptibility-weighted contrast-enhanced perfusion MR imaging. Radiology. 2009;253:486–96.
108. Aronen HJ, Gazit IE, Louis DN, et al. Cerebral blood volume maps of gliomas: comparison with tumor grade and histologic findings. Radiology. 1994;191:41–51.
109. Aronen HJ, Pardo FS, Kennedy DN, et al. High microvascular blood volume is associated with high glucose uptake and tumor angiogenesis in human gliomas. Clin Cancer Res. 2000;6:2189–200.
110. Knopp EA, Cha S, Johnson G, et al. Glial neoplasms: dynamic contrast-enhanced T2*-weighted MR imaging. Radiology. 1999;211:791–8.
111. Shin JH, Lee HK, Kwun BD, et al. Using relative cerebral blood flow and volume to evaluate the histopathologic grade of cerebral gliomas: preliminary results. AJR Am J Roentgenol. 2002;179:783–9.
112. Bisdas S, Kirkpatrick M, Giglio P, Welsh C, Spampinato MV, Rumboldt Z. Cerebral blood volume measurements by perfusion-weighted MR imaging in gliomas: ready for prime time in predicting short-term outcome and recurrent disease? AJNR Am J Neuroradiol. 2009;30:681–8.
113. Law M, Young RJ, Babb JS, et al. Gliomas: Predicting Time to Progression or Survival with Cerebral Blood Volume Measurements at Dynamic Susceptibility-weighted Contrast-enhanced Perfusion MR Imaging. Radiology. 2008;247:490–8. doi:10.1148/radiol.2472070898.
114. Danchaivijitr N, Waldman AD, Tozer DJ, et al. Low-grade gliomas: do changes in rCBV measurements at longitudinal perfusion-weighted MR imaging

predict malignant transformation? Radiology. 2008; 247:170–8.
115. Caseiras GB, Chheang S, Babb J, et al. Relative cerebral blood volume measurements of low-grade gliomas predict patient outcome in a multi-institution setting. Eur J Radiol. 2010;73:215–20.
116. Patankar TF, Haroon HA, Mills SJ, et al. Is volume transfer coefficient (K(trans)) related to histologic grade in human gliomas? AJNR Am J Neuroradiol. 2005;26:2455–65.
117. Law M, Yang S, Babb JS, et al. Comparison of cerebral blood volume and vascular permeability from dynamic susceptibility contrast-enhanced perfusion MR imaging with glioma grade. AJNR Am J Neuroradiol. 2004;25:746–55.
118. Zhang N, Zhang L, Qiu B, Meng L, Wang X, Hou BL. Correlation of volume transfer coefficient K(trans) with histopathologic grades of gliomas. J Magn Reson Imaging. 2012;36:355–63.
119. Nguyen TB, Cron GO, Mercier JF, et al. Diagnostic accuracy of dynamic contrast-enhanced MR imaging using a phase-derived vascular input function in the preoperative grading of gliomas. AJNR Am J Neuroradiol. 2012;33:1539–45.
120. Foottit C, Cron GO, Hogan MJ, Nguyen TB, Cameron I. Determination of the venous output function from MR signal phase: feasibility for quantitative DCE-MRI in human brain. Magn Reson Med. 2010;63:772–81.
121. Cron GO, Foottit C, Yankeelov TE, Avruch LI, Schweitzer ME, Cameron I. Arterial input functions determined from MR signal magnitude and phase for quantitative dynamic contrast-enhanced MRI in the human pelvis. Magn Reson Med. 2011;66:498–504.
122. Awasthi R, Rathore RK, Soni P, et al. Discriminant analysis to classify glioma grading using dynamic contrast-enhanced MRI and immunohistochemical markers. Neuroradiology. 2012;54:205–13.
123. Chenevert TL, Stegman LD, Taylor JM, et al. Diffusion magnetic resonance imaging: an early surrogate marker of therapeutic efficacy in brain tumors. J Natl Cancer Inst. 2000;92:2029–36.
124. Sugahara T, Korogi Y, Kochi M, et al. Usefulness of diffusion-weighted MRI with echo-planar technique in the evaluation of cellularity in gliomas. J Magn Reson Imaging. 1999;9:53–60.
125. Kono K, Inoue Y, Nakayama K, et al. The role of diffusion-weighted imaging in patients with brain tumors. AJNR Am J Neuroradiol. 2001;22:1081–8.
126. Mills SJ, Soh C, Rose CJ, et al. Candidate biomarkers of extravascular extracellular space: a direct comparison of apparent diffusion coefficient and dynamic contrast-enhanced MR imaging-derived measurement of the volume of the extravascular extracellular space in glioblastoma multiforme. AJNR Am J Neuroradiol. 2010;31:549–53.
127. Weber MA, Zoubaa S, Schlieter M, et al. Diagnostic performance of spectroscopic and perfusion MRI for distinction of brain tumors. Neurology. 2006;66: 1899–906.
128. Weber MA, Thilmann C, Lichy MP, et al. Assessment of irradiated brain metastases by means of arterial spin-labeling and dynamic susceptibility-weighted contrast-enhanced perfusion MRI: initial results. Invest Radiol. 2004;39:277–87.
129. Canale S, Rodrigo S, Tourdias T, et al. Grading of adults primitive glial neoplasms using arterial spin-labeled perfusion MR imaging. J Neuroradiol. 2011;38:207–13.
130. Hirai T, Kitajima M, Nakamura H, et al. Quantitative blood flow measurements in gliomas using arterial spin-labeling at 3T: intermodality agreement and inter- and intraobserver reproducibility study. AJNR Am J Neuroradiol. 2011;32:2073–9.
131. van Westen D, Petersen ET, Wirestam R, et al. Correlation between arterial blood volume obtained by arterial spin labelling and cerebral blood volume in intracranial tumours. MAGMA. 2011;24:211–23.
132. Law M, Cha S, Knopp EA, Johnson G, Arnett J, Litt AW. High-grade gliomas and solitary metastases: differentiation by using perfusion and proton spectroscopic MR imaging. Radiology. 2002;222:715–21.
133. Young GS, Setayesh K. Spin-echo echo-planar perfusion MR imaging in the differential diagnosis of solitary enhancing brain lesions: distinguishing solitary metastases from primary glioma. AJNR Am J Neuroradiol. 2009;30:575–7.
134. Liao W, Liu Y, Wang X, et al. Differentiation of primary central nervous system lymphoma and high-grade glioma with dynamic susceptibility contrast-enhanced perfusion magnetic resonance imaging. Acta Radiol. 2009;50:217–25.
135. Saloner D, Uzelac A, Hetts S, Martin A, Dillon W. Modern meningioma imaging techniques. J Neurooncol. 2010;99:333–40.
136. Martin AJ, Cha S, Higashida RT, et al. Assessment of vasculature of meningiomas and the effects of embolization with intra-arterial MR perfusion imaging: a feasibility study. AJNR Am J Neuroradiol. 2007;28:1771–7.
137. Zhang H, Rodiger LA, Shen T, Miao J, Oudkerk M. Preoperative subtyping of meningiomas by perfusion MR imaging. Neuroradiology. 2008;50: 835–40.
138. Arai M, Kashihara K, Kaizaki Y. Enhancing gliotic cyst wall with microvascular proliferation adjacent to a meningioma. J Clin Neurosci. 2006;13:136–9.
139. Nakano T, Asano K, Miura H, Itoh S, Suzuki S. Meningiomas with brain edema: radiological characteristics on MRI and review of the literature. Clin Imaging. 2002;26:243–9.
140. Yang S, Law M, Zagzag D, et al. Dynamic contrast-enhanced perfusion MR imaging measurements of endothelial permeability: differentiation between atypical and typical meningiomas. AJNR Am J Neuroradiol. 2003;24:1554–9.
141. Kelly PJ, Daumas-Duport C, Scheithauer BW, Kall BA, Kispert DB. Stereotactic histologic correlations of computed tomography- and magnetic resonance imaging-defined abnormalities in patients with glial neoplasms. Mayo Clin Proc. 1987;62:450–9.

142. Kelly PJ, Daumas-Duport C, Kispert DB, Kall BA, Scheithauer BW, Illig JJ. Imaging-based stereotaxic serial biopsies in untreated intracranial glial neoplasms. J Neurosurg. 1987;66:865–74.
143. Lev MH, Rosen BR. Clinical applications of intracranial perfusion MR imaging. Neuroimaging Clin N Am. 1999;9:309–31.
144. Macdonald DR, Cascino TL, Schold Jr SC, Cairncross JG. Response criteria for phase II studies of supratentorial malignant glioma. J Clin Oncol. 1990;8:1277–80.
145. Henegar MM, Moran CJ, Silbergeld DL. Early postoperative magnetic resonance imaging following nonneoplastic cortical resection. J Neurosurg. 1996;84:174–9.
146. Kumar AJ, Leeds NE, Fuller GN, et al. Malignant gliomas: MR imaging spectrum of radiation therapy- and chemotherapy-induced necrosis of the brain after treatment. Radiology. 2000;217:377–84.
147. Ulmer S, Braga TA, Barker 2nd FG, Lev MH, Gonzalez RG, Henson JW. Clinical and radiographic features of peritumoral infarction following resection of glioblastoma. Neurology. 2006;67:1668–70.
148. Finn MA, Blumenthal DT, Salzman KL, Jensen RL. Transient postictal MRI changes in patients with brain tumors may mimic disease progression. Surg Neurol. 2007;67:246–50. discussion 250.
149. Valk PE, Dillon WP. Radiation injury of the brain. AJNR Am J Neuroradiol. 1991;12:45–62.
150. Hu LS, Baxter LC, Smith KA, et al. Relative cerebral blood volume values to differentiate high-grade glioma recurrence from posttreatment radiation effect: direct correlation between image-guided tissue histopathology and localized dynamic susceptibility-weighted contrast-enhanced perfusion MR imaging measurements. AJNR Am J Neuroradiol. 2009; 30:552–8.
151. Hopewell JW, Calvo W, Jaenke R, Reinhold HS, Robbins ME, Whitehouse EM. Microvasculature and radiation damage. Recent Results Cancer Res. 1993;130:1–16.
152. Wesseling P, Ruiter DJ, Burger PC. Angiogenesis in brain tumors; pathobiological and clinical aspects. J Neurooncol. 1997;32:253–65.
153. Oh BC, Pagnini PG, Wang MY, et al. Stereotactic radiosurgery: adjacent tissue injury and response after high-dose single fraction radiation: Part I–Histology, imaging, and molecular events. Neurosurgery. 2007;60:31–44. discussion 44–35.
154. Hazle JD, Jackson EF, Schomer DF, Leeds NE. Dynamic imaging of intracranial lesions using fast spin-echo imaging: differentiation of brain tumors and treatment effects. J Magn Reson Imaging. 1997;7:1084–93.
155. Narang J, Jain R, Arbab AS, et al. Differentiating treatment-induced necrosis from recurrent/progressive brain tumor using nonmodel-based semiquantitative indices derived from dynamic contrast-enhanced T1-weighted MR perfusion. Neuro Oncol. 2011; 13:1037–46.
156. Ozsunar Y, Mullins ME, Kwong K, et al. Glioma recurrence versus radiation necrosis? A pilot comparison of arterial spin-labeled, dynamic susceptibility contrast enhanced MRI, and FDG-PET imaging. Acad Radiol. 2010;17:282–90.
157. Stupp R, Hegi ME, Mason WP, et al. Effects of radiotherapy with concomitant and adjuvant temozolomide versus radiotherapy alone on survival in glioblastoma in a randomised phase III study: 5-year analysis of the EORTC-NCIC trial. Lancet Oncol. 2009;10:459–66.
158. Stupp R, Mason WP, van den Bent MJ, et al. Radiotherapy plus concomitant and adjuvant temozolomide for glioblastoma. N Engl J Med. 2005;352:987–96.
159. Clarke JL, Chang S. Pseudoprogression and pseudoresponse: challenges in brain tumor imaging. Curr Neurol Neurosci Rep. 2009;9:241–6.
160. Brandes AA, Franceschi E, Tosoni A, et al. MGMT Promoter Methylation Status Can Predict the Incidence and Outcome of Pseudoprogression After Concomitant Radiochemotherapy in Newly Diagnosed Glioblastoma Patients. J Clin Oncol. 2008;26:2192–7. doi:10.1200/JCO.2007.14.8163.
161. van Nifterik KA, van den Berg J, van der Meide WF, et al. Absence of the MGMT protein as well as methylation of the MGMT promoter predict the sensitivity for temozolomide. Br J Cancer. 2010;103: 29–35.
162. Prados MD. Treatment strategies for patients with recurrent brain tumors. Semin Radiat Oncol. 1991;1:62–8.
163. Hegi ME, Diserens AC, Gorlia T, et al. MGMT gene silencing and benefit from temozolomide in glioblastoma. N Engl J Med. 2005;352:997–1003.
164. Young RJ, Gupta A, Shah AD, et al. Potential utility of conventional MRI signs in diagnosing pseudoprogression in glioblastoma. Neurology. 2011;76:1918–24.
165. Mangla R, Singh G, Ziegelitz D, et al. Changes in relative cerebral blood volume 1 month after radiation-temozolomide therapy can help predict overall survival in patients with glioblastoma. Radiology. 2010;256:575–84.
166. Kong DS, Kim ST, Kim EH, et al. Diagnostic dilemma of pseudoprogression in the treatment of newly diagnosed glioblastomas: the role of assessing relative cerebral blood flow volume and oxygen-6-methylguanine-DNA methyltransferase promoter methylation status. AJNR Am J Neuroradiol. 2011;32:382–7.
167. Shiroishi MS, Jones JGA, Ozhand A, et al. Dynamic contrast-enhanced and dynamic susceptibility contrast MR imaging evaluation of true early progression versus pseudoprogression in patients with high-grade gliomas. In:Proceedings of the American Society of Neuroradiology. Seattle, WA, 2011
168. Wen PY, Macdonald DR, Reardon DA, et al. Updated response assessment criteria for high-grade gliomas: response assessment in neuro-oncology working group. J Clin Oncol. 2010;28:1963–72.

169. Pope WB, Hessel C. Response assessment in neuro-oncology criteria: implementation challenges in multicenter neuro-oncology trials. AJNR Am J Neuroradiol. 2011;32:794–7.
170. Price RE, Langford LA, Jackson EF, Stephens LC, Tinkey PT, Ang KK. Radiation-induced morphologic changes in the rhesus monkey (Macaca mulatta) brain. J Med Primatol. 2001;30:81–7.
171. Ljubimova NV, Levitman MK, Plotnikova ED, Eidus L. Endothelial cell population dynamics in rat brain after local irradiation. Br J Radiol. 1991;64:934–40.
172. Pena LA, Fuks Z, Kolesnick RN. Radiation-induced apoptosis of endothelial cells in the murine central nervous system: protection by fibroblast growth factor and sphingomyelinase deficiency. Cancer Res. 2000;60:321–7.
173. Li YQ, Chen P, Haimovitz-Friedman A, Reilly RM, Wong CS. Endothelial apoptosis initiates acute blood-brain barrier disruption after ionizing radiation. Cancer Res. 2003;63:5950–6.
174. Wenz F, Rempp K, Hess T, et al. Effect of radiation on blood volume in low-grade astrocytomas and normal brain tissue: quantification with dynamic susceptibility contrast MR imaging. Am J Roentgenol. 1996;166:187–93.
175. Lee MC, Cha S, Chang SM, Nelson SJ. Dynamic susceptibility contrast perfusion imaging of radiation effects in normal-appearing brain tissue: changes in the first-pass and recirculation phases. J Magn Reson Imaging. 2005;21:683–93.
176. Cao Y, Tsien CI, Sundgren PC, et al. Dynamic contrast-enhanced magnetic resonance imaging as a biomarker for prediction of radiation-induced neurocognitive dysfunction. Clin Cancer Res. 2009;15:1747–54.
177. Pope WB, Lai A, Nghiemphu P, Mischel P, Cloughesy TF. MRI in patients with high-grade gliomas treated with bevacizumab and chemotherapy. Neurology. 2006;66:1258–60. doi:10.1212/01.wnl.0000208958.29600.87.
178. Norden AD, Young GS, Setayesh K, et al. Bevacizumab for recurrent malignant gliomas: efficacy, toxicity, and patterns of recurrence. Neurology. 2008;70:779–87.
179. Gerstner ER, Chen PJ, Wen PY, Jain RK, Batchelor TT, Sorensen G. Infiltrative patterns of glioblastoma spread detected via diffusion MRI after treatment with cediranib. Neuro Oncol. 2010;12:466–72.
180. Pope WB, Kim HJ, Huo J, et al. Recurrent glioblastoma multiforme: ADC histogram analysis predicts response to bevacizumab treatment. Radiology. 2009;252:182–9.
181. Sorensen AG, Batchelor TT, Zhang WT, et al. A "vascular normalization index" as potential mechanistic biomarker to predict survival after a single dose of cediranib in recurrent glioblastoma patients. Cancer Res. 2009;69:5296–300.
182. Brandsma D, van den Bent MJ. Pseudoprogression and pseudoresponse in the treatment of gliomas. Curr Opin Neurol. 2009;22:633–8.
183. Wetzel SG, Cha S, Johnson G, et al. Relative cerebral blood volume measurements in intracranial mass lesions: interobserver and intraobserver reproducibility study. Radiology. 2002;224:797–803.
184. Law M, Young R, Babb J, Pollack E, Johnson G. Histogram analysis versus region of interest analysis of dynamic susceptibility contrast perfusion MR imaging data in the grading of cerebral gliomas. AJNR Am J Neuroradiol. 2007;28:761–6.
185. Emblem KE, Scheie D, Due-Tonnessen P, et al. Histogram analysis of MR imaging-derived cerebral blood volume maps: combined glioma grading and identification of low-grade oligodendroglial subtypes. AJNR Am J Neuroradiol. 2008;29:1664–70.
186. Galban CJ, Chenevert TL, Meyer CR, et al. The parametric response map is an imaging biomarker for early cancer treatment outcome. Nat Med. 2009;15:572–6.
187. Tsien C, Galban CJ, Chenevert TL, et al. Parametric response map as an imaging biomarker to distinguish progression from pseudoprogression in high-grade glioma. J Clin Oncol. 2010;28:2293–9.
188. Arllinghaus LR, Yankeelov TE. Diffusion-weighted MRI. In: Yankeelov TE, Pickens DR, Price RR, editors. Quantitative MRI in cancer. Boca Raton, FL: CRC Press; 2012.
189. Moffat BA, Chenevert TL, Lawrence TS, et al. Functional diffusion map: a noninvasive MRI biomarker for early stratification of clinical brain tumor response. Proc Natl Acad Sci U S A. 2005;102:5524–9.
190. Gerstner ER, Sorensen AG. Diffusion and diffusion tensor imaging in brain cancer. Semin Radiat Oncol. 2011;21:141–6.
191. Sorensen AG. Perfusion MR, imaging: moving forward. Radiology. 2008;249:416–7.
192. Geer CP, Simonds J, Anvery A, et al. Does MR perfusion imaging impact management decisions for patients with brain tumors? A prospective study. AJNR Am J Neuroradiol. 2012;33:556–62.
193. Smith JJ, Sorensen AG, Thrall JH. Biomarkers in imaging: realizing radiology's future. Radiology. 2003;227:633–8.
194. Clarke LP, Croft BS, Nordstrom R, Zhang H, Kelloff G, Tatum J. Quantitative imaging for evaluation of response to cancer therapy. Transl Oncol. 2009;2:195–7.
195. Buckler AJ, Bresolin L, Dunnick NR, Sullivan DC. A collaborative enterprise for multi-stakeholder participation in the advancement of quantitative imaging. Radiology. 2011;258:906–14.

Diffusion Tensor Imaging: Introduction and Applications to Brain Tumor Characterization

2

Sumei Wang, Sungheon Kim, and Elias R. Melhem

Introduction

Brain tumors are the second leading cause of cancer-related deaths in children and adults younger than 39 years old, and they affect adults of all ages. The total number of newly diagnosed primary malignant or nonmalignant brain tumors was estimated to be 64,530 in 2004–2007, with 24,070 being malignant and 40,470 being nonmalignant, according to the Central Brain Tumor Registry of the United States (CBTRUS) [1]. Although the long-term survival of patients with brain tumors has been considerably improved over the last two or three decades, death still occurs in a significant proportion of the patients. In particular, glioblastoma, the most malignant primary brain tumor, presents a major challenge with a median survival time of only 12.2–18.2 months [2].

S. Wang, M.D. (✉)
Division of Neuroradiology, Department of Radiology, Hospital of the University of Pennsylvania, 219 Dulles Building, 3400 Spruce St., Philadelphia, PA 19104, USA
e-mail: Sumei.Wang@uphs.upenn.edu

S. Kim, Ph.D.
Department of Radiology, Center for Biomedical Imaging, New York University School of Medicine, New York, NY 10016, USA

E.R. Melhem, M.D., Ph.D.
Department of Diagnostic Radiology and Nuclear Medicine, University of Maryland School of Medicine, Baltimore, MD 21201, USA

Brain tumor malignancy or grade is generally assessed according to World Health Organization (WHO) criteria, taking into account the cellularity, mitotic activity, endothelial proliferation, and necrosis [3]. Brain tumors consist of a variety of subtypes with a wide range of histopathology, molecular and genetic profile, clinical spectrum, and treatment options and outcome. The most common primary brain tumors in adults are glioblastomas and meningiomas. Brain metastases outnumber primary brain tumors in adults owing to high incidence of systemic cancer. Accurate diagnosis and grading of brain tumors are often crucial as the management and prognosis of different types of tumors are substantially different [4–6]. Pathological analysis of biopsy samples is the current gold standard for tumor grading. However, biopsy has limitations attributable to sampling error (e.g., missing the most malignant part) and is not always feasible (e.g., tumor in the brain stem).

Conventional MRI can display the anatomical appearance of brain tumor, but fails to provide physiologic and functional information that is crucial for tumor grading, predicting clinical outcome and response to therapy. Over the past few years, diffusion tensor imaging (DTI) has been increasingly used to study pathologic changes in brain tumors [7–10]. Various DTI metrics can be derived from the imaging data to provide information about the orientation and architecture of tissue microstructure at the voxel level. In this chapter, we briefly explain the DTI technique, followed by application of various DTI metrics in brain tumor characterization.

J.J. Pillai (ed.), *Functional Brain Tumor Imaging*, DOI 10.1007/978-1-4419-5858-7_2,

Basic Principles of Diffusion Tensor Imaging

Water molecules, the principle components of the brain, are in constant motion caused by random thermal fluctuation. By applying a pair of dephasing and rephrasing magnetic field gradients, MR imaging may be sensitized to the motion (diffusion) in the direction of the field gradient. This gradient pulse configuration is often known as diffusion weighting [11]. The degree of diffusion weighting is described by the *b* value, a parameter that is determined by the amplitude and timing of diffusion gradients. The measurement of signal loss or attenuation is a function of the diffusivity in a chosen direction as shown below:

$$S = S_0 e^{-bD} \tag{2.1}$$

where S is the diffusion-weighted signal, S_0 is the signal without diffusion weighting, and D is the estimated diffusivity or apparent diffusion coefficient (ADC). Acquiring diffusion-weighted images with at least two different b values allows the determination of the diffusivity for each image voxel.

In white matter, diffusion is anisotropic, as axonal membranes and myelin sheaths restrict and/or hinder this molecular motion in a particular direction. Apparent diffusivity of water is generally higher in directions parallel to fiber tracts than in the perpendicular direction [12]. Three-dimensional probability distribution of diffusivity can be described by a diffusion tensor ellipsoid with three eigenvectors and the corresponding eigenvalues (λ_1, λ_2, and λ_3). The eigenvector associated with the largest eigenvalue denotes the predominant orientation of fibers in a given imaging voxel. If a particular voxel has a high degree of anisotropy, one of the eigenvalues will be much higher than the other two.

Most commonly used indices for diffusion tensor are mean diffusivity (MD) and fractional anisotropy (FA) [13], which can be calculated according to (2.2) and (2.3), respectively:

$$MD = (\lambda_1 + \lambda_2 + \lambda_3)/3 \tag{2.2}$$

$$FA = \sqrt{\frac{3}{2}} \sqrt{\frac{(\lambda_1 - \bar{\lambda})^2 + (\lambda_2 - \bar{\lambda})^2 + (\lambda_3 - \bar{\lambda})^2}{\lambda_1^2 + \lambda_2^2 + \lambda_3^2}} \tag{2.3}$$

where $\bar{\lambda}$ denotes mean of the three eigenvalues. MD is a measure of the directionally averaged magnitude of diffusion and is related to cell density, size, and parenchyma permeability. FA represents the degree of diffusion anisotropy, and reflects the degree of alignment of cellular structure [13].

Although FA is a good indicator of diffusion anisotropy, it does not provide information on the shape of the diffusion ellipsoid. For example, it cannot distinguish a flat ellipsoid from an oblong one. Westin et al. [14] have modeled diffusion anisotropy using a set of three basic metrics that depend on the shape of the diffusion tensor: linear anisotropy coefficient (CL) where diffusion is mainly along the direction corresponding to the largest eigenvalue; planar anisotropy coefficient (CP) where diffusion is mainly restricted to the plane spanned by the two eigenvectors with the two largest eigenvalues; and spherical anisotropy coefficient (CS), which indicates isotropic diffusion. The CL, CP, and CS values can be calculated using the following equations:

$$CL = (\lambda_1 - \lambda_2)/(\lambda_1 + \lambda_2 + \lambda_3) \tag{2.4}$$

$$CP = 2(\lambda_2 - \lambda_3)/(\lambda_1 + \lambda_2 + \lambda_3) \tag{2.5}$$

$$CS = 3\lambda_3/(\lambda_1 + \lambda_2 + \lambda_3) \tag{2.6}$$

The CL, CP, and CS values lie in the range from 0 to 1 and the sum of these three metrics is equal to 1 (Fig. 2.1).

Each anisotropy measure shows unique features in different regions of white matter. These differences arise from the relative contribution of the linear, planar, and spherical shape components of the diffusion tensor. Linear ellipsoid is typically found in regions with parallel arrangement, such as corpus callosum and pyramidal tract. Planar ellipsoid corresponds to regions of fibers with different orientations, or bundles of fibers that are randomly oriented in a plane, such as centrum semiovale and subcortical white matter regions. The gray matter appears isotropic with high CS [15]. These studies suggest that tensor shape measurements allow one to explore the tissue microstructural difference.

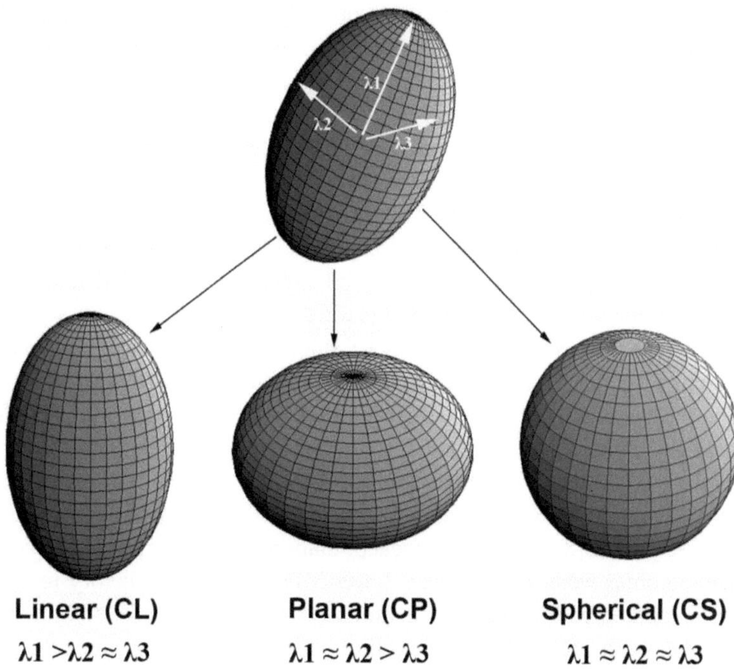

Fig. 2.1 Three shapes of diffusion ellipsoid

Application to Brain Tumor Characterization

Water diffusion is affected by tissue constitutes, such as macromolecules, membranes, and organelles, as well as by tissue microstructure and organization. From the metrics derived from DTI, one can infer information about the brain tissue that cannot be obtained using conventional MRI. In brain tumors, microstructural tissue characteristics vary significantly between tumor types, including the cellularity, presence of tumor necrosis, fibrous tissue within tumors, tumor infiltration, and so forth. DTI is a promising tool for detecting such microscopic difference in tumors.

Most of DTI studies in brain tumors focused on the analysis of different parts within the tumor using various DTI metrics. But it is often helpful to measure reactive and infiltrative changes in the tissue surrounding the tumor. The neoplastic mass can be generally subdivided into two regions: the solid part of the tumor and central necrotic or cystic part of the tumor. Similarly, the peritumoral edematous region can be separated into two regions: proximal region surrounding the enhancing part of the tumor potentially including infiltrative tumor cells, and more distal region mainly comprising vasogenic edema. These four subregions of a neoplasm can be substantially different from each other in terms of their DTI metrics. A variety of methods to analyze diffusion information have been proposed and range from simple mean/median value to histogram analysis over the selected regions of interest (ROIs). Systematic analysis of various DTI metrics including tensor shape measures from these different areas may provide a robust way for characterization of brain neoplasms.

Mean Diffusivity and Tumor Cellularity

Of all the histologic features used in tumor classification, cellularity has been the main target of assessment with DTI. MD measures the magnitude of diffusion within cerebral tissues. The higher the tumor cellularity, the lower the MD value due to decrease in the extracellular space (i.e., increased hindrance to extracellular water diffusion, assuming that the intracellular water diffusion is restricted) [12, 16]. This inverse correlation between MD and cellularity has been reported in both glial [9] and nonglial tumors [17].

MD values have been used in differentiating tumor grades [7, 8, 18, 19] and types [8, 20–22], however, with mixed results. Some reports have suggested that mean MD [20, 23, 24], minimum MD [7] [25], or MD ratio [18, 19] is helpful for grading and tumor differentiation, while others indicated the limited use of MD in the differentiation of neoplasms [8, 26–28]. Those studies in which MD was found useful have generally observed lower diffusivities in high-grade or more cellular tumors. It has been accepted that primary cerebral lymphomas and medulloblastomas have lower MD values because of densely packed cells in these tumors [8, 17]. Also atypical or malignant meningiomas were found to have lower MD values compared with typical meningiomas [18, 19, 29]. However, MD itself is very limited in ++ tumor classification with low sensitivity and specificity [21, 22]. Besides cellularity, other factors such as extracellular matrix, viscosity, and mucins may also affect the measurement of MD [30, 31].

MD has also been used to monitor tumor treatment response. In most malignant tumors, successful treatment is reflected by increases in MD values. This may be due to the cellular death and vascular changes in response to treatment. Results from animal models [32] and clinical studies [33] provide supportive evidence for the use of MD as a responsive biomarker. A novel method called functional diffusion mapping (fDM) has been introduced to map voxel-by-voxel changes of apparent diffusivity over time [2, 34].

Diffusion Anisotropy of Tumor

FA is the most commonly used anisotropy index. FA reflects the degree of alignment of tissue microstructure, and as such its use may not be limited to the white matter tracts alone [12]. Regions of relatively high anisotropy have been reported in brain abscesses [35], glioblastomas [36, 37], and areas of hemorrhage [38], indicating that the tissues other than the white matter can also have preferentially oriented structures.

In contrast to MD, the relationship between FA and tumor cellularity is unclear, as both positive [36, 37, 39] and negative [9, 40] correlation has been reported. While Inoue et al. [41] stated that FA values of low-grade gliomas were significantly lower than those of high-grade gliomas, Stadlbauer et al. [9] reported lower FA values in high-grade gliomas. A recent study reported that mean and maximal FA from the solid part of the tumor are useful in grading nonenhancing gliomas [26]. For tumor type differentiation, Wang W et al. [42] and Reiche et al. [43] reported lower FA from the enhancing regions of glioblastomas compared with brain metastases, whereas Wang S et al. [22] observed higher FA in the enhancing regions of glioblastomas than in those of metastases. One likely reason for these contradictory results is the lack of standardized methods, both for acquisition as well as postprocessing and selection of ROI. It has also been demonstrated by Wang et al. [21] that FA in glioblastomas is higher than that in both brain metastases and primary cerebral lymphomas (Figs. 2.2, 2.3, 2.4, and 2.5). Among these three tumor types, lymphomas have the highest cellularity, followed by glioblastomas and brain metastases [44–46]. These findings indicate that diffusion anisotropy may not directly correlate with tumor cellularity. It has been reported that FA of tumor can be affected by several factors including extracellular-to-intracellular space ratio, extracellular matrix, tortuosity, and vascularity [30, 31]. Further study is warranted to help understand the underlying tumor microstructure contributing to FA.

Shape-Based Diffusion Tensor Metrics

Information on the geometric nature of diffusion tensor provides further differentiation of tumor types based on tensor shape in addition to FA [14, 15, 47]. Both CL and CP values contribute to FA observed in tissue and their relative values indicate the shape of diffusion ellipsoid [15]. Anisotropy changes within and surrounding the tumor have been demonstrated in animal studies, indicating that tensor shape is related to the macroscopic organization of tumor cells [48–50].

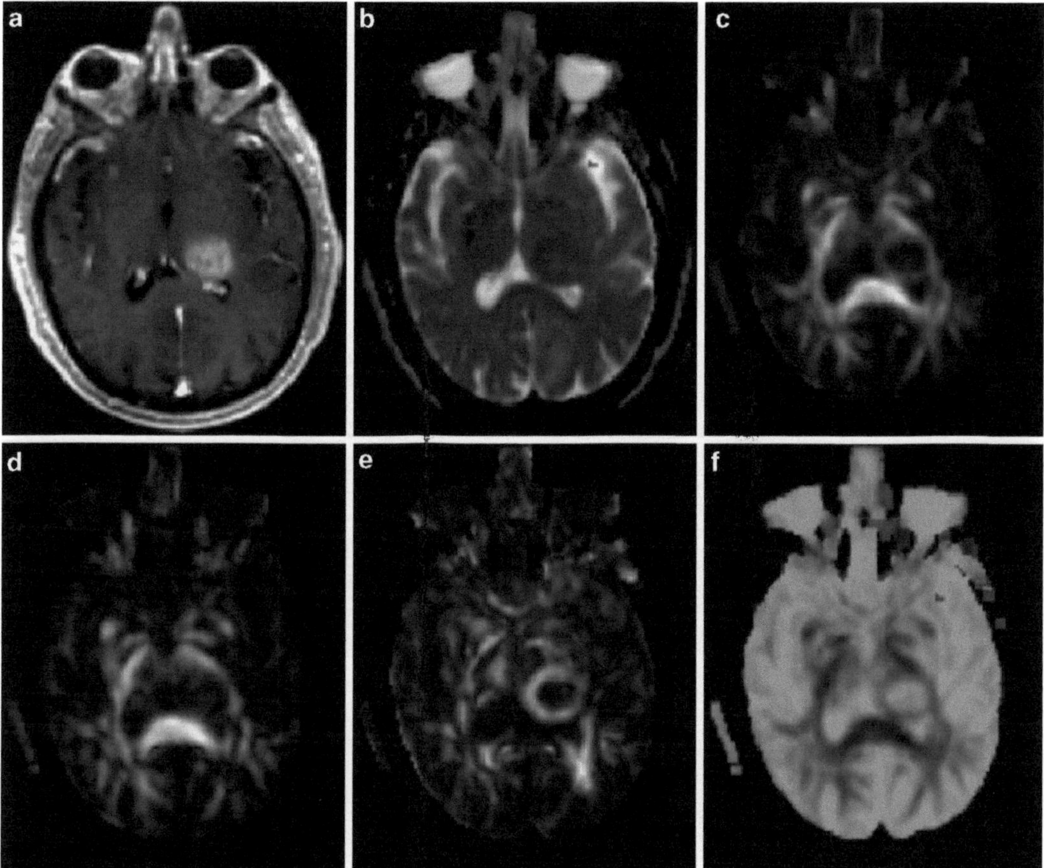

Fig. 2.2 A 71-year-old male with a glioblastoma in the *left* thalamus. Axial contrast-enhanced T1-weighted image (**a**) shows solid enhancement. MD map (**b**) shows restricted diffusion of the enhancing part ($0.75\times10^{-3}/\mathrm{mm}^2/\mathrm{s}$). FA (**c**), CL (**d**), and CP (**e**) from the enhancing part (0.18, 0.15, and 0.15, respectively) are higher than those for brain metastasis (Fig. 2.3) and primary cerebral lymphoma (PCL, Fig. 2.4). CS (**f**) from the enhancing portion (0.68) is lower compared with brain metastasis and PCL. Reprinted and modified with permission from Wang et al. [21]

The types of the tumor, the degree of invasiveness, and growth rate can affect the diffusion properties [49, 50]. Tensor shape measurements have also been used to characterize pathologic changes in the human brain. Zhang et al. [47] reported lower CL in brain metastases than in contralateral normal brain. Elevated FA and CP along with decreased CS were observed in fibroblastic meningiomas compared with other subtypes of meningiomas [29, 51, 52]. Kumar et al. [53] reported high CP and low CL in the abscess cavity compared with normal white matter, thus distinguishing true from pseudo white matter tracts. It has also been reported that epidermoid cysts have high CP [54] and tuberculomas showed lower CL, CP, and higher CS [55] compared with normal white matter. Wang et al. [21] also demonstrated higher FA, CL, and CP from the enhancing part of glioblastomas in comparison to both brain metastases and primary cerebral lymphomas (Figs. 2.2, 2.3, 2.4, and 2.5). These results suggest that tensor shape measurements provide additional information about tissue characteristics, which may further aid in tumor classification.

A ring with high CP has been reported in glioblastomas, brain metastases, and meningiomas. While the potential reason for the observation of this ring remains speculative, its presence may reflect compression of surrounding tissue by the tumor [47, 52].

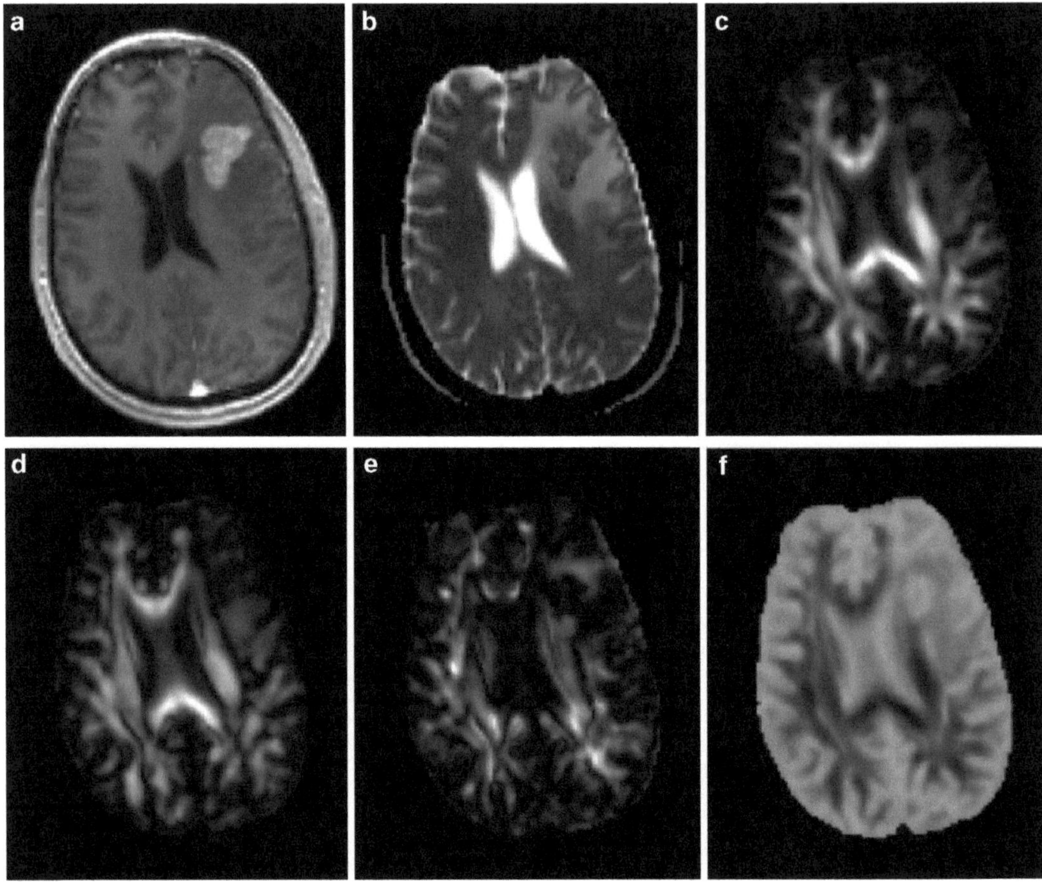

Fig. 2.3 A 53-year-old male with metastatic lung adenocarcinoma in the *left* frontal lobe. Axial contrast-enhanced T1-weighted (**a**) shows a solid enhancing lesion. MD map (**b**) shows restricted diffusion of the enhancing part ($0.95 \times 10^{-3}/\text{mm}^2/\text{s}$). Lower FA (**c**), CL (**d**), and CP (**e**) are noticed from the enhancing part (0.10, 0.08, and 0.09, respectively) relative to normal-appearing white matter compared with the glioblastoma. CS (**f**) appearance looks similar to glioblastoma (Fig. 2.2f), but has a higher value (0.82)

DTI and Tumor Infiltration

Peritumoral region is usually defined as the area of abnormality surrounding the enhancing part of the tumor. In metastatic brain tumors or noninfiltrative primary tumors such as meningiomas, peritumoral edema is widely regarded as vasogenic edema. In this region, increased extracellular water is present due to leakage of plasma from altered tumor capillaries. Also this region does not include any tumor cells. In gliomas, however, the peritumoral region includes both vasogenic edema and infiltrating tumor cells.

Investigators have tried to use DTI to differentiate tumor-infiltrated edema from pure vasogenic edema [20, 22, 24], which may be beneficial for accurate preoperative diagnosis of glioblastomas and metastases. Lu et al. [20] reported a significant difference between tumor-infiltrated edema and pure vasogenic edema using a parameter called "tumor infiltration index," which measures departure from a linear relationship between MD and FA. These authors also reported higher MD in metastasis compared to glioblastomas. However, other studies demonstrated lower MD and minimum MD or MD ratio in the peritumoral region of metastases compared to that of glioblastomas [24, 56]. In contrast, van Westen et al. [57] reported no difference in MD and FA values in the peritumoral region of glioblastomas, metastases, and meningiomas. Recently, Kinoshita et al. [58] claimed that "tumor infiltration index" could

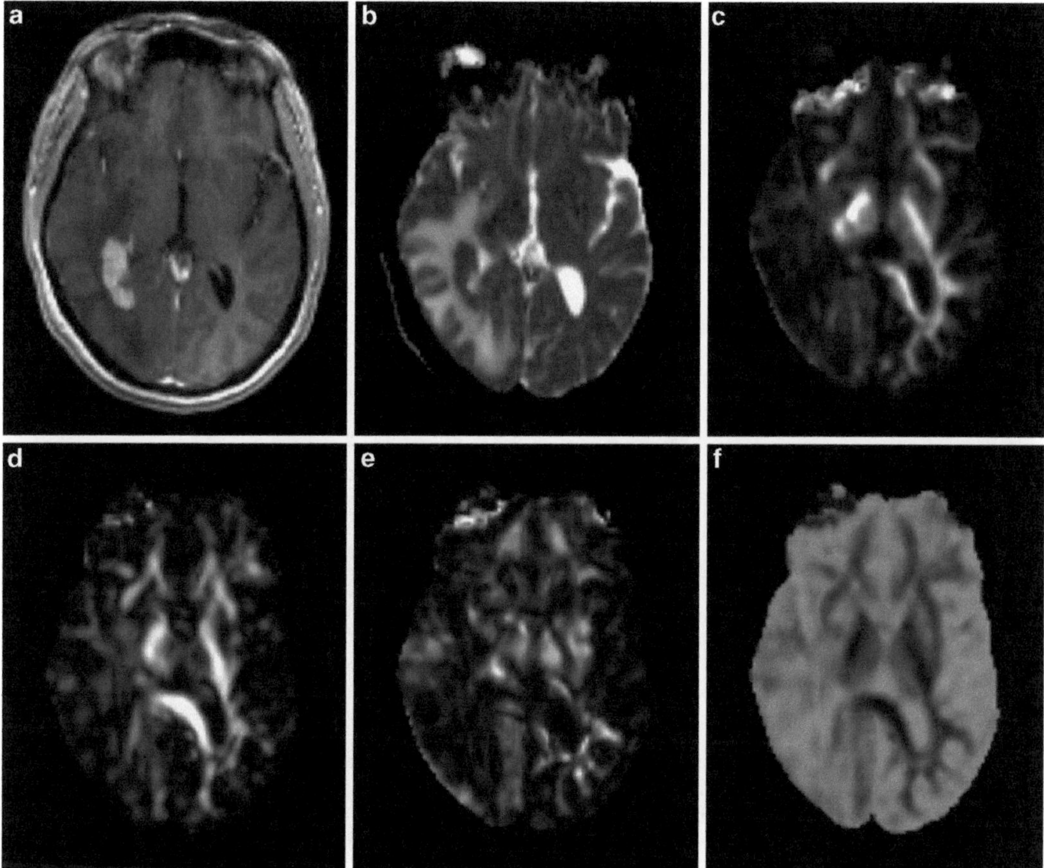

Fig. 2.4 A 58-year-old female with primary cerebral diffuse large B cell lymphoma in the *right* peritrigonal area. Axial contrast-enhanced T1-weighted (**a**) shows a solid enhancing lesion with extensive edema. MD map (**b**) shows restricted diffusion of the enhancing part (0.80×10^{-3}/mm^2/s). Lower FA (**c**), CL (**d**), and CP (**e**) are noticed from the enhancing part (0.08, 0.08, and 0.06, respectively) relative to normal-appearing white matter compared with the glioblastoma. CS (**f**) from the enhancing part appears higher (0.85) compared with glioblastoma

not differentiate vasogenic edema from tumor-infiltrated edema. The difference in defining the ROIs for the peritumoral region in these studies may in part be responsible for the discrepancy. A number of studies have focused on the area close to the enhancing region (peritumoral region) either by manually placing a number of small ROIs around the tumor [23, 24] or by using a band of arbitrarily chosen thickness around the tumor [28, 59]. In the study reported by Wang et al. [22], the peritumoral areas were further subdivided into immediate peritumoral region and distant peritumoral region with the hypothesis that the immediate peritumoral region may have a higher degree of tumor infiltration in glioblastomas. There was a significant difference in FA, CL, and CP between glioblastomas and metastases in the immediate peritumoral region. In the distant peritumoral region, only FA and CP measurements reached significant difference between the two tumor types [22]. While statistical significance was observed, the overall sensitivity, specificity, and accuracy for all the DTI metrics in the peritumoral areas were lower than in the enhancing part of the tumor. Since the edematous region contains areas of increased extracellular water, tumor infiltration, and varying fractional composition of normal white/gray matter, it is difficult to determine which factor dominates the DTI metrics. These confounding factors may further explain the conflicting reports of DTI characteristics in the peritumoral regions.

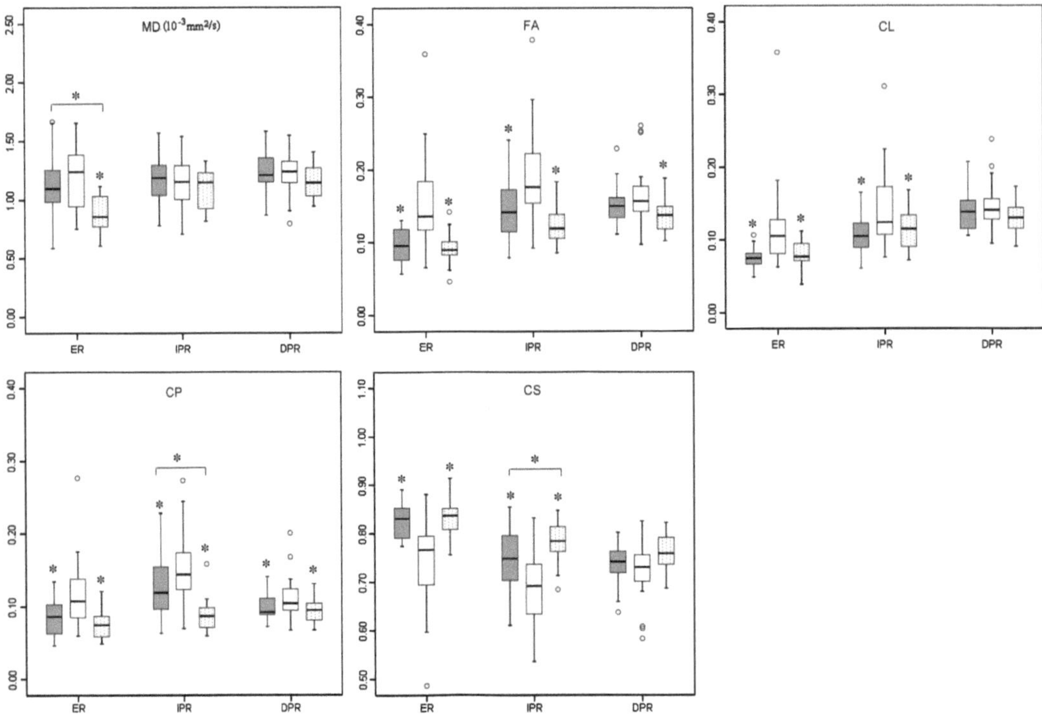

Fig. 2.5 Box plots of diffusion characteristics in brain metastases (*gray*), glioblastomas (*white*), and primary cerebral lymphomas (PCLs, *dotted*). The solid line inside the box represents the median value, while the edges represent the 25th and 75th percentiles. Straight line (*bars*) on each box indicates the range of data distribution. *Circles* represent outliers (values more than 1.5 box length from the 75th/25th percentile). *Above *gray* or *dotted box* indicates significant difference ($p<0.05$) for glioblastomas *vs.* metastases or glioblastomas vs. PCLs, respectively. *Above a *horizontal line* between *gray* and *dotted boxes* indicates significant difference ($p<0.05$) between metastases and PCLs. ER: enhancing region. IPR: immediate peritumoral region. DPR: distant peritumoral region. Reprinted and modified with permission from Wang et al. [21]

Histogram Analysis of DTI

Many of the challenges in use of DTI for characterizing brain tumors stem from the heterogeneity within or across tumor types. Standard ROI summary statistics of mean or median, however, do not address tumor spatial heterogeneity. The degree of tumor heterogeneity typically correlates with the tumor grade. The higher the heterogeneity, the more malignant the tumor is. Use of histogram for studying distributions of different parameters provides a better assessment of tissue heterogeneity, and is thus more objective and may result in higher reproducibility.

Histogram analysis of perfusion parameters has been successfully used in brain tumor classification [60–62]. Histogram-derived parameters varied in different studies, including mean, variance, peak height position, peak width, skewness, and kurtosis. But histogram analysis in DTI has not been well documented. Tozer et al. [63] reported that low-grade oligodendrogliomas are more homogeneous and showed lower MD compared with low-grade astrocytomas. Jakab et al. [61] recently reported that using histogram bins from FA, axial diffusivity, DWI, and B0 maps can differentiate low-grade from high-grade gliomas. MD histogram analysis has also been used to predict response to treatment in patients with recurrent GBM [64]. Minimum MD values have been found to be prognostic of outcomes in gliomas [65]. Recently, Wang et al. [66] have utilized histogram to quantify the diffusion data in meningiomas. Four histogram parameters, mean, variance, skewness, and kurtosis, were extracted from the enhancing part of the tumor. Their result indicated that histogram analysis of eigenvalue skewness can help differentiate atypical from typical meningiomas. Among typical meningiomas, histogram analysis of tensor shape measurements can distinguish fibroblastic from other subtype meningiomas [66].

Combined DTI Metrics for Classification

DTI provides a number of parameters about the shape, magnitude, and degree of diffusion anisotropy, which may be used to differentiate different tumor types. However, these parameters, by themselves individually, have a limited role in tumor classification. Wang et al. have previously reported that the single best predictor for differentiation between glioblastomas and brain metastases is FA, with a sensitivity of 89 %, specificity of 80 %, and AUC of 0.90 [22]. Accurate characterization of complicated tissue, such as a tumor, may require two or more imaging parameters. To date, only a limited number of studies have investigated the role of DTI parameters in combination for tumor classification. One study suggested that a combination of minimum MDs and difference of MD facilitates more accurate grading of astrocytomas than either parameter measured individually [7], whereas another study indicated that a combination of mean FA and maximum FA improves the diagnostic accuracy of nonenhencing gliomas [26]. Wang et al. have previously reported that a multivariate logistic regression analysis can determine an optimal combination of DTI parameters to differentiate glioblastomas from brain metastases and primary cerebral lymphomas [21, 22]. Their results indicated that the best model to distinguish glioblastomas from non-glioblastomas consisted of MD, CS (or FA) from the enhancing region, and rCBV from the immediate peritumoral region, resulting in an AUC of 0.938. The best predictor to differentiate primary cerebral lymphomas from brain metastases comprised MD from the enhancing region and CP from the immediate peritumoral region with AUC of 0.909 (Fig. 2.6).

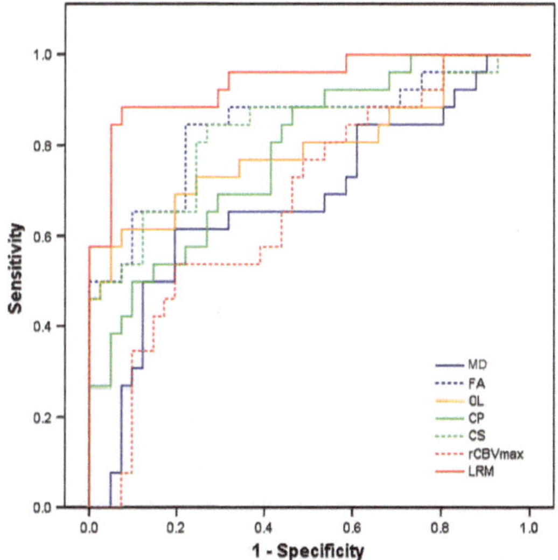

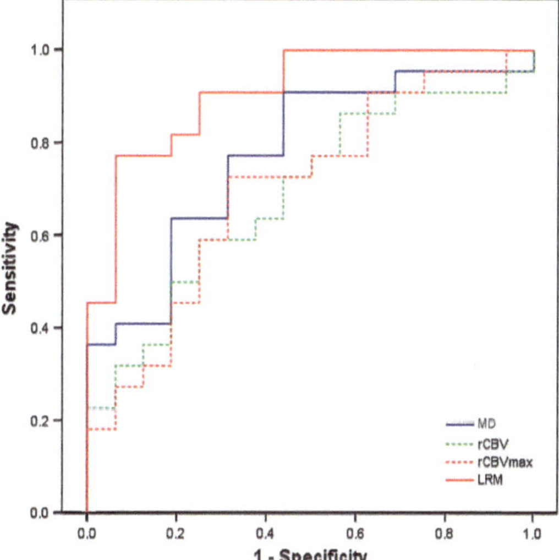

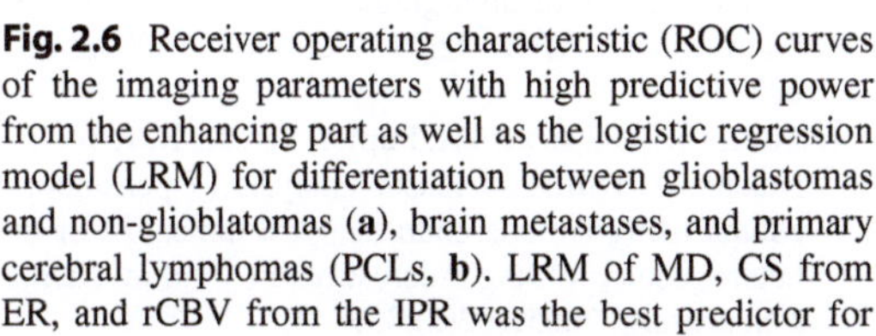
Fig. 2.6 Receiver operating characteristic (ROC) curves of the imaging parameters with high predictive power from the enhancing part as well as the logistic regression model (LRM) for differentiation between glioblastomas and non-glioblatomas (**a**), brain metastases, and primary cerebral lymphomas (PCLs, **b**). LRM of MD, CS from ER, and rCBV from the IPR was the best predictor for differentiation of glioblastomas from non-glioblastomas with area under the curve (AUC) of 0.938 (**a**), whereas combination of MD from the ER and CP from the IPR was the best model for distinguishing lymphomas from metastases with AUC of 0.909 (**b**). Reprinted and modified with permission from Wang et al. [21]

Conclusion

As reviewed in this chapter, a number of studies have demonstrated the high potential of DTI as a promising tool to study microstructural differences among different tumor types and grades. DTI metrics, such as MD, FA, CL, CP, and CS, can be used individually or in combination for brain tumor characterization. Further investigations on a larger patient population and histological validation will be necessary to determine the underlying tissue properties associated with DTI measures and to improve the robustness of these parameters in differentiating tumor types. With the recent development of new techniques, such as diffusion kurtosis imaging (DKI) and diffusion spectrum imaging (DSI), the clinical significance of diffusion imaging in brain tumor will be further established and acknowledged.

References

1. Central Brain Tumor Registry of the United States. Statistical report: primary brain and central nervous system tumors diagnosed in the United States, 2004–2007. Central Brain Tumor Registry of the United States. 2011.
2. Chenevert TL, Ross BD. Diffusion imaging for therapy response assessment of brain tumor. Neuroimaging Clin N Am. 2009;19(4):559–71.
3. Louis DN, Ohgaki H, Wiestler OD, et al. The 2007 WHO classification of tumours of the central nervous system. Acta Neuropathol. 2007;114(2):97–109.
4. Batchelor T, Loeffler JS. Primary CNS lymphoma. J Clin Oncol. 2006;24(8):1281–8.
5. Giese A, Westphal M. Treatment of malignant glioma: a problem beyond the margins of resection. J Cancer Res Clin Oncol. 2001;127(4):217–25.
6. Soffietti R, Ruda R, Mutani R. Management of brain metastases. J Neurol. 2002;249(10):1357–69.
7. Murakami R, Hirai T, Sugahara T, et al. Grading astrocytic tumors by using apparent diffusion coefficient parameters: superiority of a one- versus two-parameter pilot method. Radiology. 2009;251(3): 838–45.
8. Yamasaki F, Kurisu K, Satoh K, et al. Apparent diffusion coefficient of human brain tumors at MR imaging. Radiology. 2005;235(3):985–91.
9. Stadlbauer A, Ganslandt O, Buslei R, et al. Gliomas: histopathologic evaluation of changes in directionality and magnitude of water diffusion at diffusion-tensor MR imaging. Radiology. 2006;240(3):803–10.
10. Al-Okaili RN, Krejza J, Woo JH, et al. Intraaxial brain masses: MR imaging-based diagnostic strategy—initial experience. Radiology. 2007;243(2):539–50.
11. Melhem ER, Mori S, Mukundan G, Kraut MA, Pomper MG, van Zijl PC. Diffusion tensor MR imaging of the brain and white matter tractography. AJR Am J Roentgenol. 2002;178(1):3–16.
12. Beaulieu C. The basis of anisotropic water diffusion in the nervous system—a technical review. NMR Biomed. 2002;15(7–8):435–55.
13. Basser PJ, Pierpaoli C. Microstructural and physiological features of tissues elucidated by quantitative-diffusion-tensor MRI. J Magn Reson B. 1996;111(3): 209–19.
14. Westin CF, Maier SE, Mamata H, Nabavi A, Jolesz FA, Kikinis R. Processing and visualization for diffusion tensor MRI. Med Image Anal. 2002;6(2): 93–108.
15. Alexander AL, Hasan K, Kindlmann G, Parker DL, Tsuruda JS. A geometric analysis of diffusion tensor measurements of the human brain. Magn Reson Med. 2000;44(2):283–91.
16. Chenevert TL, Sundgren PC, Ross BD. Diffusion imaging: insight to cell status and cytoarchitecture. Neuroimaging Clin N Am. 2006;16(4):619–32. viii-ix.
17. Guo AC, Cummings TJ, Dash RC, Provenzale JM. Lymphomas and high-grade astrocytomas: comparison of water diffusibility and histologic characteristics. Radiology. 2002;224(1):177–83.
18. Nagar VA, Ye JR, Ng WH, et al. Diffusion-weighted MR imaging: diagnosing atypical or malignant meningiomas and detecting tumor dedifferentiation. AJNR Am J Neuroradiol. 2008;29(6):1147–52.
19. Toh CH, Castillo M, Wong AM, et al. Differentiation between classic and atypical meningiomas with use of diffusion tensor imaging. AJNR Am J Neuroradiol. 2008;29(9):1630–5.
20. Lu S, Ahn D, Johnson G, Law M, Zagzag D, Grossman RI. Diffusion-tensor MR imaging of intracranial neoplasia and associated peritumoral edema: introduction of the tumor infiltration index. Radiology. 2004; 232(1):221–8.
21. Wang S, Kim S, Chawla S, et al. Differentiation between glioblastomas, solitary brain metastases, and primary cerebral lymphomas using diffusion tensor and dynamic susceptibility contrast-enhanced MR imaging. AJNR Am J Neuroradiol. 2011;32(3):507–14.
22. Wang S, Kim S, Chawla S, et al. Differentiation between glioblastomas and solitary brain metastases using diffusion tensor imaging. Neuroimage. 2009; 44(3):653–60.
23. Lu S, Ahn D, Johnson G, Cha S. Peritumoral diffusion tensor imaging of high-grade gliomas and metastatic brain tumors. AJNR Am J Neuroradiol. 2003;24(5): 937–41.
24. Morita K, Matsuzawa H, Fujii Y, Tanaka R, Kwee IL, Nakada T. Diffusion tensor analysis of peritumoral edema using lambda chart analysis indicative of the heterogeneity of the microstructure within edema. J Neurosurg. 2005;102(2):336–41.

25. Lee EJ, Lee SK, Agid R, Bae JM, Keller A, Terbrugge K. Preoperative grading of presumptive low-grade astrocytomas on MR imaging: diagnostic value of minimum apparent diffusion coefficient. AJNR Am J Neuroradiol. 2008;29(10):1872–7.
26. Liu X, Tian W, Kolar B, et al. MR diffusion tensor and perfusion-weighted imaging in preoperative grading of supratentorial nonenhancing gliomas. Neuro Oncol. 2011;13(4):447–55.
27. Calli C, Kitis O, Yunten N, Yurtseven T, Islekel S, Akalin T. Perfusion and diffusion MR imaging in enhancing malignant cerebral tumors. Eur J Radiol. 2006;58(3):394–403.
28. Oh J, Cha S, Aiken AH, et al. Quantitative apparent diffusion coefficients and T2 relaxation times in characterizing contrast enhancing brain tumors and regions of peritumoral edema. J Magn Reson Imaging. 2005;21(6):701–8.
29. Jolapara M, Kesavadas C, Radhakrishnan VV, et al. Role of diffusion tensor imaging in differentiating subtypes of meningiomas. J Neuroradiol. 2010;37(5): 277–83.
30. Zamecnik J. The extracellular space and matrix of gliomas. Acta Neuropathol. 2005;110(5): 435–42.
31. Vargova L, Homola A, Zamecnik J, Tichy M, Benes V, Sykova E. Diffusion parameters of the extracellular space in human gliomas. Glia. 2003;42(1):77–88.
32. McConville P, Hambardzumyan D, Moody JB, et al. Magnetic resonance imaging determination of tumor grade and early response to temozolomide in a genetically engineered mouse model of glioma. Clin Cancer Res. 2007;13(10):2897–904.
33. Moffat BA, Chenevert TL, Lawrence TS, et al. Functional diffusion map: a noninvasive MRI biomarker for early stratification of clinical brain tumor response. Proc Natl Acad Sci U S A. 2005;102(15): 5524–9.
34. Padhani AR, Liu G, Koh DM, et al. Diffusion-weighted magnetic resonance imaging as a cancer biomarker: consensus and recommendations. Neoplasia. 2009;11(2):102–25.
35. Wang S, Wolf RL, Woo JH, et al. Actinomycotic brain infection: registered diffusion, perfusion MR imaging and MR spectroscopy. Neuroradiology. 2006;48(5): 346–50.
36. Beppu T, Inoue T, Shibata Y, et al. Measurement of fractional anisotropy using diffusion tensor MRI in supratentorial astrocytic tumors. J Neurooncol. 2003;63(2):109–16.
37. Beppu T, Inoue T, Shibata Y, et al. Fractional anisotropy value by diffusion tensor magnetic resonance imaging as a predictor of cell density and proliferation activity of glioblastomas. Surg Neurol. 2005;63(1):56–61. discussion 61.
38. Haris M, Gupta RK, Husain N, Hasan KM, Husain M, Narayana PA. Measurement of DTI metrics in hemorrhagic brain lesions: possible implication in MRI interpretation. J Magn Reson Imaging. 2006;24(6): 1259–68.
39. Kinoshita M, Hashimoto N, Goto T, et al. Fractional anisotropy and tumor cell density of the tumor core show positive correlation in diffusion tensor magnetic resonance imaging of malignant brain tumors. NeuroImage. 2008;43:29–35.
40. Toh CH, Castillo M, Wong AM, et al. Primary cerebral lymphoma and glioblastoma multiforme: differences in diffusion characteristics evaluated with diffusion tensor imaging. AJNR Am J Neuroradiol. 2008;29(3):471–5.
41. Inoue T, Ogasawara K, Beppu T, Ogawa A, Kabasawa H. Diffusion tensor imaging for preoperative evaluation of tumor grade in gliomas. Clin Neurol Neurosurg. 2005;107(3):174–80.
42. Wang W, Steward CE, Desmond PM. Diffusion tensor imaging in glioblastoma multiforme and brain metastases: the role of p, q, L, and fractional anisotropy. AJNR Am J Neuroradiol. 2009;30(1):203–8.
43. Reiche W, Schuchardt V, Hagen T, Il'yasov KA, Billmann P, Weber J. Differential diagnosis of intracranial ring enhancing cystic mass lesions–role of diffusion-weighted imaging (DWI) and diffusion-tensor imaging (DTI). Clin Neurol Neurosurg. 2010;112(3):218–25.
44. Koeller KK, Smirniotopoulos JG, Jones RV. Primary central nervous system lymphoma: radiologic-pathologic correlation. Radiographics. 1997;17(6):1497–526.
45. Rees JH, Smirniotopoulos JG, Jones RV, Wong K. Glioblastoma multiforme: radiologic-pathologic correlation. Radiographics. 1996;16(6):1413–38. quiz 1462–1413.
46. Zhang M, Olsson Y. Hematogenous metastases of the human brain—characteristics of peritumoral brain changes: a review. J Neurooncol. 1997;35(1):81–9.
47. Zhang S, Bastin ME, Laidlaw DH, Sinha S, Armitage PA, Deisboeck TS. Visualization and analysis of white matter structural asymmetry in diffusion tensor MRI data. Magn Reson Med. 2004;51(1):140–7.
48. Kim S, Pickup S, Hsu O, Poptani H. Diffusion tensor MRI in rat models of invasive and well-demarcated brain tumors. NMR Biomed. 2008;21(3):208–16.
49. Lope-Piedrafita S, Garcia-Martin ML, Galons JP, Gillies RJ, Trouard TP. Longitudinal diffusion tensor imaging in a rat brain glioma model. NMR Biomed. 2008;21(8):799–808.
50. Zhang J, van Zijl PC, Laterra J, et al. Unique patterns of diffusion directionality in rat brain tumors revealed by high-resolution diffusion tensor MRI. Magn Reson Med. 2007;58(3):454–62.
51. Kashimura H, Inoue T, Ogasawara K, et al. Prediction of meningioma consistency using fractional anisotropy value measured by magnetic resonance imaging. J Neurosurg. 2007;107(4):784–7.
52. Tropine A, Dellani PD, Glaser M, et al. Differentiation of fibroblastic meningiomas from other benign subtypes using diffusion tensor imaging. J Magn Reson Imaging. 2007;25(4):703–8.
53. Kumar M, Gupta RK, Nath K, et al. Can we differentiate true white matter fibers from pseudofibers inside a brain abscess cavity using geometrical diffusion

tensor imaging metrics? NMR Biomed. 2007;21(6): 581–8.
54. Santhosh K, Thomas B, Radhakrishnan VV, et al. Diffusion tensor and tensor metrics imaging in intracranial epidermoid cysts. J Magn Reson Imaging. 2009;29(4):967–70.
55. Gupta RK, Haris M, Husain N, Saksena S, Husain M, Rathore RK. DTI derived indices correlate with immunohistochemistry obtained matrix metalloproteinase (MMP-9) expression in cellular fraction of brain tuberculoma. J Neurol Sci. 2008;275(1–2):78–85.
56. Lee EJ, Lee EJ, Lee EJ, Terbrugge K, Mikulis D, et al. Diagnostic value of peritumoral minimum apparent diffusion coefficient for differentiation of glioblastoma multiforme from solitary metastatic lesions. AJR Am J Roentgenol. 2011;196(1):71–6.
57. van Westen D, Latt J, Englund E, Brockstedt S, Larsson EM. Tumor extension in high-grade gliomas assessed with diffusion magnetic resonance imaging: values and lesion-to-brain ratios of apparent diffusion coefficient and fractional anisotropy. Acta Radiol. 2006;47(3):311–9.
58. Kinoshita M, Goto T, Okita Y, et al. Diffusion tensor-based tumor infiltration index cannot discriminate vasogenic edema from tumor-infiltrated edema. J Neurooncol. 2010;96(3):409–15.
59. Law M, Cha S, Knopp EA, Johnson G, Arnett J, Litt AW. High-grade gliomas and solitary metastases: differentiation by using perfusion and proton spectroscopic MR imaging. Radiology. 2002;222(3):715–21.
60. Emblem KE, Nedregaard B, Nome T, et al. Glioma grading by using histogram analysis of blood volume heterogeneity from MR-derived cerebral blood volume maps. Radiology. 2008;247(3):808–17.
61. Jakab A, Molnar P, Emri M, Berenyi E. Glioma grade assessment by using histogram analysis of diffusion tensor imaging-derived maps. Neuroradiology. 2011; 53(7):483–91. Epub 2010 Sep 21.
62. Kim HS, Kim JH, Kim SH, Cho KG, Kim SY. Posttreatment high-grade glioma: usefulness of peak height position with semiquantitative MR perfusion histogram analysis in an entire contrast-enhanced lesion for predicting volume fraction of recurrence. Radiology. 2010;256(3):906–15.
63. Tozer DJ, Jager HR, Danchaivijitr N, et al. Apparent diffusion coefficient histograms may predict low-grade glioma subtype. NMR Biomed. 2007;20(1): 49–57.
64. Pope WB, Kim HJ, Huo J, et al. Recurrent glioblastoma multiforme: ADC histogram analysis predicts response to bevacizumab treatment. Radiology. 2009; 252(1):182–9.
65. Pope WB, Lai A, Mehta R, et al. Apparent diffusion coefficent histogram analysis stratifies progression-free survival in newly diagnosed bevacizumab-treated glioblastoma. AJNR Am J Neuroradiol. 2011;32(5): 882–9.
66. Wang S, Kim S, Zhang Y, et al. Determination of grade and subtype of meningiomas by using histogram analysis of diffusion-tensor Imaging metrics. Radiology. 2012;262:584–92.

Diagnosis and Characterization of Brain Tumors: MR Spectroscopic Imaging

3

Peter B. Barker

Introduction

In vivo proton magnetic resonance spectroscopy (MRS) was first demonstrated to be feasible in vivo in the human brain in the mid-1980s [1], and the first example of it being applied to human brain tumors following soon after in 1989 [2]. It was already apparent from this paper that brain tumors had greatly different metabolite profiles compared to normal tissue, and that differences in spectra may exist between different brain lesions of different pathologies. Since that time, there has been steady progress in the use of MRS and the related technique of magnetic resonance spectroscopic imaging (MRSI) for the clinical evaluation of human brain tumors [3].

This chapter briefly reviews the information content of in vivo proton MRS of the human brain and appropriate techniques for use in the study of brain tumors, and then discusses some common clinical applications of MRS in the diagnosis and categorization.

P.B. Barker, D.Phil. (✉)
Department of Radiology, Johns Hopkins University School of Medicine, Park 367B, 600 N. Wolfe Street, Baltimore, MD 21287, USA
e-mail: pbarker2@jhmi.edu

Meet the Metabolites

A short echo time spectrum from the normal human brain is shown in Fig. 3.1. The most prominent peak in the adult human brain is from *N*-acetyl aspartate (NAA) which resonates at 2.0 ppm on the chemical shift scale. There is good evidence that NAA is primarily located in neurons and axons, and not in glial cells, so NAA is often referred to as a "neuronal" or a "neuroaxonal" marker; NAA is nearly always found to be reduced in brain tumors, as tumor cells invade or replace normal brain tissue.

Other prominent peaks in the spectrum of Fig. 3.1 include "choline" (Cho—actually a composite peak consisting of several different Cho-containing compounds, in particular glycerophosphocholine (GPC) and phosphocholine (PC)) at 3.2 ppm, and "creatine" (actually the combination of both creatine and phosphocreatine (PCr)) at 3.0 ppm on the chemical shift scale. The Cho signal is often found to be increased in brain tumors, particularly those which are non-necrotic and of high grade. The increase in Cho is believed to be related to a number of factors, including increased tumor cell density, increased membrane turnover, and altered Cho metabolism, in particular increased synthesis of PC in tumor cells [4, 5]. The combined increase in Cho and decrease in NAA thus leads to a decreased ratio of NAA/Cho in nearly all brain tumors, although this pattern is not particularly specific, since many other neuropathologies may also have reduced NAA/Cho [3].

J.J. Pillai (ed.), *Functional Brain Tumor Imaging*, DOI 10.1007/978-1-4419-5858-7_3,

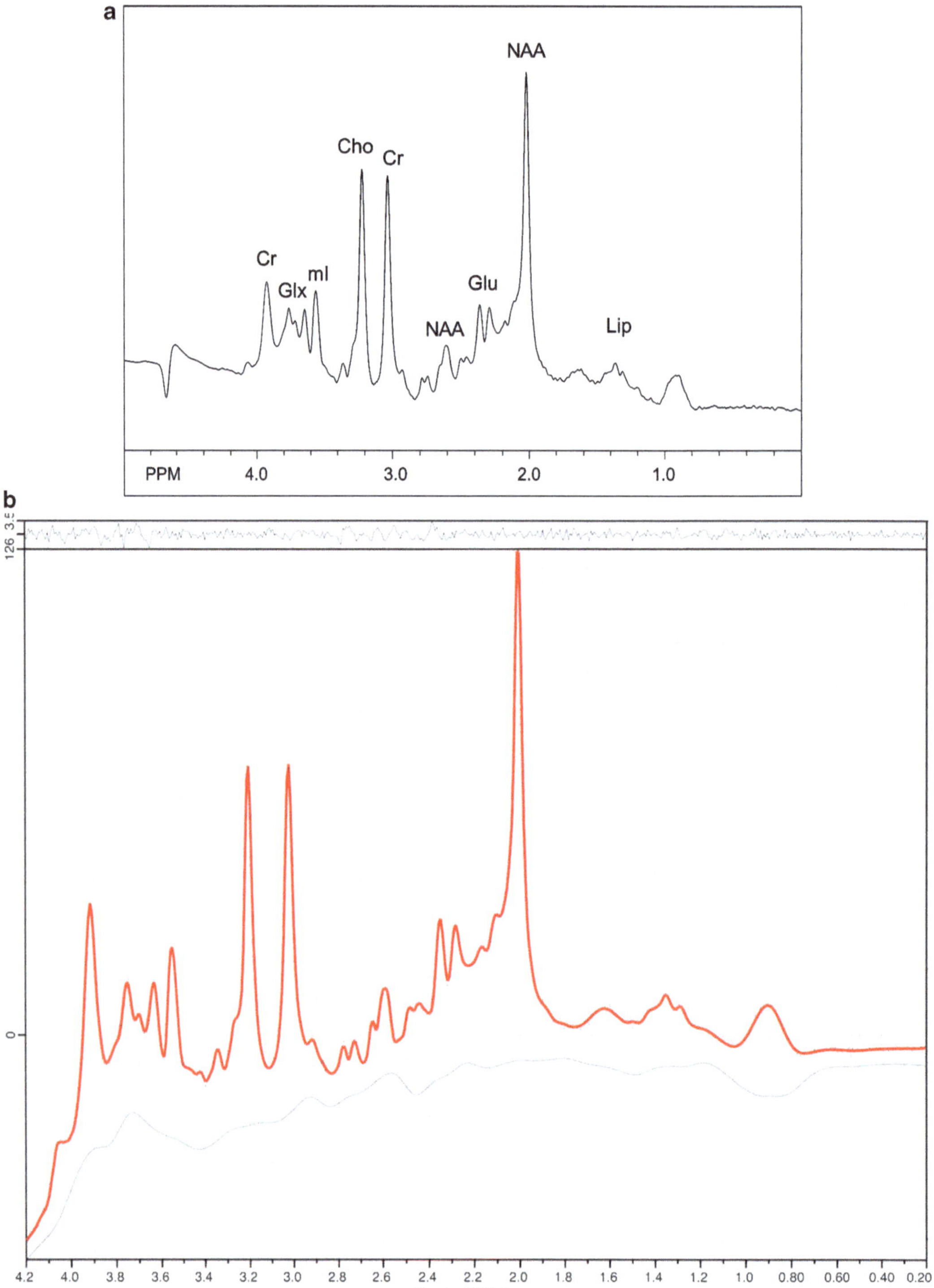

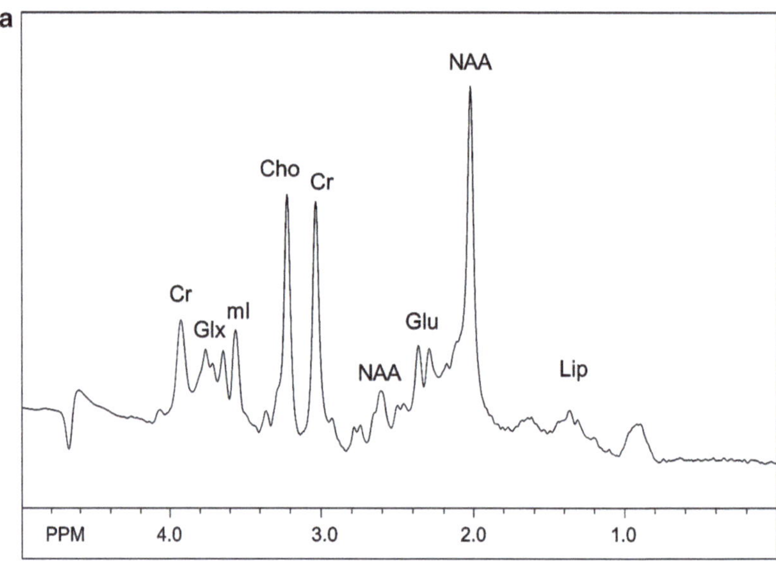

Fig. 3.1 (**a**) A short echo time (TE 31 ms) PRESS spectrum recorded from the anterior cingulate gyrus of a normal adult human brain at 3 T. Peak assignments are as follows: NAA—*N*-acetylaspartate, Cho—choline-containing compounds, Cr—creatine, mI—*myo*-inositol, Glu—glutamate, Glx—glutamate and glutamine, Lip—Lipid. (**b**) LCModel analysis of the spectrum shown in (**a**)—the *red line* is the result of the fitting algorithm, the *lower black line* the fitted baseline, and the *upper black line* is the difference between the fit and experimental data

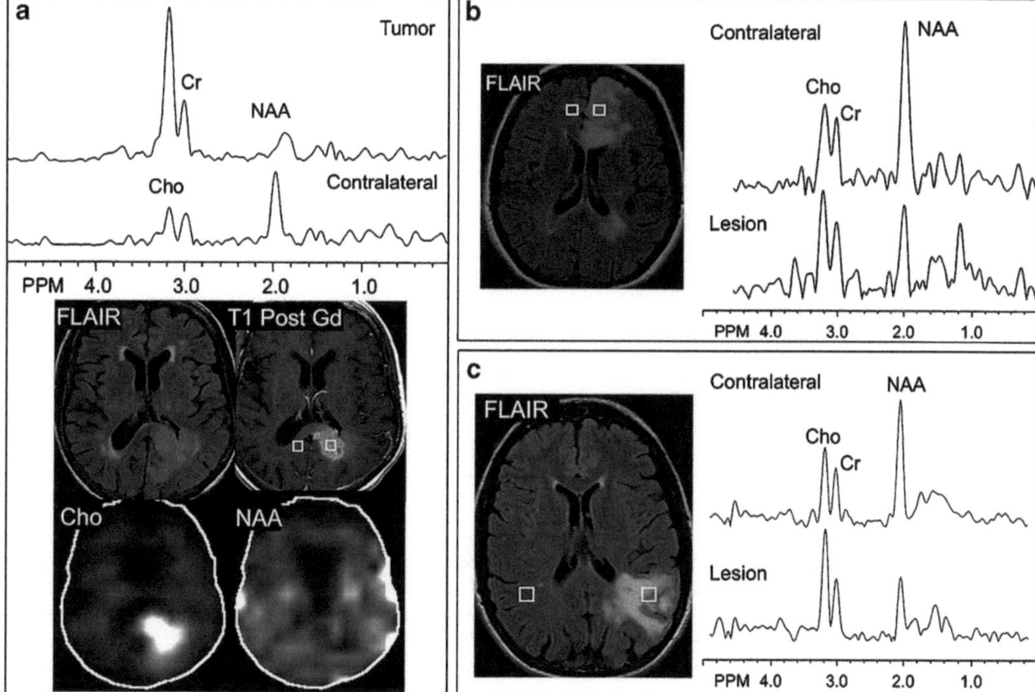

Fig. 3.2 Representative brain tumor spectra and spectroscopic images (1.5 T, TE 280 ms) from three different human brain tumors: (**a**) a glioblastoma multiforme (GBM) involving the splenium of the corpus callosum, showing high Cho and low NAA compared to the contralateral hemisphere, (**b**) a left frontal grade II oligodendroglioma, which has decreased NAA and near-normal Cho, and (**c**) a left parietal primary central nervous system (CNS) lymphoma which has an elevated Cho signal and decreased NAA

Other metabolic alterations in brain tumors that may be detected by in vivo MRS include increases in *myo*-inositol (mI) which resonates at about 3.5 ppm, a cyclic sugar alcohol that has been proposed as a glial cell marker [6], particularly in low-grade gliomas [7]; increases in alanine (~1.5 ppm) in meningiomas [8]; and increases or decreases in creatine. Since abnormal glycolysis and/or hypoxia and necrosis are also commonly associated with brain tumors, it is also not uncommon to observe increases in lactate (1.3 ppm) in some cases [9]. Tumor necrosis is also associated with increases in mobile lipid signals that can be detected by MRS [10] at various frequencies in the spectrum, but most notably at 1.3 and 0.9 ppm. Examples of the different spectral patterns from human brain tumors are shown in Fig. 3.2.

Other compounds that may be detected by in vivo MRS include glutamate (Glu) and glutamine (Gln), often expressed as their sum "Glx" (i.e., Glu + Gln) since they are hard to separate, particularly at 1.5 T, although at higher field strengths (3 or 7 T) it is possible to measure the individual components with reasonable accuracy [11]. There is interest in the roles of Glu as a promotor of tumor cell growth and invasion of surrounding brain tissue [12], a cause of seizures related to tumors [13], and also as a possible therapeutic target [14]. Gln is believed to be an important source of nitrogen for tumor growth, and is involved in tumor cell signaling pathways [15, 16]. However, to date there have been relatively few studies of these compounds in vivo in human brain tumors using MRS.

Although they are relatively rare observations, peaks from the TCA-cycle intermediates are occasionally observed in human brain tumors by MRS. Succinate, a singlet resonance at about 2.4 ppm, has been reported both in treatment-naive

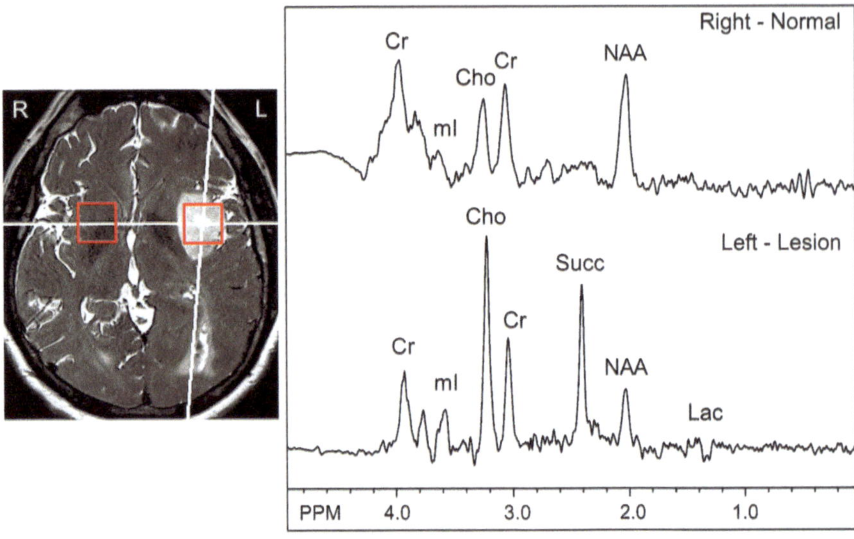

Fig. 3.3 An untreated, left insular presumed low-grade glioma seen on T_2-weighted MRI, which has an elevated signal at 2.4 ppm which is assigned to succinate (Succ), a tricarboxylic acid (TCA) cycle. The lesion also has a large reduction in NAA, and moderate increases in Cho and Lac (inverted doublet at ~1.3 ppm) compared to the contralateral hemisphere (which has slightly larger linewidths due to field inhomogeneity). There is also an incidental left parietal hemorrhage. Spectra recorded at 3.0 T using TR 2000 and TE 135 ms

gliomas as well as post-radiation therapy [17], although the significance of this finding is currently unclear (Fig. 3.3). It has also been observed in some brain abscesses [18]. Also, citrate has been observed in certain pediatric brain tumors (a complex multiplet around 2.6 ppm), in particular low-grade astrocytomas that exhibit malignant progression [19].

Finally, recent work has also shown that it is possible to detect the compound 2-hydroxyglutarate (2HG) in grade 2 and grade 3 gliomas which exhibit mutations of isocitrate dehydrogenase (IDH) [20, 21]; this may be of importance since these tumors have been reported to be associated with longer survival times compared to the phenotype without such mutations.

Methodological Considerations

While many of the early MRS studies of brain tumors used single-voxel (SV) MRS (i.e., spectra typically recorded from a single, typically ~8 cm^3 cube of tissue within the brain) [2, 22], it soon became apparent that spectral patterns in many cases varied from one part of the lesion to another, and for this reason tumors are best studied using methods ("multi-voxel" MRS, also known as "chemical shift imaging" (CSI) or MRSI) that map out the spatial distribution of these compounds throughout the lesion and surrounding areas. MRSI, primarily based on the Cho signal, is particularly essential for mapping out the distribution of the density of tumor cells within the lesion [3, 23–27], and distinguishing regions of active tumor, necrosis, and edema, all of which have different spectral patterns. MRSI therefore should be considered the preferred modality (vs. SV-MRS) for brain tumor imaging in most cases, although in some instances SV-MRS may be more practical, for instance, lesions in difficult locations for MRSI, such as pontine gliomas, skull base, or inferior frontal lobe lesions, or in non-compliant patients and/or when time is short.

SV-MRS is traditionally performed with pulse sequences known as "PRESS" or "STEAM," which are robust [3], single-shot localization techniques that generally give excellent quality

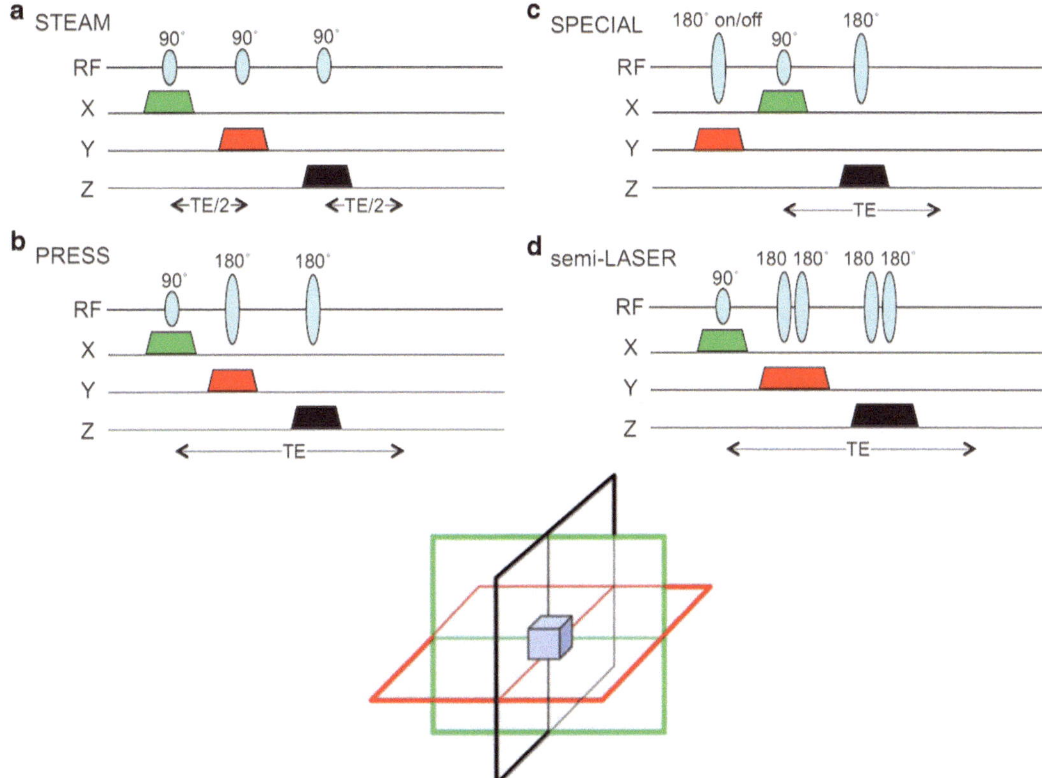

Fig. 3.4 Pulse sequences used for spatial localization in MRS: (**a**) STEAM, (**b**) PRESS, (**c**) SPECIAL, and (**d**) semi-LASER. All sequences utilize slice-selective pulses with gradients applied in three orthogonal directions; for clarity, only slice selection gradients are shown, without refocusing lobes or crusher gradients. In (**c**) two scans are subtracted with the adiabatic inversion pre-pulse "on" and "off," respectively. In (**d**), each of the four 180° are frequency-swept, adiabatic pulses. Each has its own advantages and disadvantages which are listed in Table 3.1

spectra (Fig. 3.4). PRESS usually has higher signal-to-noise ratios (SNR), while STEAM can be used to record spectra with very short echo times (TE), which improves the precision of measuring compounds with coupled spin systems such as Glu or mI. More recently, other sequences have been introduced for SV-MRS, including the "semi-LASER" (sLASER) sequence [28, 29] which is similar to PRESS, but uses high-bandwidth adiabatic refocusing pulses to achieve excellent slice profiles, even if transmit power is not optimally set, and the "SPECIAL" pulse sequence [30] which offers the SNR of PRESS while also allowing very short TEs to be used (like STEAM). A summary of the relative advantages and disadvantages of each sequence is given in Table 3.1. All of these sequences are used in

Table 3.1 Comparison of single-voxel MRS localization sequences

Sequence	Advantages	Disadvantages
STEAM	Short TE, low SAR, good slice profiles of 90° pulses	Lower SNR
PRESS	Better SNR than STEAM	Longer minimum TE, higher SAR
SPECIAL	Good SNR, short TE	Possible artifacts since localization depends on subtraction of two scans
Semi-LASER	Good SNR, good slice profiles, adiabatic pulses are B1 insensitive	High SAR, longer minimum TE

SAR specific absorption rate, *SNR* signal-to-noise ratio

combination with optimized, frequency-selective pre-pulses to saturate the brain water signal [31] [32], which, since brain water is approximately 50 M, is approximately three orders of magnitude larger than the metabolites to be observed, which are in the mM concentration range.

The concept of chemical shift imaging can be traced back to the original paper by Brown et al. [33] in 1982 which demonstrated that an array of spatially localized spectra could be reconstructed by the application of a pulse sequence with phase-encoding gradients applied in that direction prior to turning on the receiver (Fig. 3.5). Since that original paper, there has been a continuous development and refinement of MRSI methods for localization in multiple dimensions within the human brain, with increasing spatial coverage and resolution and decreasing scan times [3]. A commonly used technique in the clinic is 2D-PRESS-MRSI [34], which combines excitation of a fairly large region of the brain using the PRESS sequence (but avoiding regions of the scalp with large lipid signals) with phase-encoding in two dimensions to map out the distribution of metabolites within the PRESS voxel. An example of PRESS-MRSI is shown in Fig. 3.6. 3D-PRESS-MRSI [35] has also been used in the study of brain tumors, which importantly allows localization to be extended to three dimensions; however this technique

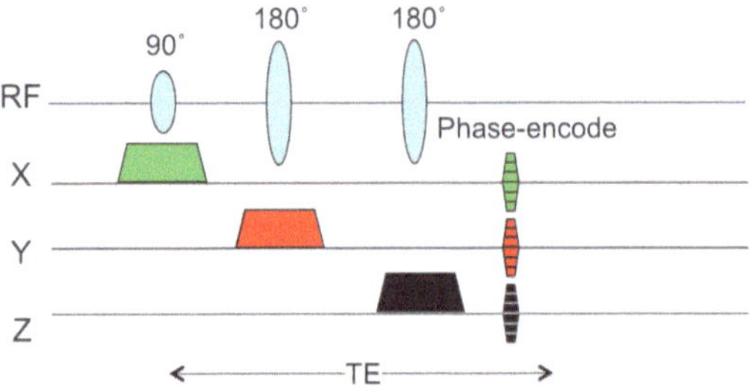

Fig. 3.5 MRSI pulse sequence based on the PRESS pulse sequence. In this case the PRESS sequence excites a relatively large volume of brain tissue, which is then sub-divided into smaller regions by the application of phase-encoding gradients in one, two, or three dimensions

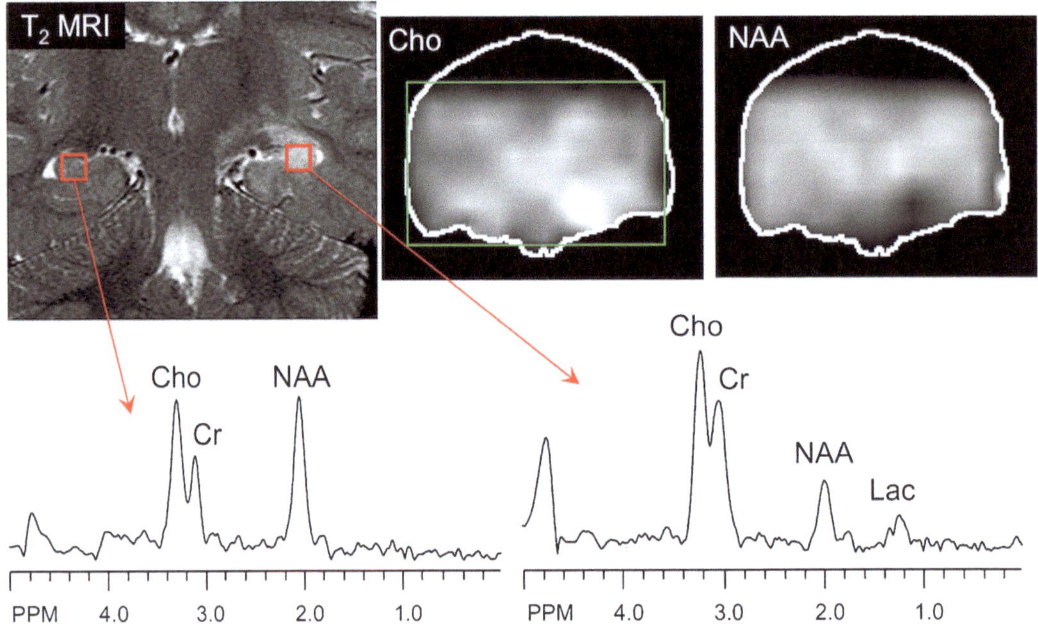

Fig. 3.6 Example of 2D-PRESS-MRSI (1.5 T, TR 2000, TE 280 ms) in the coronal plane in a patient with a lesion of the left hippocampus seen on T_2-weighted MRI. The lesion is characterized by increased choline, creatine, and lactate and decreased NAA compared to the normal contralateral left hippocampus, as seen in both the selected hippocampal spectra and reconstructed Cho and NAA images, consistent with either a glioma or viral encephalitis

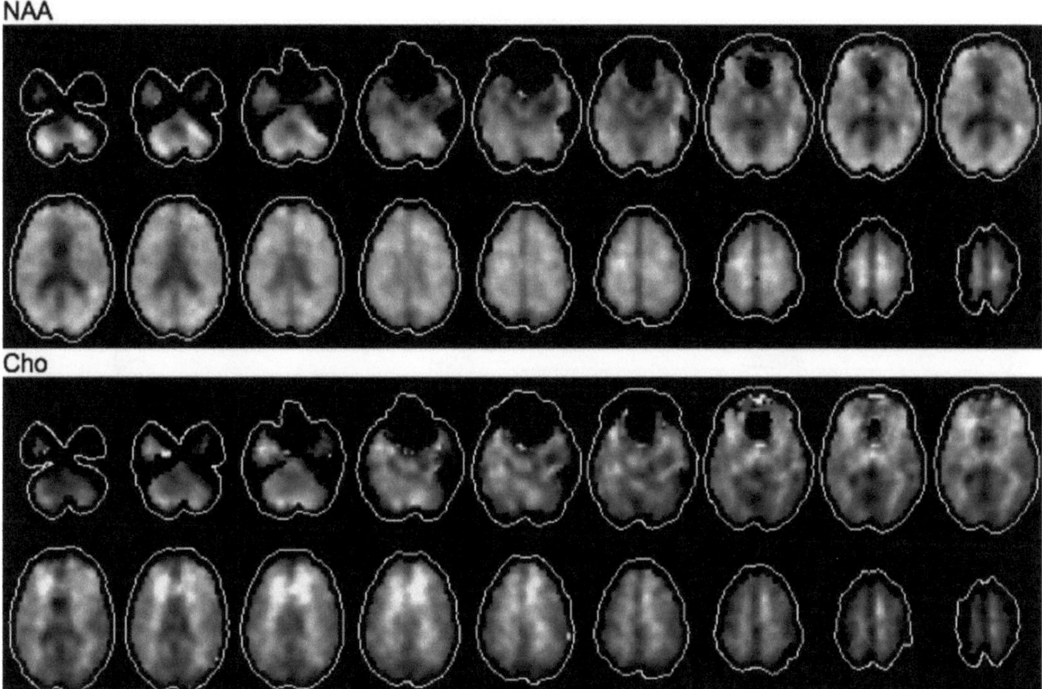

Fig. 3.7 An example of NAA and choline images reconstructed from a 3 T EPSI acquisition with whole-brain coverage in a normal adult volunteer. Scan parameters include 0.5 cm^3 voxel size, TE 26 ms, GRAPPA acceleration factor of 2, scan time 16 min, 32-channel head coil

becomes very time-consuming if high spatial resolution and coverage are required. Other problems with PRESS-based MRSI include difficulties in covering to the edges of the brain, as well as left–right and anterior–posterior differences in spectra towards the edges of the PRESS voxel, due to the finite bandwidth of the slice-selective radio-frequency (RF) pulses.

For these reasons, there continues to be development of other approaches to MRSI, including the use of slice- or slab-selective excitation (to reach the edges of the brain) as well as multi-slice [36] or 3D encoding to increase coverage, even up to whole brain [37]. Since extended coverage also implies long scan times, methods have been developed to reduce MRSI scan times, for instance using multi-echo approaches [38], parallel imaging (SENSE, GRAPPA) [39–42], or echo-planar spectroscopic imaging (EPSI) [37, 43]. EPSI is a particularly promising methodology since it offers an order of magnitude speedup (reduction) in scan time, without sacrificing spectral quality, and appears to be the most practical way of achieving whole-brain coverage. An example of a short TE whole-brain EPSI scan recorded on a 3 T system with a 32-channel head coil is shown in Fig. 3.7. However, there have been few applications of this methodology to brain tumors to date, most likely because of its current lack of commercial availability.

Finally, there are certain compounds that are present in the brain at low mM concentrations which are potentially detectable by MRS, but which are difficult to quantify by conventional techniques because their signals overlap with those of the compounds present at higher concentrations—examples of these include the inhibitory transmitter γ-aminobutyric acid (GABA) [44], and the antioxidant glutathione (GSH). In these cases, a methodology known as "spectral-editing" makes use of the specific properties of the coupled spin system to be

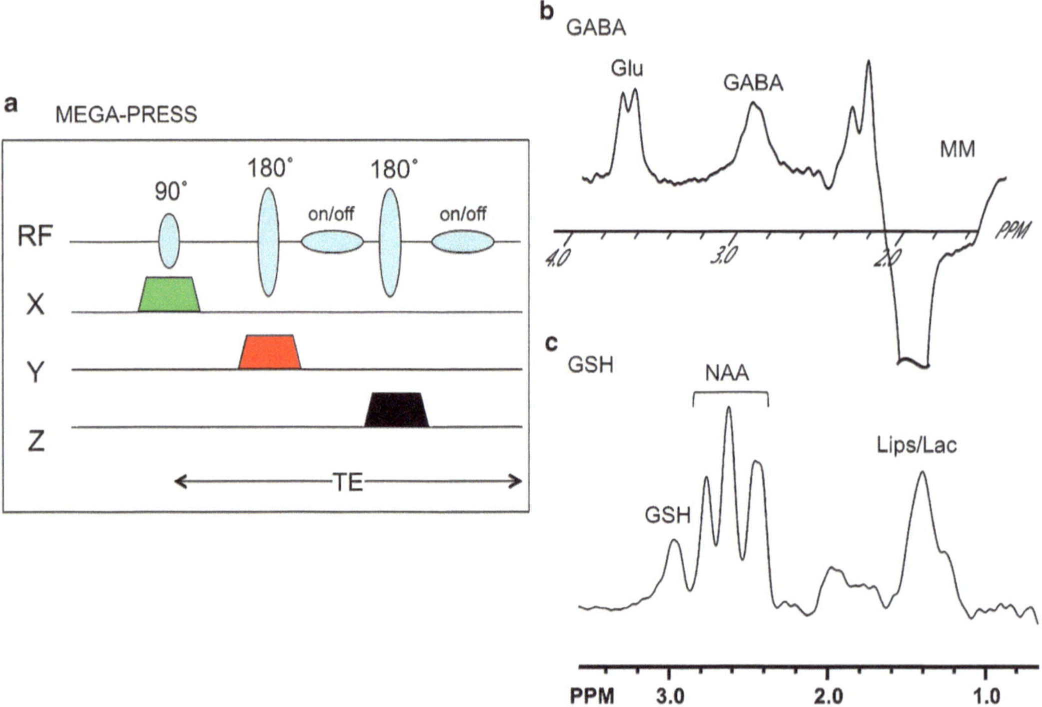

Fig. 3.8 (**a**) MEGA-PRESS pulse sequence for spectral editing—the standard PRESS sequence (Fig. 3.4) is modified to include a pair of frequency-selective editing pulses during the TE time period which can be used to select specific spin systems such as (**b**) GABA or (**c**) glutathione (GSH). Edited spectra are shown at 3 T in a normal adult volunteer. In (**b**), in addition to the GABA peak at 3.0 ppm, other peaks co-edit from glutamate and macromolecules. In (**c**), in addition to the GSH peak at 2.9 ppm, other peaks co-edit from NAAG and lipids/lactate

detected to selectively observe the desired compound, suppressing the signals from the higher concentration, overlapping compounds. One editing sequence increasingly being used for this purpose is the SV MEGA-PRESS sequence [45]; examples of this sequence for GABA and GSH in normal brain are shown in Fig. 3.8. Again, to date, there have been few studies of these compounds yet in human brain tumors, most likely because of lack of commercial availability of MEGA-PRESS sequence. However, MEGA-PRESS has been successfully used to observe 2HG in tumors with IDH1 and IDH2 mutations (Fig. 3.9) [21].

Equally as important as the pulse sequence used to record the data is the software used for data analysis. Ideally, fully automated spectral curve-fitting algorithms should be used to provide a quantitative estimate of each metabolite concentration [46]. An example of one such analysis package ("LCModel") is shown in Fig. 3.1 [46]. However, although such software exists and is often used in clinical research studies, it is little utilized in routine clinical practice, where visual interpretation (as in most radiological readings) is most common. Other commonly used metrics include ratios of metabolites such as NAA/Cho, NAA/Cr, Cho/Cr, and mI/Cr. While these can be helpful, they can also be ambiguous or difficult to interpret when both metabolites change at the same time. For this reason, a better approach is often to compare the metabolite level in the tumor with that of the same metabolite in a normal brain region, for instance the mirror image location in the contralateral hemisphere, if available [47]. These measurements are often referred to as "normalized." Sometimes, unfortunately, a contralateral reference normal region is not available for comparison (e.g., midline lesions such as pontine gliomas), in which case a knowledge of

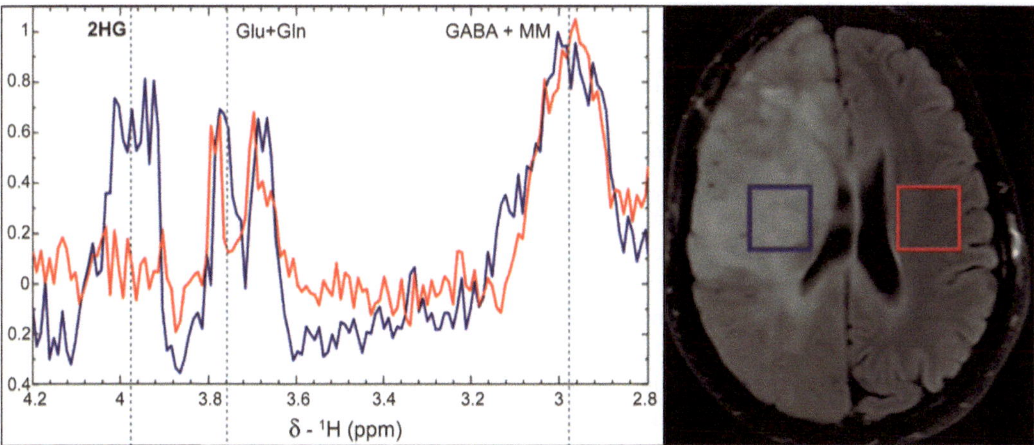

Fig. 3.9 Detection of 2-hydroxyglutarate (2-HG) in vivo in a secondary glioblastoma with an $IDH1_{R132H}$ mutation using the MEGA-PRESS pulse sequence. Edited spectra from both the lesion and normal brain show co-edited signals from glutamate, glutamine, and GABA; however only the spectrum from the lesion shows a peak from 2-HG at about 3.9 ppm. Adapted from Andronesi et al., Science Translational Medicine, 116(4), 1–10, 2012

normal age- and regional-related spectral variations in normal control subjects is essential for proper interpretation.

Tumor Grading and Diagnosis

While conventional MRI is exquisitely sensitive for the detection of lesions within the brain, its actual specificity is quite low, in that lesions of similar MRI appearance may have quite different underlying pathophysiology. Since the pathophysiology determines the appropriate course of treatment, it is very important to establish an accurate diagnosis as early as possible, preferably before a biopsy is performed. MRS may help narrow the range of differential diagnoses, but also suffers itself from a relative lack of specificity.

Since high-grade brain tumors are usually treated more aggressively than low-grade, the planning of a surgical biopsy may be assisted by knowledge of tumor grade, and location of the most aggressive region of tumor growth. Several studies in astrocytomas have found a positive correlation between Cho levels and tumor grade [9, 23, 48], which is consistent with more aggressive tumors having higher membrane turnover and cellular density. However, some studies have found that high-grade tumors (e.g., grade IV glioblastoma multiforme (GBM)) actually have lower levels of Cho than grade II or grade III astrocytomas [22]. This may be due to the presence of necrosis in high-grade tumors, particularly those with necrotic cores sampled by SV MRS, since necrosis is associated with low levels of all metabolites [47, 49]. Since tumors are commonly heterogenous, with, in addition to necrosis, proliferative rims and invasion of surrounding brain tissue, the spectrum may vary greatly depending on the region that is sampled, and for this reason high-resolution MRSI is the preferred technique to be used [50]. Hence, the region of interest chosen for analysis will have a large influence on the results, and, as stated above, MRSI is generally considered preferable since it allows metabolic heterogeneity to be evaluated, and the voxel with the maximum Cho signal to be chosen for analysis and/or targeted for biopsy [51]. The importance of choosing the correct region of interest was illustrated in a combined MRSI/arterial spin-labeling (ASL) study; in regions with elevated flow, Cho (as well as glutamate plus glutamine (Glx), and lactate plus lipid) was found to be higher in high-grade compared to low-grade gliomas [52], whereas no significant metabolic differences were found between grades in normal or hypoperfused tumor regions. Despite these findings, overlap in Cho values between grades generally precludes the use of MRSI for accurate grading; however, at least in astrocytomas, a near-normal Cho level (compared to normal brain) is likely to be of low grade, whereas a markedly elevated Cho level is most likely to be of high grade. Exceptions do exist, and high Cho (or lactate) levels in pediatric brain tumors such as pilocytic astrocytoma [53, 54] and certain oligodendrogliomas for instance do not necessarily imply that they are high-grade, malignant lesions [55].

Several groups have investigated the use of pattern recognition of proton MRS or MRSI spectra to diagnose different tumor types [56–60]. However, probably because of lesion heterogeneity, overlap between different tumor types, and also the dependence of the spectral appearance on data collection and analysis techniques, these methods have not entered into clinical practise. In most cases, therefore, it is unlikely that MRS by itself can diagnose a specific brain lesion, but rather it may be used as an adjunct technique that may contribute to narrowing the range of differential diagnoses that are being considered on the basis of MRI, clinical, and other information. For instance, high Cho levels are typically seen in non-necrotic high-grade brain tumors (for instance anaplastic astrocytoma, GBM, primary CNS lymphoma), while necrotic GBM and metastases are characterized by low levels of all metabolites and increased lipids.

MRSI of peri-enhancing brain regions may also be useful for discriminating solitary metastases from primary brain tumors; gliomas are often invasive lesions which show elevated Cho in surrounding tissue, whereas metastatic lesions tend to be more encapsulated and do not typically show high Cho signals or other abnormalities outside the region of enhancement [61, 62]. Metastatic lesions and glioblastomas nearly always show elevated lipid peaks; thus, if the lesion has high Cho but does not contain lipid signals, a grade III anaplastic astrocytoma should be considered more likely [63].

Neoplastic vs. Non-neoplastic Lesions

A confident diagnosis of a lesion as nonmalignant is important, since a brain biopsy (with its associated risks) can be avoided in these patients. Examples of non-neoplastic lesions that may mimic tumors are infectious, ischemic, and demyelinating lesions (e.g., tumefactive demyelination). Since tumors typically exhibit elevated Cho and decreased NAA, the greatest benefit of adding MRS to a clinical examination may be in including (or excluding) diagnoses with markedly different spectroscopic patterns, for instance acute or semi-acute strokes usually do not have increased Cho (but will have decreased NAA and often increased lactate). Conversely, differentiation between tumors and acute demyelinating lesions is difficult based on MRS, as both typically present with elevated Cho and decreased NAA, as well as often increased lactate probably due to inflammation [64].

Several studies have evaluated the utility of ^{1}H MRS to differentiate between tumors and non-neoplastic lesions [65–69], or compared spectroscopic characteristics of specific groups of neoplastic and non-neoplastic lesions [70–72]. In a long TE MRSI study of 69 brain lesions, a discriminant index based on the ratios NAA/Cho, NAA/Cr, as well as the Cho and NAA signal areas normalized to the contralateral hemisphere correctly classified 84 % of the lesions [73]. There were five cases of tumors misclassified as non-neoplastic lesions (four grade II, one grade III) and six non-neoplastic lesions classified as tumors (including demyelinating lesions, and gliosis). If just using individual measurements, the best classifier was the NAA/Cho ratio, with a cutoff value of 0.61 (lower than 0.61 corresponding to tumor) [73]. In another study [74], SV MRS of 84 solid brain masses (68 grade II and III gliomas, and 16 "pseudo"-tumors, who on final diagnosis has diagnoses of infarct, multiple sclerosis, or inflammatory changes) was performed at both short (30 ms) and long TE (136 ms). Presence of tumor was indicated when mI/NAA ratio (obtained at short TE) was greater than 0.9 and when Cho/NAA ratio (obtained at the long TE) was greater than 1.9 [48], and accuracy of classification was also around 80 %. Of course, MRS is never performed in isolation, but is always part of a larger clinical evaluation, including conventional contrast-enhanced MRI, as well as diffusion and perfusion MRI. A recent review article described how to incorporate the information from MRS into this larger dataset in order to distinguish low-grade and high-grade neoplasia, metastatic disease, lymphoma, tumefactive demyelination, abscess, and encephalitis [75]. The diagnostic strategy was tested on 40 patients who had complete data from all modalities, and it was found that the accuracy, sensitivity, and specificity for differentiating between tumors and non-neoplastic lesions were 90, 97, and 67 %, respectively [75, 76].

On MRS, brain abscesses usually exhibit very different patterns from those seen in neoplastic lesion. Abscesses usually have low levels of Cho, Cr, and NAA, and increased signals from amino acids that are rarely seen in neoplasia, e.g., alanine, acetate, acetoacetate, and succinate, depending on the origin of the primary infection [18, 77].

Prognosis

Despite advances in both imaging and therapy, long-term prognosis for patients with high-grade gliomas remains poor. However, survival time is variable, and is an important information for patients and their families alike. Various studies have evaluated the role of MRSI in prediction of survival in patients with GBM [78–80]. In one study, pretreatment MRSI combined with conventional MRI and diffusion and perfusion MRI was examined for its ability to predict survival [79]. It was found that shorter survival was associated with the volume of tissue with abnormally high Cho/NAA ratio, as well as other parameters such as volumes of contrast-enhancing tissue, and tissue with low ADC values. High lactate and lipid levels were also associated with shorter survival times [79]. In another study, MRSI was performed after surgery but before administration of adjuvant radiation treatment and chemotherapy [78]. As in the previous study, high Cho/NAA ratios and lactate and lipid signals were associated with shorter survival times [78].

In other studies, an inverse relationship between Cho/Cr ratio and survival time was detected in seven patients with gliomatosis cerebri, examined before treatment [81]. In another pretreatment study of 51 supratentorial gliomas, four MRSI indices (maximum values of Cho/Cr, Lac/Cr, total number of voxels with decreased NAA/Cr (<2/3rd of the contralateral NAA/Cr value), and the number of voxels with Lac/Cr ratios ≥1) measured in the area of abnormal MRI signal were significant predictors of survival [82]. Finally, multivariate analysis of spectra of 21 patients with brain metastases differentiated between patients surviving 5 months or more from those with shorter survival times [83].

However, not all studies have found associations between metabolic indices and prognosis; for instance, in 16 immunocompromised patients with primary CNS lymphoma, no pretreatment metabolite measure (including lactate and lipid) was found to correlate with either overall or progression-free survival, although changes with treatment were observed [84]. In another prospective ^{1}H MRS study, 50 patients with newly diagnosed low-grade gliomas (WHO grade II) evaluated prior to surgery showed no relationship between Cho and Cr levels in the tumor and survival, although this finding may be due to the relatively small number of patients who died at the time this study was concluded [85]. The same study did however find a correlation between the normalized Cr level and survival time, with higher Cr corresponded to shorter survival time.

Several studies have also examined the prognostic value of spectroscopy in pediatric brain tumors. In a ^{1}H MRSI study of 76 children with brain tumors, a low value (<1.8) of an index including choline and lactate + lipid levels, normalized to contralateral Cr, was found to be a strong predictor of survival [86]. In another study of children with recurrent gliomas, a high Cho/NAA ratio was associated with decreased survival [87].

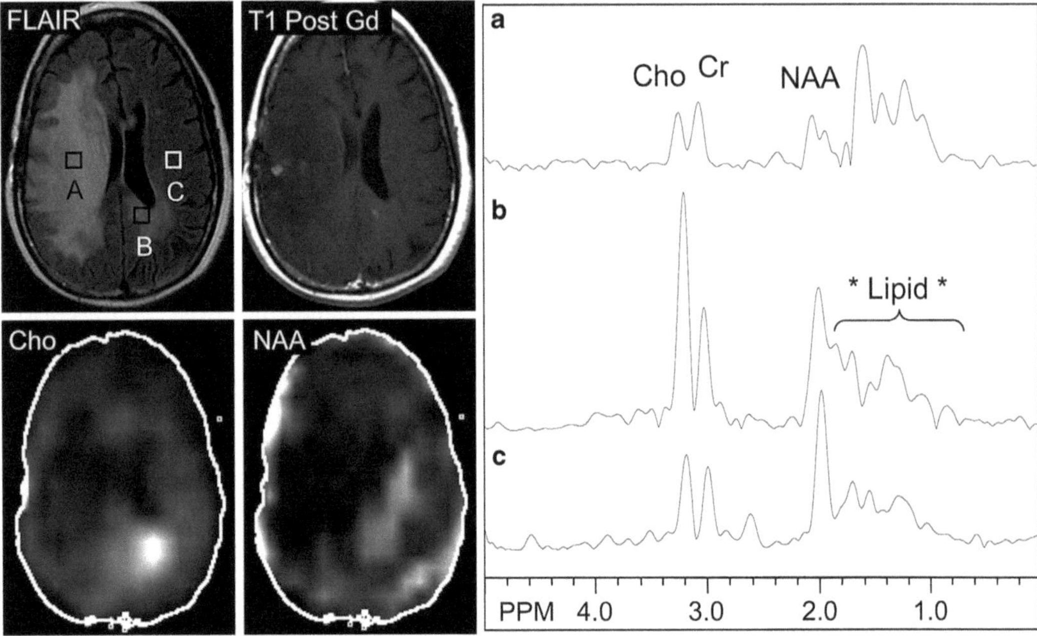

Fig. 3.10 1.5 T MRSI (TE 280 ms) in a patient with high-grade glioma being evaluated for radiation necrosis or tumor recurrence. Conventional T_2-weighted FLAIR MRI shows a large region of hyperintensity in the right hemisphere with minimal mass effect, and T_1-weighted MRI post Gd shows a few enhancing nodules. On MRSI, Cho and NAA are both lower in the lesion in the right hemisphere (**a**) compared to normal brain (**c**), consistent with radiation necrosis; however, Cho is elevated in the left parietal white matter and splenium of the corpus callosum (**b**)

Treatment Planning and Monitoring

A potential major role for MRSI is in treatment planning and monitoring of tumor response to therapy. This topic is covered in detail in Chap. 9, so it is discussed only briefly here. In regard to treatment planning, either for surgery or targeted radiotherapy, a limitation of conventional MRI (as mentioned above) is its lack of specificity. For instance, contrast-enhancement due to blood–brain barrier breakdown can occur both in necrotic tissue and in actively growing tumor, while T_2-hyperintense tissue may be either invasive tumor or peri-tumoral edema. High-resolution MRSI-based mapping of regional Cho levels may assist in differentiating active tumor from necrosis or edema, and therefore assist in treatment planning, as well as in follow-up of response to treatment. Only active tumor is expected to show elevated Cho signals; both edema and necrosis are expected to have normal or lower Cho [10, 49, 88]. An example of MRSI in a patient with both recurrent tumor and necrosis (in different regions) post surgery and chemo- and radiotherapy is shown in Fig. 3.10. The results from a recent phase II prospective trial of Gamma Knife stereotactic radiosurgery (SRS) in 35 patients with GBM showed that survival could be increased (compared to historical controls) by boosting radiation dose to regions of high tumor activity, as defined by a Cho/NAA ratio of >2 [89]. The authors concluded that these results were encouraging, and could form the basis of a future multi-site trial of MRS-guided SRS.

Standard treatment for high-grade gliomas includes surgery, chemotherapy with temozolomide, and a course of radiation therapy. Anti-angiogenic treatment with bevacizumab is also being increasingly used in the USA. Usually, imaging is performed at regular intervals (e.g., every 3 months) to monitor the effects of treatment and possible disease recurrence. Ideally, accurate imaging biomarkers are needed to determine early in the course of the disease if a treatment scheme should be continued, adapted, or changed completely [90]. In this regard, conventional MRI has a limited role because of its lack of specificity, particularly in the anti-angiogenic era, where contrast-enhancement and edema may be markedly reduced even in the presence of residual or recurrent tumor (termed "pseudo-response") [91]. "Pseudo-progression" (increased enhancement and edema) can also occur at early time points in patients who ultimately have a good treatment response [92]; clearly additional imaging markers are urgently needed in these scenarios.

Proton MRSI measurements of Cho show promise in this regard; for instance, an MRSI study in 31 patients treated with radiation for intracranial tumor reported a sensitivity of 85 % and a specificity of 69 % to differentiate between recurrent tumor and radiation necrosis based on the Cho/NAA ratio [93]. However, another MRSI study combined with diagnosis via image-guided biopsy specimens revealed overlap in normalized Cho levels (and lipid) with tumor/radiation necrosis and either tumor or radiation necrosis, although good separation between pure necrosis and pure tumor was achieved based on normalized Cho levels [10]. In a recent study comparing SV-MRS, MRSI, perfusion, and diffusion for the differentiation between posttreatment effects and recurrent tumor, MRSI Cho/Cr and Cho/NAA ratios outperformed both perfusion (CBV) and diffusion (ADC) measures, as well as SV-MRS Cho ratio measures, illustrating the importance of spatial sampling using MRSI [94]. Another study [95] of previously treated glioma patients was also encouraging for the use of MRS to distinguish recurrent tumor from necrosis, with superior positive and negative predictive values to both PET and conventional contrast-enhanced MRI, although relatively few details of the MRS procedures were included in this paper.

Radiotherapy planning involves a careful balance between maximizing dose to the tumor while limiting the effects on surrounding brain tissue. Long-term radiation injury is particularly an issue for treatment of malignancies in children, where long-term deleterious effects on the developing brain can lead to cognitive deficits and other complications [96]. MRS has been shown to be able to detect the effects of radiation on normal brain, and may have some role in monitoring radiation injury. The most commonly reported changes following radiation are decreases in NAA [97], which can be detected 1 to 4 months after radiation in non-tumoral regions receiving between 20 and 50 Gy [98], as well as decreases in Cho [96].

Recently, the use of MRSI has been reported for the monitoring of tumor response to intra-arterial bevacizumab [99]. In this phase I trial, it appears that the Cho/NAA ratio may be helpful in monitoring tumor response (most tumors showed a decrease in Cho/NAA 3–5 weeks post treatment); however correlation with clinical or other measures of outcome was not performed.

Conclusion

As described above, multiple studies indicate the potential value of MRSI to aid in the differential diagnosis of brain lesions, as well as to assist in the guidance and monitoring of response to treatment. Since MRSI can be performed at the same time as routine brain MRI, and does not require any specialized hardware, in principle it should be straightforward to incorporate MRSI into the routine evaluation of patients with brain tumors. However, at present this goal is only achieved in a relatively small number of academic medical centers; there are several reasons for this, including the length of time required to perform, process, and interpret MRSI data; the lack of widespread technologist and radiologist training in MRSI; the lack of standardization of acquisition and analysis techniques; and the rather suboptimal commercially available protocols to perform MRSI (compared to current state-of-the-art research MRSI techniques). Other problems include the lack of powerful, easy-to-use analysis software interfaced with clinical PAC systems for the analysis and display of MRSI data. Each of these problems is potentially soluble, but will require a concerted effort from clinicians, commercial vendors, and researchers alike. Larger, multi-site clinical trials of MRSI methodology are also required to convince referring clinicians (oncologists, neurosurgeons) and funding agencies of the value of MRSI for the evaluation of brain tumors, and its relative value compared to other modalities, such as other advanced MRI techniques, or PET.

References

1. Frahm J. Localized Proton Spectroscopy using stimulated echoes. J Magn Reson. 1987;72:502–8.
2. Bruhn H, Frahm J, Gyngell ML, et al. Noninvasive differentiation of tumors with use of localized H-1 MR spectroscopy in vivo: initial experience in patients with cerebral tumors. Radiology. 1989;172:541–8.
3. Barker PB, Lin DD. In vivo proton MR spectroscopy of the human brain. Prog NMR Spect. 2006;49: 99–128.
4. Gupta RK, Cloughesy TF, Sinha U, et al. Relationships between choline magnetic resonance spectroscopy, apparent diffusion coefficient and quantitative histopathology in human glioma. J Neurooncol. 2000;50: 215–26.
5. Aboagye EO, Bhujwalla ZM. Malignant transformation alters membrane choline phospholipid metabolism of human mammary epithelial cells. Cancer Res. 1999;59:80–4.
6. Brand A, Richter-Landsberg C, Leibfritz D. Multinuclear NMR studies on the energy metabolism of glial and neuronal cells. Dev Neurosci. 1993;15: 289–98.
7. Castillo M, Smith JK, Kwock L. Correlation of myo-inositol levels and grading of cerebral astrocytomas. AJNR Am J Neuroradiol. 2000;21:1645–9.
8. Demir MK, Iplikcioglu AC, Dincer A, Arslan M, Sav A. Single voxel proton MR spectroscopy findings of typical and atypical intracranial meningiomas. Eur J Radiol. 2006;60:48–55.
9. Arnold DL, Shoubridge EA, Villemure JG, Feindel W. Proton and phosphorus magnetic resonance spectroscopy of human astrocytomas in vivo. Preliminary observations on tumor grading. NMR Biomed. 1990; 3:184–9.
10. Rock JP, Hearshen D, Scarpace L, et al. Correlations between magnetic resonance spectroscopy and image-guided histopathology, with special attention to radiation necrosis. Neurosurgery. 2002;51:912–9. discussion 919–920.
11. Tkac I, Andersen P, Adriany G, Merkle H, Ugurbil K, Gruetter R. In vivo 1H NMR spectroscopy of the human brain at 7 T. Magn Reson Med. 2001;46: 451–6.
12. de Groot J, Sontheimer H. Glutamate and the biology of gliomas. Glia. 2011;59:1181–9.
13. Sontheimer H. Glutamate and tumor-associated epilepsy. Oncotarget. 2011;2:823–4.
14. Grossman SA, Ye X, Chamberlain M, et al. Talampanel with standard radiation and temozolomide in patients with newly diagnosed glioblastoma: a multicenter phase II trial. J Clin Oncol. 2009;27: 4155–61.
15. Medina MA, Sanchez-Jimenez F, Marquez J, Rodriguez Quesada A, Nunez de Castro I. Relevance of glutamine metabolism to tumor cell growth. Mol cell biochem. 1992;113:1–15.
16. DeBerardinis RJ, Cheng T. Q's next: the diverse functions of glutamine in metabolism, cell biology and cancer. Oncogene. 2010;29:313–24.
17. Yeung DK, Chan Y, Leung S, Poon PM, Pang C. Detection of an intense resonance at 2.4 ppm in 1H MR spectra of patients with severe late-delayed, radiation-induced brain injuries. Magnetic resonance in medicine : official journal of the Society of Magnetic Resonance in Medicine/Society of. Magn Reson Med. 2001;45:994–1000.
18. Remy C, Grand S, Lai ES, et al. 1H MRS of human brain abscesses in vivo and in vitro. Magn Reson Med. 1995;34:508–14.
19. Bluml S, Panigrahy A, Laskov M, et al. Elevated citrate in pediatric astrocytomas with malignant progression. Neuro-Oncology. 2011;13:1107–17.
20. Dang L, White DW, Gross S, et al. Cancer-associated IDH1 mutations produce 2-hydroxyglutarate. Nature. 2009;462:739–44.
21. Choi C, Ganji SK, DeBerardinis RJ, et al. 2-hydroxyglutarate detection by magnetic resonance spectroscopy in IDH-mutated patients with gliomas. Nat Med. 2012;18:624–9.
22. Howe FA, Barton SJ, Cudlip SA, et al. Metabolic profiles of human brain tumors using quantitative in vivo 1H magnetic resonance spectroscopy. Magn Reson Med. 2003;49:223–32.
23. Hourani R, Horska A, Albayram S, et al. Proton magnetic resonance spectroscopic imaging to differentiate between nonneoplastic lesions and brain tumors in children. Journal of magnetic resonance imaging : JMRI. 2006;23:99–107.
24. Graves EE, Nelson SJ, Vigneron DB, et al. Serial proton MR spectroscopic imaging of recurrent malignant gliomas after gamma knife radiosurgery. AJNR Am J Neuroradiol. 2001;22:613–24.
25. McKnight TR, von dem Bussche MH, Vigneron DB, et al. Histopathological validation of a three-dimensional magnetic resonance spectroscopy index as a predictor of tumor presence. J Neurosurg. 2002;97:794–802.
26. Nelson SJ. Multivoxel magnetic resonance spectroscopy of brain tumors. Mol Cancer Ther. 2003;2: 497–507.
27. Nelson SJ, Graves E, Pirzkall A, et al. In vivo molecular imaging for planning radiation therapy of gliomas: an application of 1H MRSI. J Magn Reson Imaging. 2002;16:464–76.
28. Scheenen TW, Klomp DW, Wijnen JP, Heerschap A. Short echo time 1H-MRSI of the human brain at 3T with minimal chemical shift displacement errors using adiabatic refocusing pulses. Magn Reson Med. 2008;59:1–6.

29. Oz G, Tkac I. Short-echo, single-shot, full-intensity proton magnetic resonance spectroscopy for neurochemical profiling at 4 T: validation in the cerebellum and brainstem. Magn Reson Med. 2011;65:901–10.
30. Mlynarik V, Gambarota G, Frenkel H, Gruetter R. Localized short-echo-time proton MR spectroscopy with full signal-intensity acquisition. Magn Reson Med. 2006;56:965–70.
31. Haase A, Frahm J, Hanicke W, Matthei D. 1H NMR chemical shift selective imaging. Phys Med Biol. 1985;30:341–4.
32. Tkac I, Starcuk Z, Choi IY, Gruetter R. In vivo 1H NMR spectroscopy of rat brain at 1 ms echo time. Magn Reson Med. 1999;41:649–56.
33. Brown TR, Kincaid BM, Ugurbil K. NMR chemical shift imaging in three dimensions. Proc Natl Acad Sci U S A. 1982;79:3523–6.
34. Moonen CTW, Sobering G, van Zijl PCM, Gillen J, von Kienlin M, Bizzi A. Proton spectroscopic imaging of human brain. J Magn Reson. 1992;98:556–75.
35. Vigneron D, Bollen A, McDermott M, et al. Three-dimensional magnetic resonance spectroscopic imaging of histologically confirmed brain tumors. Magn Reson Imaging. 2001;19:89–101.
36. Duyn JH, Gillen J, Sobering G, van Zijl PC, Moonen CT. Multisection proton MR spectroscopic imaging of the brain. Radiology. 1993;188:277–82.
37. Ebel A, Soher BJ, Maudsley AA. Assessment of 3D proton MR echo-planar spectroscopic imaging using automated spectral analysis. Magn Reson Med. 2001; 46:1072–8.
38. Duyn JH, Moonen CT. Fast proton spectroscopic imaging of human brain using multiple spin-echoes. Magn Reson Med. 1993;30:409–14.
39. Dydak U, Weiger M, Pruessmann KP, Meier D, Boesiger P. Sensitivity-encoded spectroscopic imaging. Magn Reson Med. 2001;46:713–22.
40. Bonekamp D, Smith MA, Zhu H, Barker PB. Quantitative SENSE-MRSI of the human brain. Magn reson imaging. 2010;28:305–13.
41. Banerjee S, Ozturk-Isik E, Nelson SJ, Majumdar S. Elliptical magnetic resonance spectroscopic imaging with GRAPPA for imaging brain tumors at 3 T. Magn reson imaging. 2009;27:1319–25.
42. Banerjee S, Ozturk-Isik E, Nelson SJ, Majumdar S. Fast magnetic resonance spectroscopic imaging at 3 Tesla using autocalibrating parallel technique. Conference proceedings : Annual International Conference of the IEEE Engineering in Medicine and Biology Society IEEE Engineering in Medicine and Biology Society Conference 2006;1:1866–1869
43. Posse S, Tedeschi G, Risinger R, Ogg R, Le Bihan D. High speed 1H spectroscopic imaging in human brain by echo planar spatial-spectral encoding. Magn Reson Med. 1995;33:34–40.
44. Puts NA, Edden RA. In vivo magnetic resonance spectroscopy of GABA: a methodological review. Prog Nucl Magn Reson Spectrosc. 2012;60:29–41.
45. Mescher M, Merkle H, Kirsch J, Garwood M, Gruetter R. Simultaneous in vivo spectral editing and water suppression. NMR Biomed. 1998;11:266–72.
46. Provencher SW. Estimation of metabolite concentrations from localized in vivo proton NMR spectra. Magn Reson Med. 1993;30:672–9.
47. Rabinov JD, Lee PL, Barker FG, et al. In vivo 3-T MR spectroscopy in the distinction of recurrent glioma versus radiation effects: initial experience. Radiology. 2002;225:871–9.
48. Gill SS, Thomas DG, Van Bruggen N, et al. Proton MR spectroscopy of intracranial tumours: in vivo and in vitro studies. J Comput Assist Tomogr. 1990; 14:497–504.
49. Preul MC, Leblanc R, Caramanos Z, Kasrai R, Narayanan S, Arnold DL. Magnetic resonance spectroscopy guided brain tumor resection: differentiation between recurrent glioma and radiation change in two diagnostically difficult cases. Can J Neurol Sci. 1998;25:13–22.
50. Ricci PE, Pitt A, Keller PJ, Coons SW, Heiserman JE. Effect of voxel position on single-voxel MR spectroscopy findings. AJNR Am J neuroradiol. 2000;21: 367–74.
51. Senft C, Hattingen E, Pilatus U, et al. Diagnostic value of proton magnetic resonance spectroscopy in the noninvasive grading of solid gliomas: comparison of maximum and mean choline values. Neurosurgery. 2009;65:908–13. discussion 913.
52. Chawla S, Wang S, Wolf RL, et al. Arterial spin-labeling and MR spectroscopy in the differentiation of gliomas. AJNR Am J Neuroradiol. 2007;28:1683–9.
53. Hwang JH, Egnaczyk GF, Ballard E, Dunn RS, Holland SK, Ball Jr WS. Proton MR spectroscopic characteristics of pediatric pilocytic astrocytomas. AJNR Am J Neuroradiol. 1998;19:535–40.
54. Panigrahy A, Krieger MD, Gonzalez-Gomez I, et al. Quantitative short echo time 1H-MR spectroscopy of untreated pediatric brain tumors: preoperative diagnosis and characterization. AJNR Am J Neuroradiol. 2006;27:560–72.
55. Fulham MJ, Bizzi A, Dietz MJ, et al. Mapping of brain tumor metabolites with proton MR spectroscopic imaging: clinical relevance. Radiology. 1992; 185:675–86.
56. Tate AR, Griffiths JR, Martinez-Perez I, et al. Towards a method for automated classification of 1H MRS spectra from brain tumours. NMR Biomed. 1998;11:177–91.
57. Tate AR, Majos C, Moreno A, Howe FA, Griffiths JR, Arus C. Automated classification of short echo time in in vivo 1H brain tumor spectra: a multicenter study. Magn reson Med. 2003;49:29–36.
58. Wright AJ, Fellows G, Byrnes TJ, et al. Pattern recognition of MRSI data shows regions of glioma growth that agree with DTI markers of brain tumor infiltration. Magn Reson Med. 2009;62:1646–51.
59. Preul MC, Caramanos Z, Collins DL, et al. Accurate, noninvasive diagnosis of human brain tumors by using proton magnetic resonance spectroscopy. Nat Med. 1996;2:323–5.
60. De Edelenyi FS, Rubin C, Esteve F, et al. A new approach for analyzing proton magnetic resonance spectroscopic images of brain tumors: nosologic images. Nat Med. 2000;6:1287–9.

61. Fan G, Sun B, Wu Z, Guo Q, Guo Y. In vivo single-voxel proton MR spectroscopy in the differentiation of high-grade gliomas and solitary metastases. Clin Radiol. 2004;59:77–85.
62. Chiang IC, Kuo YT, Lu CY, et al. Distinction between high-grade gliomas and solitary metastases using peritumoral 3-T magnetic resonance spectroscopy, diffusion, and perfusion imagings. Neuroradiology. 2004;46:619–27.
63. Ishimaru H, Morikawa M, Iwanaga S, Kaminogo M, Ochi M, Hayashi K. Differentiation between high-grade glioma and metastatic brain tumor using single-voxel proton MR spectroscopy. Eur Radiol. 2001;11:1784–91.
64. Saindane AM, Cha S, Law M, Xue X, Knopp EA, Zagzag D. Proton MR spectroscopy of tumefactive demyelinating lesions. AJNR Am J Neuroradiol. 2002;23:1378–86.
65. Poptani H, Kaartinen J, Gupta RK, Niemitz M, Hiltunen Y, Kauppinen RA. Diagnostic assessment of brain tumours and non-neoplastic brain disorders in vivo using proton nuclear magnetic resonance spectroscopy and artificial neural networks. J Cancer Res Clin Oncol. 1999;125:343–9.
66. Poptani H, Gupta RK, Roy R, Pandey R, Jain VK, Chhabra DK. Characterization of intracranial mass lesions with in vivo proton MR spectroscopy. AJNR Am J Neuroradiol. 1995;16:1593–603.
67. Rand SD, Prost R, Haughton V, et al. Accuracy of single-voxel proton MR spectroscopy in distinguishing neoplastic from nonneoplastic brain lesions. AJNR Am J Neuroradiol. 1997;18:1695–704.
68. Butzen J, Prost R, Chetty V, et al. Discrimination between neoplastic and nonneoplastic brain lesions by use of proton MR spectroscopy: the limits of accuracy with a logistic regression model. AJNR Am J Neuroradiol. 2000;21:1213–9.
69. Moller-Hartmann W, Herminghaus S, Krings T, et al. Clinical application of proton magnetic resonance spectroscopy in the diagnosis of intracranial mass lesions. Neuroradiology. 2002;44:371–81.
70. De Stefano N, Caramanos Z, Preul MC, Francis G, Antel JP, Arnold DL. In vivo differentiation of astrocytic brain tumors and isolated demyelinating lesions of the type seen in multiple sclerosis using 1H magnetic resonance spectroscopic imaging. Ann Neurol. 1998;44:273–8.
71. Venkatesh SK, Gupta RK, Pal L, Husain N, Husain M. Spectroscopic increase in choline signal is a non-specific marker for differentiation of infective/inflammatory from neoplastic lesions of the brain. J Magn Reson Imaging. 2001;14:8–15.
72. Vuori K, Kankaanranta L, Hakkinen AM, et al. Low-grade gliomas and focal cortical developmental malformations: differentiation with proton MR spectroscopy. Radiology. 2004;230:703–8.
73. Hourani R, Brant LJ, Rizk T, Weingart JD, Barker PB, Horska A. Can proton MR spectroscopic and perfusion imaging differentiate between neoplastic and nonneoplastic brain lesions in adults? AJNR Am J Neuroradiol. 2008;29:366–72.
74. Majos C, Aguilera C, Alonso J, et al. Proton MR spectroscopy improves discrimination between tumor and pseudotumoral lesion in solid brain masses. AJNR Am J Neuroradiol. 2009;30:544–51.
75. Al-Okaili RN, Krejza J, Wang S, Woo JH, Melhem ER. Advanced MR imaging techniques in the diagnosis of intraaxial brain tumors in adults. Radiographics. 2006;26 Suppl 1:S173–89.
76. Al-Okaili RN, Krejza J, Woo JH, et al. Intraaxial brain masses: MR imaging-based diagnostic strategy–initial experience. Radiology. 2007;243:539–50.
77. Garg M, Gupta RK. Spectroscopy in intracranial infection. In: Gillard J, Waldman A, Barker PB, editors. Clinical MR Neuroimaging: Diffusion, Perfusion and Spectroscopy. Cambridge, UK: Cambridge University Press; 2004. p. 380–406.
78. Saraswathy S, Crawford FW, Lamborn KR, et al. Evaluation of MR markers that predict survival in patients with newly diagnosed GBM prior to adjuvant therapy. J Neurooncol. 2009;91:69–81.
79. Crawford FW, Khayal IS, McGue C, et al. Relationship of pre-surgery metabolic and physiological MR imaging parameters to survival for patients with untreated GBM. J Neurooncol. 2009;91:337–51.
80. Chan AA, Lau A, Pirzkall A, et al. Proton magnetic resonance spectroscopy imaging in the evaluation of patients undergoing gamma knife surgery for Grade IV glioma. J Neurosurg. 2004;101:467–75.
81. Guzman-de-Villoria JA, Sanchez-Gonzalez J, Munoz L, et al. 1H MR spectroscopy in the assessment of gliomatosis cerebri. AJR Am J Roentgenol. 2007;188: 710–4.
82. Kuznetsov YE, Caramanos Z, Antel SB, et al. Proton magnetic resonance spectroscopic imaging can predict length of survival in patients with supratentorial gliomas. Neurosurgery. 2003;53:565–74. discussion 574–566.
83. Sjobakk TE, Johansen R, Bathen TF, et al. Metabolic profiling of human brain metastases using in vivo proton MR spectroscopy at 3T. BMC Cancer. 2007; 7:141.
84. Raizer JJ, Koutcher JA, Abrey LE, et al. Proton magnetic resonance spectroscopy in immunocompetent patients with primary central nervous system lymphoma. J Neurooncol. 2005;71:173–80.
85. Hattingen E, Raab P, Franz K, et al. Prognostic value of choline and creatine in WHO grade II gliomas. Neuroradiology. 2008;50:759–67.
86. Marcus KJ, Astrakas LG, Zurakowski D, et al. Predicting survival of children with CNS tumors using proton magnetic resonance spectroscopic imaging biomarkers. Int J Oncol. 2007;30:651–7.
87. Warren KE, Frank JA, Black JL, et al. Proton magnetic resonance spectroscopic imaging in children with recurrent primary brain tumors. J Clin Oncol. 2000;18:1020–6.
88. Law M, Cha S, Knopp EA, Johnson G, Arnett J, Litt AW. High-grade gliomas and solitary metastases: differentiation by using perfusion and proton spectroscopic MR imaging. Radiology. 2002;222: 715–21.

89. Einstein DB, Wessels B, Bangert B, et al. Phase II trial of radiosurgery to magnetic resonance spectroscopy-defined high-risk tumor volumes in patients with glioblastoma multiforme. Int J Radiat Oncol Biol Phys. 2012;84:668–74.
90. Weber MA, Giesel FL, Stieltjes B. MRI for identification of progression in brain tumors: from morphology to function. Expert Rev Neurother. 2008;8:1507–25.
91. Hygino da Cruz Jr LC, Domingues RC, Gasparetto EL, Sorensen AG. Pseudoprogression and pseudoresponse: imaging challenges in the assessment of posttreatment glioma. AJNR Am J Neuroradiol. 2011;32:1978–85.
92. Brandsma D, Stalpers L, Taal W, Sminia P, van den Bent MJ. Clinical features, mechanisms, and management of pseudoprogression in malignant gliomas. Lancet Oncol. 2008;9:453–61.
93. Smith EA, Carlos RC, Junck LR, Tsien CI, Elias A, Sundgren PC. Developing a clinical decision model: MR spectroscopy to differentiate between recurrent tumor and radiation change in patients with new contrast-enhancing lesions. AJR Am J Roentgenol. 2009; 192:W45–52.
94. Fink JR, Carr RB, Matsusue E, et al. Comparison of 3 Tesla proton MR spectroscopy, MR perfusion and MR diffusion for distinguishing glioma recurrence from posttreatment effects. J Magn reson imaging. 2012;35: 56–63.
95. Prat R, Galeano I, Lucas A, et al. Relative value of magnetic resonance spectroscopy, magnetic resonance perfusion, and 2-(18F) fluoro-2-deoxy-D-glucose positron emission tomography for detection of recurrence or grade increase in gliomas. J Clin Neurosci. 2010;17:50–3.
96. Sundgren PC. MR spectroscopy in radiation injury. AJNR Am J Neuroradiol. 2009;30:1469–76.
97. Sundgren PC, Nagesh V, Elias A, et al. Metabolic alterations: a biomarker for radiation-induced normal brain injury-an MR spectroscopy study. J Magn reson imaging. 2009;29:291–7.
98. Esteve F, Rubin C, Grand S, Kolodie H, Le Bas JF. Transient metabolic changes observed with proton MR spectroscopy in normal human brain after radiation therapy. Int J Radiat Oncol Biol Phys. 1998;40: 279–86.
99. Jeon JY, Kovanlikaya I, Boockvar JA, et al. Metabolic response of glioblastoma to superselective intra-arterial cerebral infusion of bevacizumab: a proton MR spectroscopic imaging study. AJNR Am J Neuroradiol. 2012;33:2095–102.

Part II

Physiologic Imaging for Planning and Monitoring of Therapeutic Intervention

BOLD fMRI for Presurgical Planning: Part I

4

Domenico Zacá and Jay J. Pillai

Introduction

Blood Oxygen Level Dependent functional Magnetic Resonance Imaging (BOLD fMRI) is a noninvasive brain mapping technique developed in the early nineties by Ogawa and colleagues [1]. It exploits the transient changes in regional hemodynamics accompanying brain activation to generate activation maps that can be easily displayed and fused on structural MRI images. As such BOLD fMRI provides an indirect measurement of neuronal activity.

During neuronal activation local blood flow, oxygenation and oxygen utilization increase, albeit with a 2–4 s delay after the onset of neural activation. The exact mechanism by which a hemodynamic response is elicited by neuronal activity has not been completely understood. Two approaches are currently used to elucidate the relationship between activation and hemodynamic changes: in the first one, called the metabolic pathway, the changes in blood flow (and blood volume) are thought to be induced by vasodilatory metabolites (H^+ and CO_2) released during increased aerobic metabolism. The second theory proposes that neurotransmitters released at the synapses during neuronal activity, such as glutamate, induce the release of vasodilatory mediators which in turn increase the blood flow [2].

Despite the theory adopted to explain this neurovascular coupling mechanism there is a substantial mismatch in the magnitude of change between cerebral blood flow (CBF) and oxygen consumption (as assessed by the cerebral metabolic rate of oxygen, i.e., CMRO2) (up to 100 % increase in CBF vs. up to 33 % increase in CMRO2). This results in a local increase in oxyhemoglobin concentration with a consequent decrease in deoxyhemoglobin concentration in the venules and parenchyma during activation. Since oxyhemoglobin is diamagnetic, whereas deoxyhemoglobin is paramagnetic, transient variations in the concentration of these molecules produce temporary distortion of the local magnetic field homogeneity, and this phenomenon is indeed exploited by the BOLD technique to detect eloquent cortical areas of the brain. T2* gradient echo pulse sequences with long echo times (>25 ms [milliseconds] at magnetic fields equal to or less than 3 T) are very sensitive to local magnetic field heterogeneity; in particular, the BOLD signal decreases with increasing deoxyhemoglobin and increases with decreasing deoxyhemoglobin since deoxyhemoglobin is a negative contrast agent resulting in signal loss on such heavily T2*-weighted images. Therefore BOLD

D. Zacá, Ph.D.
MR Lab, Center for Mind Brain Sciences, University of Trento, USA

J.J. Pillai, M.D. (✉)
Russell H. Morgan Dept. of Radiology and Radiological Science, Neuroradiology Division, Johns Hopkins Univ. School of Medicine and The Johns Hopkins Hospital, Baltimore, Maryland, USA
e-mail: jpillai1@jhmi.edu

J.J. Pillai (ed.), *Functional Brain Tumor Imaging*, DOI 10.1007/978-1-4419-5858-7_4,

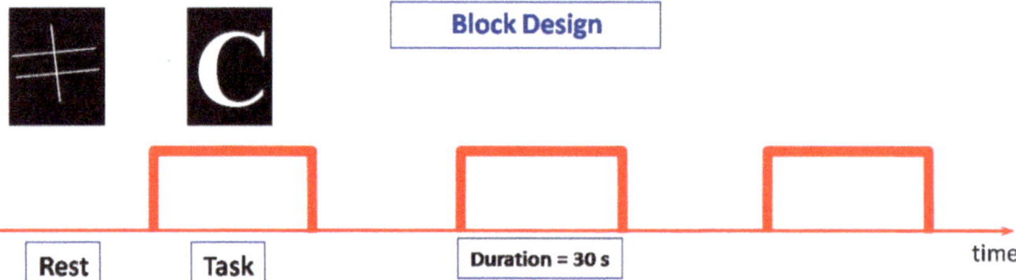

Fig. 4.1 Example of a block design silent word generation paradigm: the paradigm begins with a 30 s resting (or control) block during which the patient is asked to simply stare at abstract symbols. The following 30 s the patient is engaged in a speech production task consisting of covertly generate words beginning with the presented letter. The resting and the active block are presented in alternating fashion every 30 s for 3–4 min. The subtraction of a visual fixation task from the language active task aims to eliminate visual activation from the expressive language activation maps

fMRI reveals areas of activation in the brain by detecting the transient T2*-weighted signal increase due to the reduction in deoxyhemoglobin concentration following neuronal activation. The magnitude of the signal change, however, is only around 2–4 % compared to baseline. For this reason it is necessary to compare multiple resting and activation conditions in order to extract activation related signal, distinguishing it from noise.

fMRI studies are performed using various paradigms that require the subject or patient to perform particular well-defined cognitive, sensorimotor or visual tasks while images are acquired using a T2* gradient echo sequence with echo planar imaging (EPI) readout, a technique that allows scanning of the entire brain with a spatial resolution between 2 and 4 mm in about 2 s. Nowadays in a typical fMRI paradigm generally 100–300 imaging volumes are acquired over a period of 3–5 min.

A paradigm consists of alternating periods of an active task, involving the function that is being detected in the study, and a resting state or control task that differs from the active task only in the cognitive process of interest. It is critical to optimally design fMRI paradigms in order to generate highly specific activation maps that depict only the areas pertaining to the considered function (Fig. 4.1).

The fMRI literature distinguishes two general categories of paradigms: block design and event-related. In the block design method, the active and control tasks are presented in regular alternating epochs (blocks) and are usually labeled "on" (active) and "off" (control). The regions of the brain where there are statistically significant differences between the signal acquired during the on and off periods are considered as functionally active.

Event-related paradigms are designed presenting a single event at a time instead of epochs of multiple serial stimuli. Each event is considered separately as being time-locked to the beginning of the stimulus, and signal changes are explored in relation to the onset of the event generated by the trial.

After the image acquisition several preprocessing steps are needed before the statistical analysis that provides the activation maps can be performed. First, a four-dimensional dataset is created from the thousands of raw images where the signal time series recorded over the entire time of acquisition is reconstructed in each voxel (Fig. 4.2).

Then for each volume all the slices are temporally shifted so that they were acquired at the same time and all the volumes are registered to a reference one to correct for minor head motion. Two further preprocessing steps, not necessarily performed in all analyses, are image spatial smoothing to enhance the signal to noise ratio (SNR) and spatial normalization to a common stereotactic space for neuroanatomical labeling.

After the preprocessing, several statistical methods can be used to infer neuronal activation.

The most commonly used method is the General Linear Model (GLM) that consists of a regression analysis where the paradigm timing is convolved with an expected hemodynamic response function (HRF), and the obtained waveform (the GLM) is fitted to the acquired time series voxelwise. A map of regressors is thus

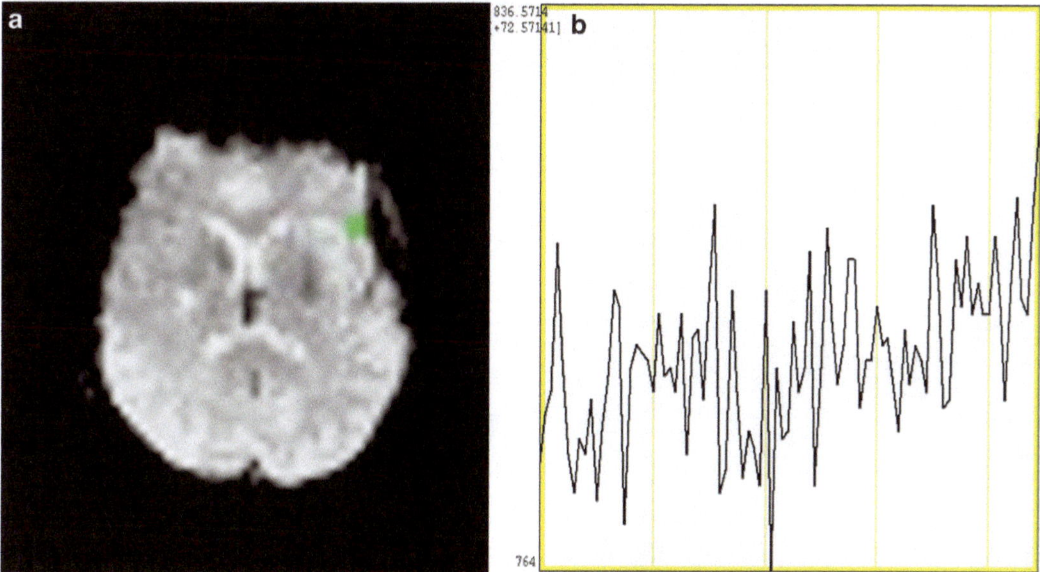

Fig. 4.2 (**a**) (*Left*) One BOLD EPI image (axial slice) as acquired and reconstructed from the scanner. In image (**b**) the time course of the signal in the voxel highlighted in *green* in (**a**) is reconstructed. Data have been processed utilizing the Analysis of Functional NeuroImages (AFNI) software package (afni.nimh.nih.gov)

obtained in each voxel with an associated statistical significance (t-value, Z-score, or p-value). These maps are thresholded at an arbitrary significance level and suprathreshold voxels are overlaid as bright clusters on anatomical images, thus forming the so-called activation maps (Fig. 4.3).

The GLM data analysis approach is the most commonly used and widely accepted method, especially in the field of clinical fMRI, because it provides activation in expected areas and with anticipated timings [3]. In the last decade several exploratory and data driven techniques (e.g., Principal Component Analysis and Independent Component Analysis) have been developed that can be used to discover brain activity without the need to make a priori assumptions regarding areas of activation or timing of the HRF [4].

Clinical fMRI

BOLD fMRI has been used in neuroscience research studies to assess a broad spectrum of brain function. Since the early 1990s when this technique was first established, investigators have progressed from the study of basic motor and visual function to the investigation of more and more complex cognitive function, including language, memory, emotion, and even abstract reasoning functions utilizing fMRI. In the last decade BOLD fMRI has evolved from a purely research imaging technique to a viable clinical technique that is mainly applied for presurgical planning in patients with brain tumors and other resectable brain lesions. However the clinical use of fMRI for presurgical planning is limited today to the detection of sensorimotor, language/speech, and vision function, with currently only limited capability for accurate assessment of memory function. The standardization of the paradigms in terms of task performed, timing parameters, and postprocessing is still an evolving process, although many language and motor activation paradigms have been reported to provide results that are concordant with those obtained using "gold-standard" electrophysiologic intraoperative mapping techniques and are currently used in many institutions [5–10].

Two Current Procedural Terminology (CPT) codes were established in January 2007 as a result of numerous single-center clinical validation studies and several landmark studies that have demonstrated the clinical impact of preoperative functional imaging on surgical planning [11, 12].

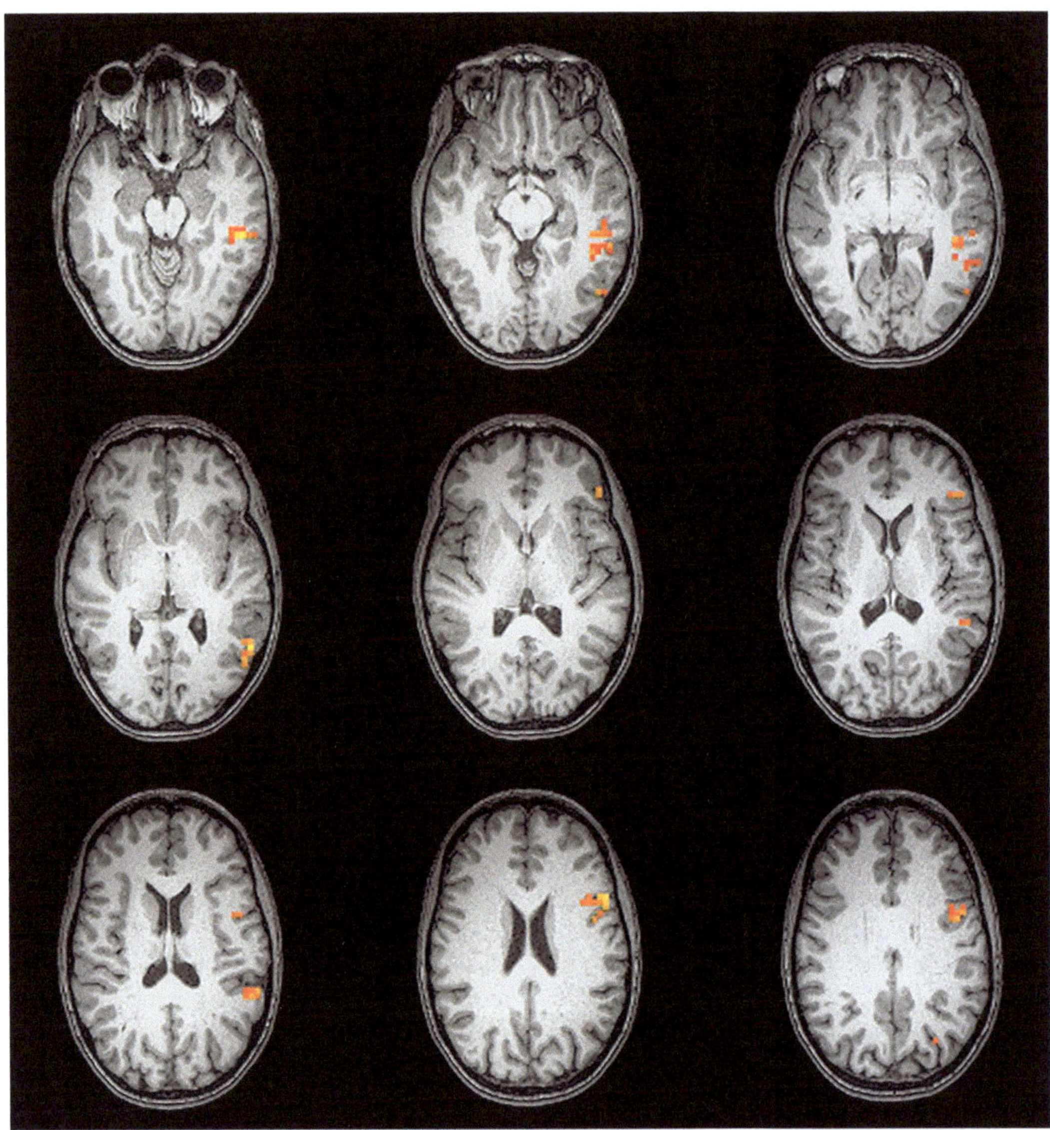

Fig. 4.3 Activation map in a right-handed normal volunteer from a sentence completion paradigm overlaid on T1 MPRAGE structural images. The bright spot pixels are the ones whose signal time series in the T2* EPI images demonstrates a statistically significant signal increase (thresholded at a *t*-value of 4.0, $p<0.0001$) corresponding to performance of the language task compared to the baseline simple fixation task. The activation is mainly localized in the left (language dominant) cerebral hemisphere

The American Society of Functional Neuroradiology (ASFNR) has been established in 2004 with the aims to promote the introduction of BOLD fMRI and other functional neuroimaging techniques, such as Diffusion Tensor Imaging (DTI) or MR spectroscopic imaging (MRSI) and MR perfusion imaging into clinical neuroradiology practice and to develop standards for their practice, including the definition of protocols for image acquisition, processing, and quality control. This last issue can be very critical in clinical fMRI because BOLD data can be degraded by artifacts of different types that in turn can affect the reliability of the activation maps. Some of these artifacts, such as minor head motion and physiological noise, are imaging session-related and can be monitored during the scan and corrected by using dedicated algorithms in postprocessing. However, when the intravoxel signal change due to gross head motion is greater than the expected BOLD effect signal change, realignment algorithms can fail. 2 mm of translational head motion in any direction and 2° of head rotation about any axis are currently considered to be the thresholds above which a motion-degraded free reconstruction of the voxel signal time series cannot be guaranteed. Most of the vendors today are able to provide devices for monitoring cardiac pulsation and/or respiratory rate as well as software to assess head motion in real time.

Other sources of artifacts might be due instead to the patient's conditions and clinical history. For example, the presence of blood products or surgical hardware in patients with previous surgery produces susceptibility artifacts that are accentuated in the BOLD fMRI images, because the sequences routinely used for fMRI are very sensitive to local magnetic field inhomogeneities. Decrease in the volume of activation in eloquent cortex adjacent to tumor has been reported that has been attributed to susceptibility artifacts [13].

Including a susceptibility-weighted imaging sequence in a fMRI protocol for presurgical planning can be helpful to determine regions of the brain where hemosiderin deposition or micromineralization exist. This is important for two reasons: (1) it helps characterize brain tumors or vascular malformations, and (2) it helps in quality control analysis of BOLD data by alerting the interpreting neuroradiologist to the possibility of false-negative activation due to excessive susceptibility artifact, which can severely impair ability to detect regional BOLD activation on GRE echoplanar images, which are particularly prone to susceptibility-related distortion.

Neurovascular uncoupling (NVU) is a further condition that could impair the detection of activation within or in spatial proximity to a brain structural lesion. As reported in the introduction of this chapter fMRI indirectly reveals neuronal activation through the detection of the increase in blood flow, volume, and oxygenation in the vessels and the parenchyma near the site of activation. However, many brain diseases (e.g., tumor, strokes, vascular malformation) are characterized by vasculature that reacts less vigorously than normal vessels to physiological stimuli. Therefore, in such conditions the BOLD signal change expected in a region of the brain activated by a particular stimulus can not be detected despite the possible presence of eloquent cortex. BOLD activation maps in these cases can be affected by type II errors (false negatives) and can misguide the neurosurgeons in the preoperative assessment of functional areas at risk of being resected during lesion resection.

Hypervascularized lesions, such as high grade gliomas or AVM, are expected to be affected by NVU because of their aberrant neovasculature [14]. In these cases regions of increased cerebral blood volume and blood flow that can be detected by MR perfusion imaging suggest the risk of NVU, and so caution should be used in the interpretation of the fMRI data in those regions.

However, cases of decreased CVR have been reported in low-grade gliomas [15], which generally do not show hyperperfusion or enhancement in postcontrast MR images. These results have been attributed to the infiltrative nature of glial tumors that compromises the neuronal contacts with the surrounding microvasculature and astrocytes, thus contributing to the attenuation of the BOLD effect.

Mapping the cerebrovascular reactivity (CVR) throughout the brain can provide a direct means of detection of NVU. CVR maps can be obtained by using a BOLD sequence itself while temporarily altering the PCO_2 level in the brain microvasculature through a hypercapnia task. Since increase in PCO_2 causes the dilation of cerebral blood vessels, without increasing the metabolic rate of brain parenchyma, and changes the deoxyhemoglobin (dHb) concentration in the cerebral vasculature, BOLD MR imaging can be used to test vascular reactivity following a hypercapnia challenge [16].

A breath-hold (BH) task and controlled CO_2 inhalation are the most commonly utilized techniques to estimate CVR in humans. A BH task does not provide any quantitative measurement of CVR; however, such a task can be easily performed and included in a clinical fMRI protocol.

A CO_2 inhalation task can directly measure CVR by recording the change in end-tidal CO_2, but it requires special equipment and dedicated personnel to be performed, and thus it is more difficult to routinely implement in a standard clinical setting.

BOLD fMRI Language Mapping for Presurgical Planning

The main goal of fMRI language mapping for presurgical planning is to provide neurosurgeons with two key bits of information: cerebral hemispheric language lateralization (dominance) and the spatial proximity of eloquent language cortical regions to potentially resectable brain lesions such as brain tumors. For this reason the paradigms designed for language mapping should elicit activation in the speech productive areas in the frontal lobe as well as the receptive language areas in the temporal and parietal lobes. The activation patterns provided by these paradigms should be limited to or predominantly involving the dominant language hemisphere, although degree of activation of contralateral hemispheric homologous regions on tasks that have been demonstrated to effectively lateralize language function is also important for surgical planning purposes. If cortical functional reorganization has occurred as a response of the brain to neoplastic infiltration of expected critical language areas, the neurosurgeon would benefit by fMRI's capability of eliciting activation in these supplementary regions that may have been recruited as an adaptive response for preservation of overall language function. The language fMRI literature reports a large variety of different paradigms that have been used both in normal subjects and in patients. In clinical fMRI block design paradigms are usually the preferred choice because they are generally easier for most patients to perform and generally produce more statistically robust results. Although event-related paradigms better reflect the hemodynamic response and are not affected by the stimulus predictability as for block design paradigms, they require longer acquisition times and have lower statistical power.

They are usually categorized into three groups: expressive, receptive, and semantic paradigms. In the following subsections the paradigms most commonly used in clinical fMRI for each category are described. The choice of the paradigms that are administered depends mainly on the location of the lesion and the patient's neurological deficits. For example if a tumor is located in the frontal lobe but does not suffer from a dense Broca's aphasia that would preclude performance of such tasks, one or more expressive paradigms should be run to localize the functional Broca's area and determine its distance from the margins of the lesion (Fig. 4.4). It is critical also to assess before the scan that the patient is not sufficiently cognitively impaired to perform a task or if such a task needs to be adapted in order to be performed by the patient; for example, the stimulus duration or frequency may need to be adjusted to account for the patient's degree of cognitive decline or slowing. A training session should be carried out by presenting the patients with stimuli that are similar to the real test stimuli and asking them to perform the paradigm. During such a session, response accuracy and latency can be assessed in order to tailor the actual paradigm that the patient performs in the scanner to the individual patient's needs and decide whether or not such a paradigm would be appropriate for such a patient.

Expressive Paradigms

Expressive paradigms are conceived and designed to elicit activation mainly in the speech production areas. Silent Word Generation, Silent Verb Generation, and Simple Object Naming are among the most used and cited verbal fluency paradigms in fMRI for presurgical mapping [17–19]. The block duration varies between 20 and 30 s and at MRI field strengths of 3 T or higher, three or four cycles of alternating control and active blocks are sufficient to provide enough statistical power for generation of robust activation maps.

In performing a silent word generation task, patients are asked to covertly generate words beginning with a presented letter during the active block, whereas for the silent verb generation task patients are asked to covertly generate verbs associated with a presented letter or word. The control block consists in both paradigms of a

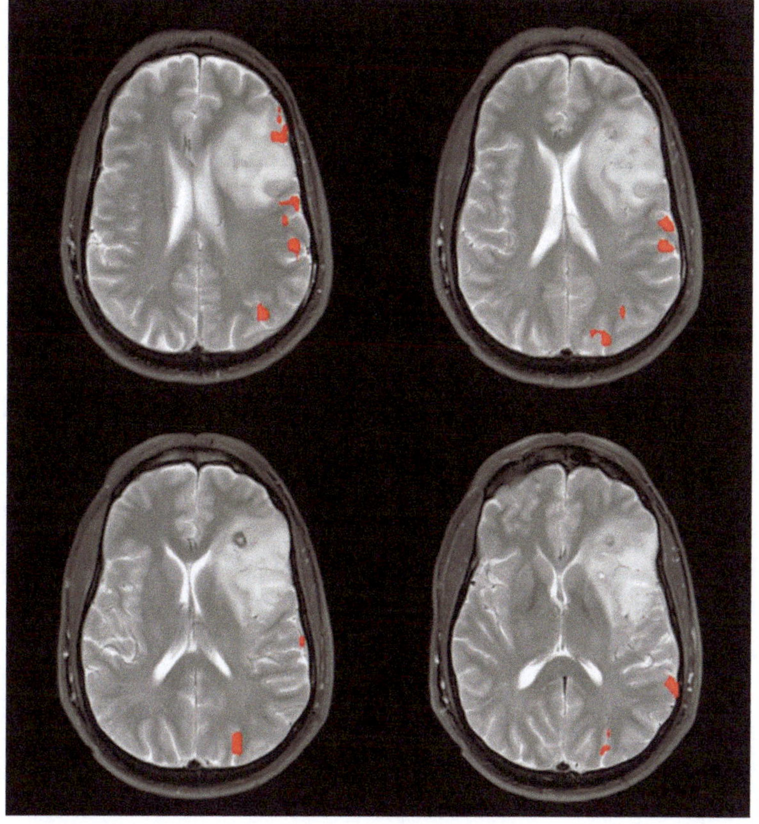

Fig. 4.4 Activation map in a patient with a left frontal lobe tumor obtained from performance of a silent word generation paradigm fused with T2 FLAIR structural images. Areas of neuronal activation are present both at the anterior and posterior margins of the lesion

simple fixation task in order to exclude the visual component from the activation maps. The stimuli for the active tasks also can be delivered aurally, and in that case the control block consists of listening to computer-generated noise or other auditory stimulus devoid of linguistic content. The pattern of activation is equivalent for these two tasks and includes the dorsolateral prefrontal cortex (DLPFC), inferior frontal gyrus (IFG), variably within cingulate language regions, supplementary motor area (SMA), premotor and motor regions and occasionally the parietal, temporal, and/or occipital cortex depending on whether auditory or visual stimuli are used. These two tasks provide robust expressive language cortical activation and effective hemispheric language lateralization, especially of frontal regions. The main disadvantage, however, is that the patient's performance cannot be objectively monitored but only assumed from patient's evaluation during a training session performed outside the scanner and patient feedback provided to the technologist immediately after completion of one of these paradigms.

During the active block of simple object naming, patients are shown an object for 2 or 3 s and asked to silently name the presented object. Again a simple fixation task makes the control block. For this paradigm robust activation is provided in the IFG (frontal operculum), DLPFC, or premotor cortex, SMA, ventral occipito-temporal cortex (VOTC), and to a variable extent within the posterior temporo-parietal language cortex. Inferior temporal gyrus (ITG) activation is also seen commonly. It is not possible to monitor the patient's performance in this task either, and in general the expected activation pattern does not allow as effective hemispheric language lateralization as with the silent word generation and silent verb generation tasks. However, this task is generally easy for most patients to perform, even those with cognitive impairment and in the pediatric population, and behaviorally it resembles confrontation naming tasks that are often performed in the operating

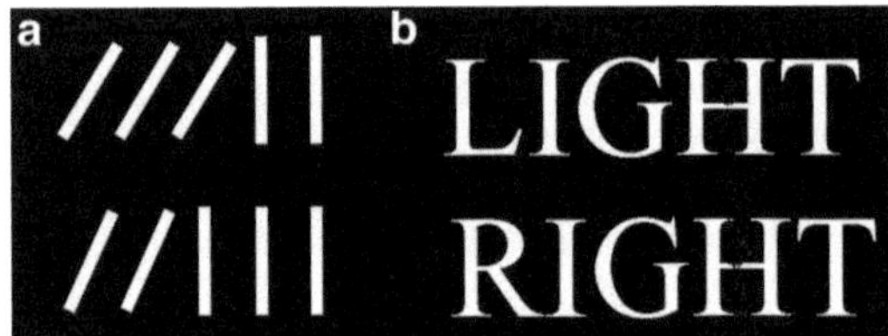

Fig. 4.5 Example of visual stimuli for a phonological (rhyming) paradigm. During the control block the patient is asked to judge whether two rows of stick figures exactly match or not (see an example in (**a**)), whereas during the active block he is asked to judge whether pairs of words rhyme or not (see an example in (**b**)). The patient's response is monitored and recorded through a button press on a keypad

room environment during awake intraoperative cortical stimulation mapping procedures.

The rhyming task, on the other hand, is an example of a phonological processing language paradigm, and as such may be categorized as an expressive language task. As implemented in most institutions, this is an example of a dual choice task, in which the patient's responses can be easily monitored. During the active block of this paradigm, pairs of words are presented every 3 or 5 s and patients are required to decide whether the word pairs rhyme or not, and are asked to press a button on a keypad in cases of affirmative responses only (Fig. 4.5b). In the control block, as implemented in our institution, two rows of stick figures are presented at the same stimulus presentation rate as the pairs of words presented in the active blocks, and patients have to judge whether the two rows exactly match or not; they are asked to press a button on a keypad in cases of affirmative responses (Fig. 4.5a).

Another version of the control block that we have used can be designed where patients are shown nonsense line drawings with a + sign in one of the lower corners of the slide. In this alternate version of the rhyming task, the subjects are instructed to press a button on the left side of keypad if the + sign is in the left corner or a button on the right if the sign is in the right corner [20].

Activation is identified in the DLPFC, IFG, and superior temporal gyrus (STG) and cortex lining the superior temporal sulcus (STS); the VOTC also demonstrates activation, typically in a left hemispheric dominant fashion corresponding to the visual word area. DLPFC and premotor/SMA activity is minimized by the control condition. Rhyming can be a challenging task for some patients to perform because of the demanding nature of the control task and role of the arcuate fasciculus in phonological processing; however, it is a very promising and effective lateralizing task and shows an activation pattern that is clearly more language-specific than that of the silent word generation task [21].

Receptive Paradigms

These paradigms are designed to identify mainly receptive language regions in the temporal and parietal lobe, such as the Wernicke's area (the posterior aspect of the left STG) and, in some cases, its right hemispheric homologue. The typical active block involves a language (reading or listening) comprehension task for 20 or 30 s alternating with a control block that in general is designed to activate all but the language areas involved in performing the active language comprehension task. The GLM analysis that looks for statistically significant difference in the signal between the control and the active block detects activation only in voxels located in specific language areas. Sentence reading or listening comprehension is a typical example of a receptive language paradigm [22]. During the active block patients are asked to read or listen to a series of sentences and decide whether each of these individually presented sentences is true or false. Patient performance is monitored by a button press response that is required in cases in which the presented sentence is true. The control block, as designed at our institution, consists of a string of nonsense symbols without any linguistic content, which the patient is asked to visually scan as if reading (serving as a control for visual processing and orthographic language processing) for the sentence reading comprehension task. Similarly, for the sentence listening comprehension task, the patient is asked to press the button on the keypad for true sentences (and not for false sentences) that are presented as auditory stimuli in the active block, but they are asked to refrain from button pressing during the control block, when they simply listen to nonsense sounds without linguistic content.

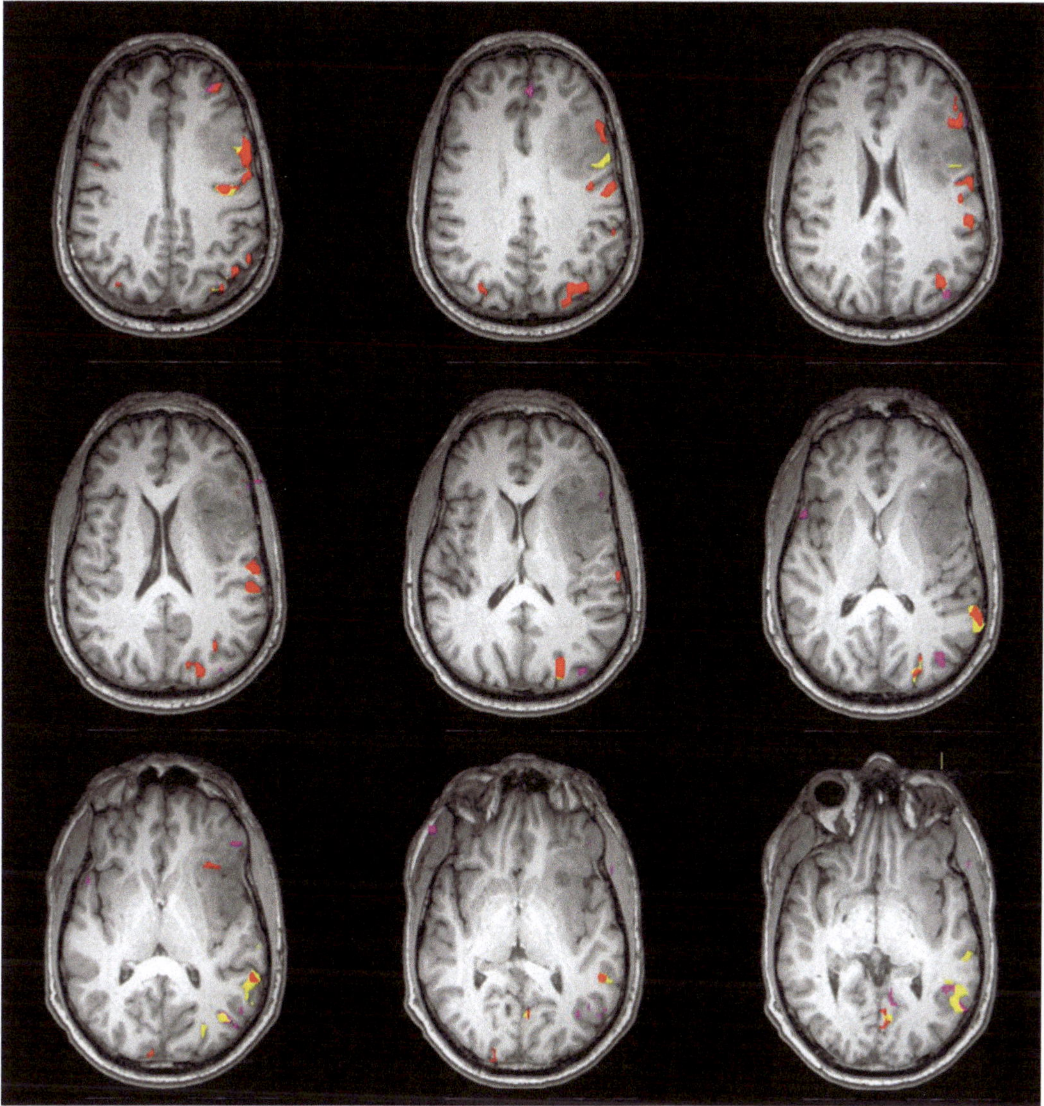

Fig. 4.6 Composite language activation map from silent word generation (color-coded as *red*), sentence completion (*yellow*), and listening comprehension tasks (magenta) in a patient presenting with a lesion in the left frontal lobe involving the frontal operculum with extension to the insular cortex and subinsular white matter. The statistical threshold was set to 0.35 cross correlation for each paradigm with three voxel clustering (spatial extent) threshold also applied. The combination of the activation from these three paradigms includes most of the typical language representation areas in the *left* (dominant hemisphere), including Wernicke's area (WA), located in the left superior temporal gyrus (STG) and Broca's area (BA) in the left inferior frontal gyrus (LIFG) as well as dorsolateral prefrontal cortex (DLPFC) and language (or pre-) SMA (supplementary motor area)

These two paradigms are not found to be effective for determining patient hemispheric language dominance, but their activation maps, when combined with the ones obtained through the use of more effectively lateralizing tasks often yield a comprehensive representation of the entire language network (Fig. 4.6) including Broca's area (BA, left IFG), Wernicke's area (WA, posterior left STG), and their right hemispheric homologues, DLPFC, ITG, middle temporal gyrus (MTG), angular (AG) and supramarginal gyrus (SMG), other parietal language cortices and SMA.

Passive story and simple word listening are two more simple receptive language paradigms that can be helpful in poorly cooperative patients [23] or in patients with temporal lobe lesions in which ITG and MTG are not sufficiently well activated on other tasks. In performing the passive story listening task, patients are simply asked to listen to a short story during the active block alternating with garbled speech (nonsense auditory stimuli) during the control block. In performing the simple word listening task, patients have to silently repeat in their minds the words they hear during the active block. The control block usually consists of a simple fixation task. Both of these tasks elicit selective activation in the temporal receptive language areas, such as the STG and cortex lining the STS, in the expected region of WA. Additionally, activation is found in the STS and MTG more anteriorly. The auditory responsive naming task is an additional receptive language paradigm that is useful for language lateralization and particularly for the localization of WA [24]. Additionally, this paradigm is able to localize the frontal speech areas because patients are required to generate a word in response to a given verbal descriptor. When presented visually, patients are asked to read the presented sentence and push the button corresponding to the correct choice (name) that matches the description. This task targets parietal cortical regions involved in reading. When presented aurally, the patient is instructed to silently generate a word that fits the auditory description. The control block consists of a resting state for the aural presentation and of fixation on a nonsense drawing for the visual presentation.

Semantic Paradigms

This category of paradigms is intended to activate both key expressive and receptive language cortices, including BA and WA. Semantic decision paradigms are very commonly used and typically require the patients to perform task such a noun to verb association (e.g., dog-barking), a word category association (e.g., apple-fruit), or an encoding decision (e.g., concrete versus abstract). Here we report two examples of how these types of paradigms can be designed. For a noun/verb association task patients are shown a pair of verbs on a line below a presented noun for each stimulus during the active block [20]. If the verb on the right is more strongly semantically associated with the presented noun, the right button is pressed, and if the verb on the left is more strongly associated with the presented noun above, the left button is pressed. For the control task, subjects are shown nonsense line drawings with a + sign in one of the lower corners of the slide. The subjects are instructed to press a button on the left side of keypad if the + sign appears in the left lower corner of the image or a button on the right if the sign appears in the right lower corner.

In a semantic encoding decision paradigm, in the active block of each cycle, the patient is asked to press a squeeze ball according to the abstract or concrete nature of the word. In the control block of the cycle, the patient is asked to press the squeeze ball depending on whether the presented word appears in upper-case or lower-case letters [25]. Sentence completion is another example of a semantic paradigm that activates both receptive and expressive language areas [26]. In the active block patients are shown sentences with blanks for the last words of each sentence and are asked to silently fill in the blanks. For the control condition patients are shown scrambled letters parsed into groups to simulate the appearance of text and are instructed to visually scan the two rows of pseudotext as if they were reading an actual sentence. This task unfortunately has the disadvantage that patient performance cannot be monitored objectively.

In functional maps obtained from performance of semantic paradigms, activation is seen consistently in the dominant cerebral hemisphere within the IFG, posterior temporal, and inferior parietal speech areas.

Clinical Validation

Language mapping by fMRI is more challenging than motor or visual mapping because of the enormous individual variability of language representation in the human brain, as well as the complexity of the language network that results in variable utilization of subnetworks for particular task performance. As such, assessment of critical eloquent cortex requires use of multiple language tasks to elicit activation throughout the global language network. Despite the importance of BA (left IFG) and WA (posterior left STG) in the classical model of language representation, considerable individual variability in localization of these functional areas has been reported [27]. Recently, a more complex "dual stream" model for language processing has been proposed that involves a dorsal stream involved in mapping sound to articulation (with connections between the STG and frontal areas via the arcuate fasciculus) and a ventral stream involved in mapping sound to meaning (which demonstrates connections between the MTG and frontal areas via the extreme capsule) [28]. This model recently has been validated in a study by using BOLD fMRI in conjunction with DTI in a study by Saur et al. [29]. Nevertheless, since the early era of functional imaging, many individual institution-based clinical validation studies have emerged that strove to compare BOLD results with those provided by the gold-standard language lateralization (the Wada test) and localization (intraoperative direct cortical simulation) techniques. fMRI yields many advantages compared to both the Wada test and intraoperative direct cortical simulation (DCS). Its noninvasiveness, repeatability, capability to potentially test many different language functions, as well as its ability to map the entire brain makes it a very attractive technique despite some of its limitations that have been previously discussed in this chapter such as NVU.

All the studies comparing preoperative BOLD imaging with the Wada test have found very high concordance (from 90 to 100 %) for lateralization between these two techniques [30–33] despite the use of different paradigms and data acquisition techniques among the cited studies. At this time, the overall consensus in the field is that BOLD fMRI is adequate for language lateralization determination but not yet for memory lateralization because memory activation studies using fMRI have not been generally reliable for accurate and consistent lateralization at the single subject level, particularly in patients with temporal lobe abnormalities such as temporal lobe epilepsy, and the few studies published to date comparing such paradigms to Wada lateralization have only evaluated small series of patients.

Numerous studies are also available that have compared the results of BOLD fMRI and DCS [26, 34–41]. The findings of these studies provided a broad spectrum of values in terms of specificity and sensitivity. Particularly, in Bizzi's study, the BOLD fMRI sensitivity varied from 59 to 100 % and specificity varied from 0 to 97 %. The effects of intraoperative brain shift, inherent differences between intraoperative mapping techniques and BOLD paradigms (i.e., the former attempts to disrupt function, while the other elicits functional activation), differences in cognitive tasks used between the operative setting and the MRI scanner, lack of standardization of both intraoperative neuropsychological testing and fMRI paradigms both within and across institutions, and the effects of anesthesia in the intraoperative setting are all likely to contribute to the overall discrepancy between the fMRI and DCS results in each study, as well as the variability of results across these studies. For these reasons, BOLD fMRI cannot be considered yet as an alternative tool to DCS. Therefore it is advisable in the future to plan multicenter studies that aim to minimize at least some of these variables by standardizing both intraoperative and fMRI protocols to better enable effective comparison.

The two techniques thus appear to have a complementary rather than an exclusive role, with DCS resulting in fewer false positives and only identifying essential but not necessarily participatory eloquent cortex, while fMRI may provide a more complete picture of global language networks with greater resultant false positives, since it cannot necessarily distinguish between essential and nonessential participatory eloquent cortex [42].

Cases Demonstrating Presurgical Language Mapping

Case 1

A 46-year-old right-handed male with a stereotactic biopsy-proven grade II oligodendroglioma presented with seizures manifesting as brief episodes of difficulty with speech production with associated transient memory difficulties, although he did not report any difficulty with reading or comprehension and did not demonstrate any gross motor or language deficit on physical examination. The patient also reported tingling and other sensory disturbances originating in his face area and often extending to involve his right upper extremity. Structural brain MR imaging revealed a left frontal opercular T2/FLAIR hyperintense nonenhancing mass resulting in expansion of the left inferior frontal gyrus, insular cortex, and subinsular white matter. See Figs. 4.4, as well as 4.6 through 4.10, for composite language activation maps that demonstrate critical activation along the

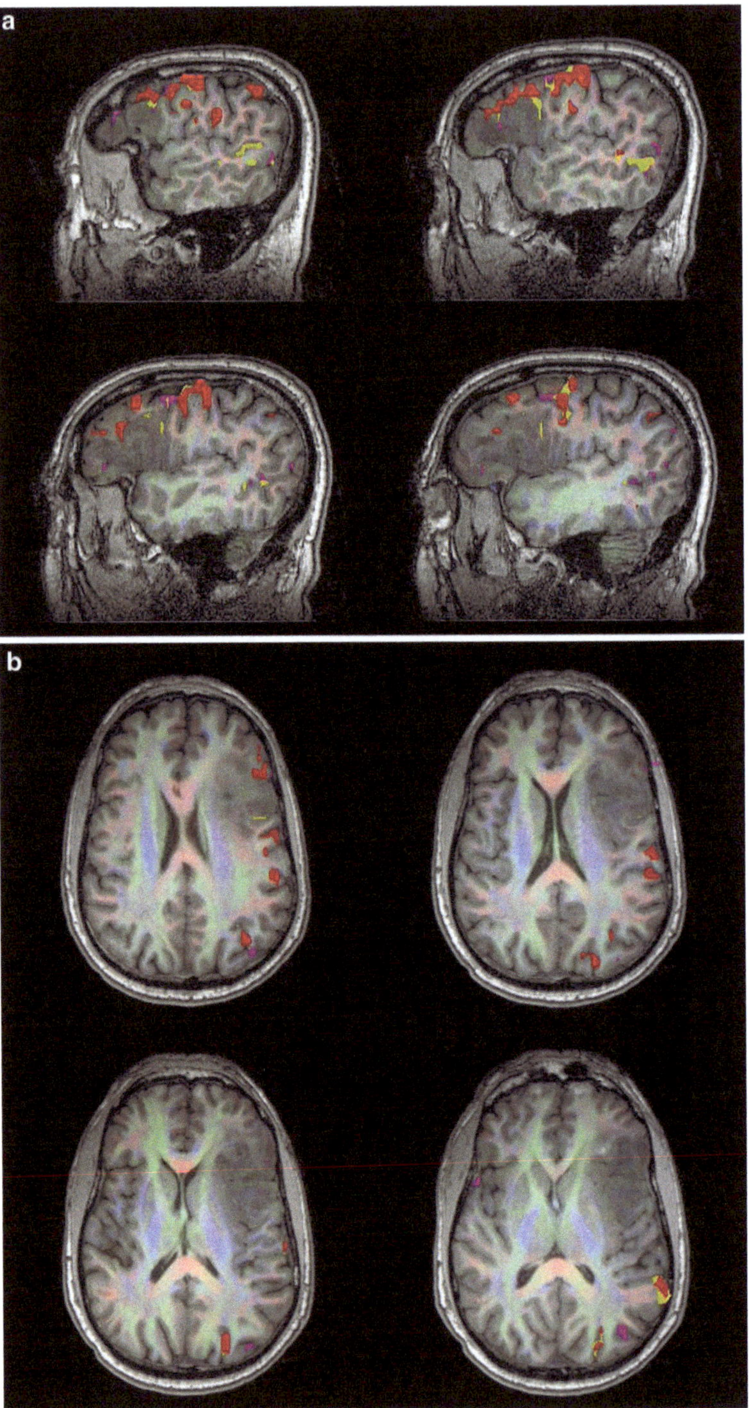

anterior and posterior margins of the tumor mass, representing eloquent cortex that is infiltrated by the tumor. In light of evidence of neurovascular uncoupling (NVU) on the breath-hold cerebrovascular reactivity maps (BH CVR), along the lateral margin of the tumor, involving the left IFG, concern existed regarding the possibility of false-negative (FN) activation within the left IFG in the expected location of Broca's area (BA). Although the sagittal images in Fig. 4.7a demonstrate activation along the superiormost cortex of the left IFG, bordering on the inferior frontal sulcus, this activation cluster appeared to blend with the dorsolateral prefrontal cortical (DLPFC) activation cluster. Thus, it was not clear whether superior displacement of BA due to the mass effect and infiltration of the left IFG was responsible for this activation pattern, or whether FN activation existed due to NVU. In other words, the absence of expected activation more inferiorly within the left IFG may represent FN or actually true negative activation (i.e., true absence of eloquent cortex in this region due to cortical reorganization or displacement). In light of this uncertainty, a recommendation was made to the referring neurosurgeon to consider doing an awake craniotomy with direct cortical stimulation mapping to identify the true location of functional BA. The patient, however, opted to not undergo surgery, in light of the determined risk to BA, but rather chose more conservative management.

Case 2

A 47-year-old male with no language or motor deficits presented with an imaging diagnosis of a left inferior temporal lobe nonenhancing T2/FLAIR hyperintense mass involving portions of the fusiform and inferior temporal gyri. He only reported a single episode of blurry vision and "flushing" sensation that led to the initial brain imaging. The neurosurgeon was primarily interested in the preoperative localization of functional Wernicke's area (WA) in order to determine its proximity to the tumor mass. As shown in Figs. 4.11a, b and 4.12, which all display composite language activation maps superimposed on coronal 3D MPRAGE or FSE T2 anatomic images, WA was identified superolateral to the tumor. As Fig. 4.12, which depicts the BOLD activation maps that have been imported into a commercial neuronavigation system, demonstrates, WA was located superolateral to the tumor mass. This led to a low horizontal surgical trajectory to the lesion in order to avoid injury to the critical receptive language area. The surgeon was able to successfully resect the lesion without any postoperative language deficits, based on this a priori knowledge of functional anatomy of WA, which was also helpful in presurgical patient counseling regarding risks and benefits of surgery.

Fig. 4.7 (**a**) Composite language activation map from a silent word generation (coded as *red*), sentence completion (*yellow*), and listening comprehension task (*magenta*) in the same patient as in Fig. 4.6, but superimposed on fractional anisotropy (FA)-weighted color directional diffusion maps that have been overlaid on 3D MPRAGE (magnetization-prepared rapid acquisition gradient echo) anatomic images. These maps follow the standard RGB convention, whereby *red* refers to preferential medial-lateral diffusion, *green* refers to preferential antero-posterior diffusion, and *blue* refers to preferential supero-inferior diffusion. These images are displayed in the sagittal plane. Note the absence of visible activation throughout most of the enlarged LIFG and apparent superior displacement of Broca's area functional activation that appears to merge with the dorsolateral prefrontal cortical (DLPFC) activation in the left middle frontal gyrus (MFG). The area of absent activation in all but the superiormost cortex of the LIFG abutting the overlying sulcus corresponds directly to the area of reduced regional cerebrovascular reactivity (CVR). (**b**) The same patient as in Fig. 4.6 and (**a**) is depicted in this figure, with composite language activation maps (using the same color-coding scheme as in (**a**)) overlaid on FA-weighted color directional diffusion maps and 3D MPRAGE anatomic images, displayed in the axial plane

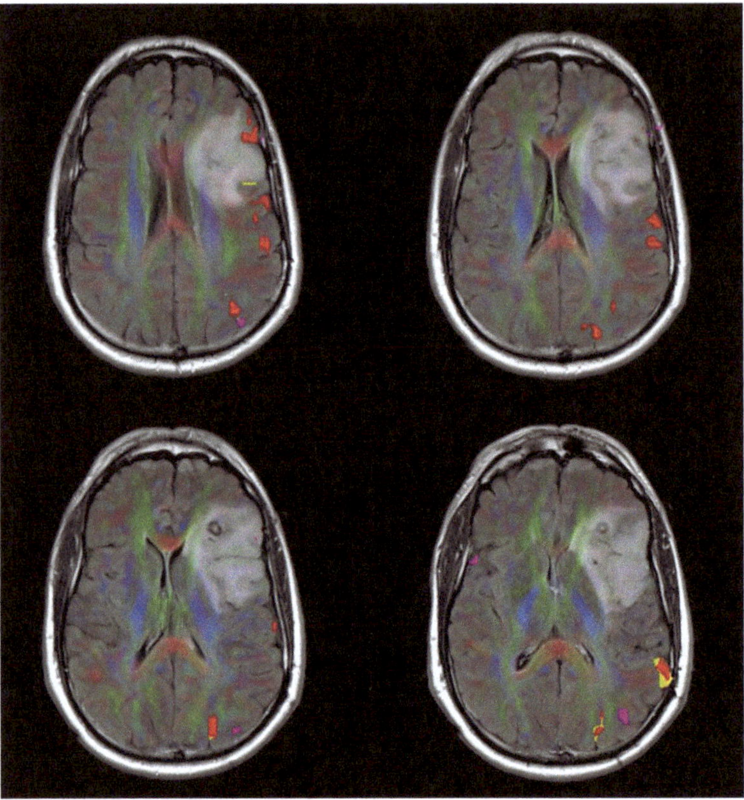

Fig. 4.8 The same patient as in Figs. 4.6 and 4.7a, b is depicted in this figure, with composite language activation maps (using the same color-coding scheme as in Fig. 4.7a) overlaid on FA-weighted color directional diffusion maps and T2 FLAIR (fluid-attenuated inversion recovery) anatomic images, displayed in the axial plane

Further Applications of Language fMRI

The lack of standardization is still one of the greatest limitations of language fMRI as well as one of its great strengths from a research standpoint. The anatomy of language appears to be much more complex and broad than that of the sensorimotor or visual system. In a recent article reviewing one hundred studies of language comprehension and production, activation has been reported in an incredibly large number of regions [43]. This makes standardization of language fMRI more difficult because it is unlikely that one or two paradigms are able to elicit activation in the entire network. However, language mapping for presurgical planning represents to date the most mature clinical application of language fMRI. Functional imaging for language mapping has been shown to be a valuable clinical tool also in different clinical scenarios. Applications include, but are not limited to, the functional characterization of brain disorders presenting abnormal activation in language eloquent cortical areas such as schizophrenia or Alzheimer's disease [44, 45], the assessment of drug action on language processing [46], the study of developmental changes in the networks of brain regions supporting language [47] and the assessment of recovery of language function following brain injuries or the development of neoplastic or epileptic lesions [48–51]. Even more interestingly, fMRI has also demonstrated changes in eloquent

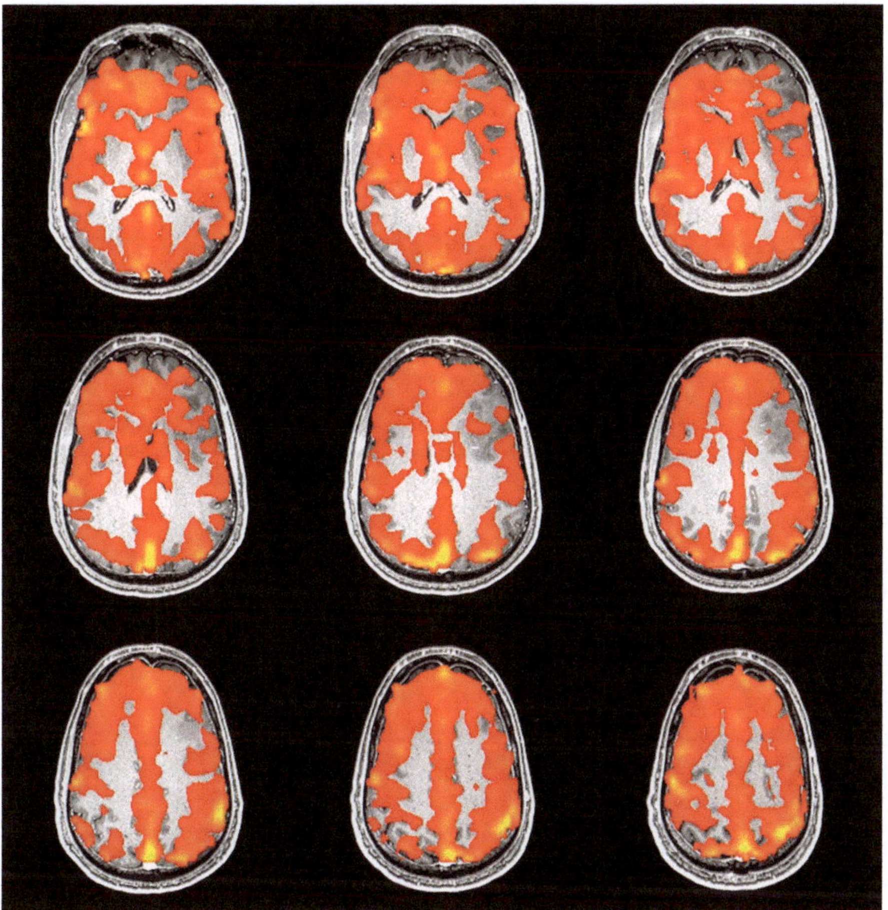

Fig. 4.9 The same patient as in Figs. 4.6, 4.7, and 4.8 is depicted in this figure, with BOLD breath hold (BH) cerebrovascular reactivity (CVR) maps displayed, overlaid on axial 3D MPRAGE anatomic images, thresholded at a value of 0.30 % BOLD signal change (increase) relative to baseline. Note the abnormally decreased regional CVR along the lateral margin of the left frontal lobe mass, within the lateral aspect of the left IFG, relative to the contralateral normal right frontal lobe. This represents an area of tumor-induced neurovascular uncoupling (NVU) and associated possibly false-negative (FN) activation

language cortex occurring as a result of actual surgical resection of diseased but, nevertheless, partially functional tissue. A recent study reports two cases of brain tumor patients who were left hemispheric language dominant preoperatively but demonstrated postsurgical decreases in language lateralization and a progressive involvement of cortical regions in the right nondominant hemisphere when the same fMRI exam was repeated in two postoperative sessions [52]. These findings were in agreement with the clinical status of the patients who recovered very well from expressive aphasia within the first 2 or 3 months after surgery. The results of fMRI are also supported by a previous study on postsurgical language plasticity in a group of brain tumor patients assessed by using DCS [53]. The authors of this study suggest that in the preoperative and immediate postoperative phases, regions of the brain adjacent to the lesion are recruited for functional compensation, whereas distant regions also in the contralateral language dominant hemisphere are involved in long-term permanent recovery.

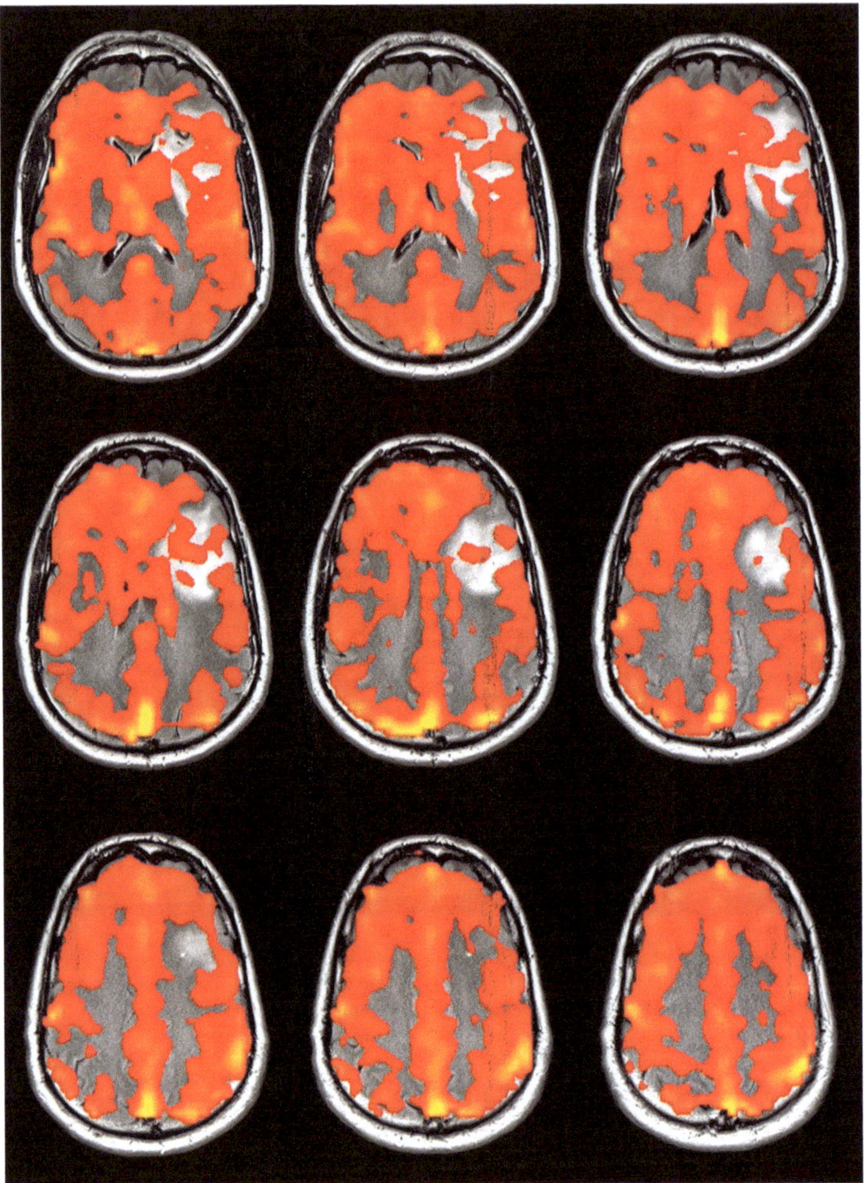

Fig. 4.10 The same patient as in Figs. 4.6, 4.7, 4.8, and 4.9 is depicted in this figure, with BOLD BH CVR maps displayed, overlaid on axial T2 FLAIR anatomic images, thresholded at a value of 0.30 % BOLD signal change (increase) relative to baseline. Note the abnormally decreased regional CVR along the lateral margin of the left frontal lobe mass, within the lateral aspect of the left IFG, relative to the contralateral normal right frontal lobe. This represents an area of tumor-induced NVU and associated possible FN activation

Resting state functional connectivity fMRI studies have begun to provide insights about the various network architectures involved in language functions, and they may provide an alternative or more likely complementary tool to task-based fMRI for presurgical planning, especially in poorly cooperative and severely cognitively impaired patients [54, 55].

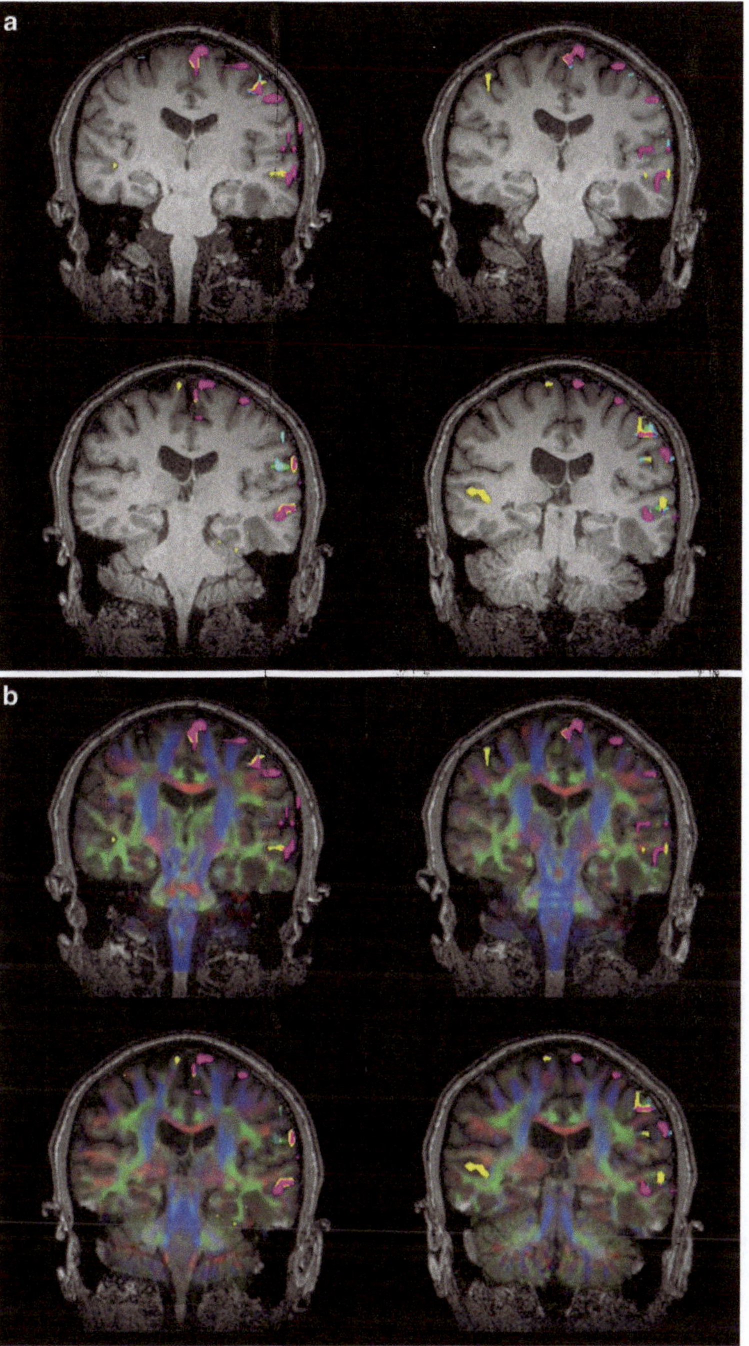

Fig. 4.11 (**a**) Coronal composite BOLD language activation maps for another patient with a left inferior temporal lobe low-grade glioma, overlaid on coronal 3D MPRAGE anatomic images. The following color-coding scheme is used for display of the four different language activation paradigms: sentence listening comprehension (LC), displayed as *magenta*, thresholded to 0.35 cross-correlation coefficient (cc); sentence completion (SC), displayed as *yellow*, thresholded to a *t*-value of 4.0; sentence reading comprehension (RC), displayed as *cyan/light blue*, thresholded to 0.40 cc; and rhyming (Rhym), displayed as green, thresholded to 0.40 cc. Note that convergent Wernicke's area (WA) activation is seen within the left STG, superolateral to the tumor. (**b**) Coronal composite BOLD language activation maps for the same patient as in (**a**), with a left inferior temporal lobe low-grade glioma, overlaid on both coronal 3D MPRAGE anatomic images and superimposed coronal FA-weighted color directional diffusion maps. The same color-coding and statistical thresholding was used as for (**a**), with display of composite language activation from the LC, RC, SC, and Rhym tasks. Note again that WA activation is present superolateral to the tumor

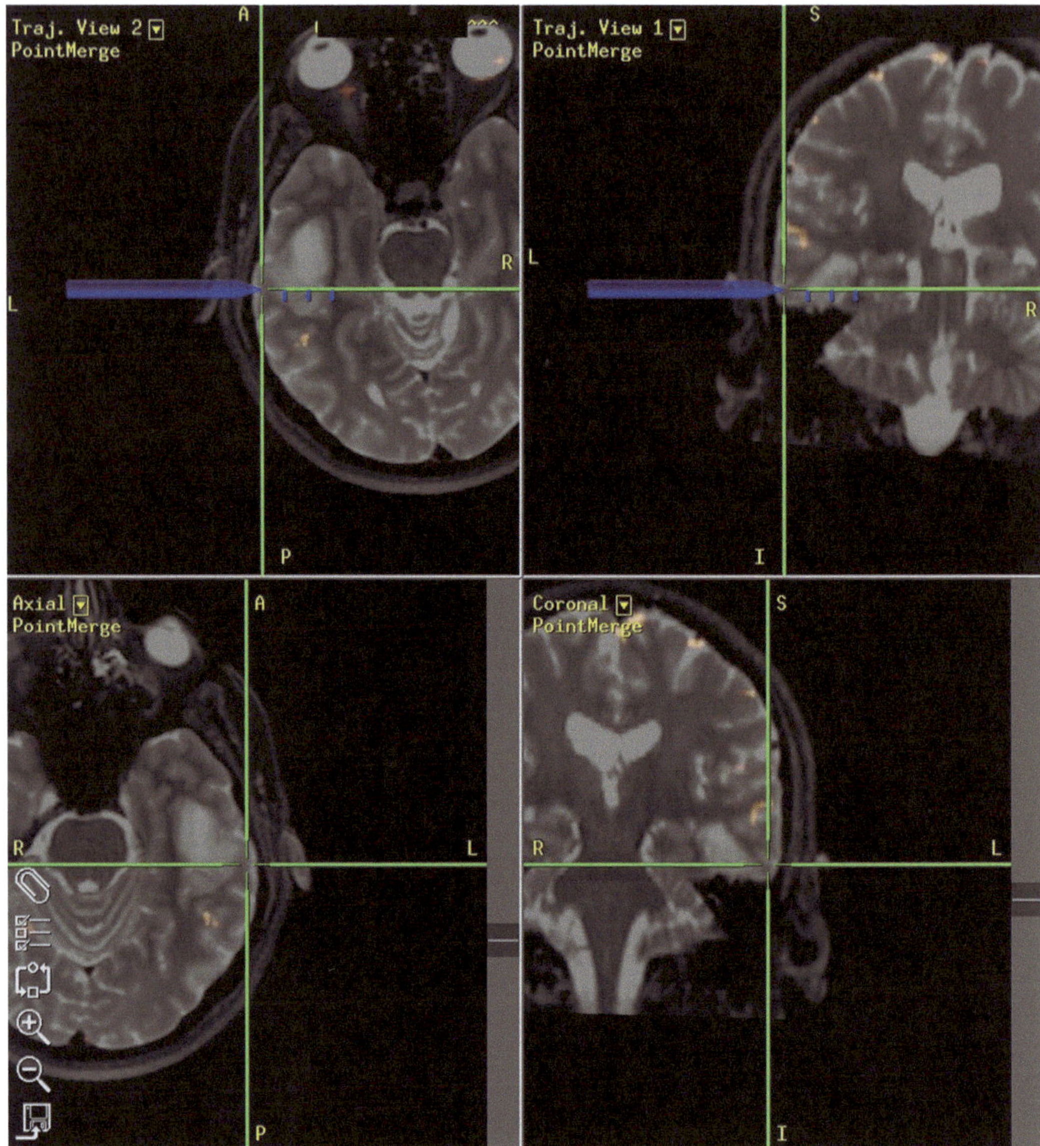

Fig. 4.12 This figure displays the same composite language activation map as in Fig. 4.11a, b, representing a composite of the individual activation maps generated from the LC, RC, SC, and Rhym tasks, but displayed using a different color-coding scheme (all displayed in Stealth Heat Spectrum orange color) and overlaid on fast spin echo (FSE) T2-weighted coronal anatomic images that have been imported into a neuronavigation system. Note that the horizontal line of the 3D cursor demonstrates the planned surgical trajectory to the tumor, which is relatively low and utilizes a lateral approach to the lesion through the left inferior temporal gyrus (ITG) in order to avoid injury to the well-depicted WA activation superolateral to the mass in the STG

Conclusion

In the current era, a growing number of neurosurgeons at academic medical centers are considering BOLD fMRI together with DTI as an indispensable tool for preoperative risk assessment, determination of the best intraoperative mapping strategy and determination of the optimal surgical trajectory in cases where the lesion resection is associated with severe risks of postoperative temporary or permanent language deficits. Several FDA-approved integrated systems are now available that provide hardware and software solutions for fMRI paradigm presentation, rapid image processing, export of postprocessed images to PACS (picture archiving and communication systems), and possibly even export of postprocessed data to neuronavigation systems. As these systems are becoming more and more streamlined and can be run by radiologic technologists, clinical functional imaging is expected to continue to grow in clinical utilization in the future.

References

1. Ogawa S, Lee TM, Kay AR, Tank DW. Brain magnetic resonance imaging with contrast dependent on blood oxygenation. Proc Natl Acad Sci USA. 1990;87:9868–72.
2. Attwell D, Iadecola C. The neural basis of functional brain imaging signals. Trends Neurosci. 2002;25:621–5.
3. Liu T, Frank L, Wong E, Buxton R. Detection power, estimation efficiency, and predictability in event-related fMRI. Neuroimage. 2001;13:759–73.
4. Calhoun VD, Adali T, Hansen LK et al. Proceedings of 4th international symposium on independent component analysis and blind signal separation (ICA2003), Nara, Japan. 2003:281–88.
5. Roux FE, Boulanouar K, Ranjeva JP, et al. Usefulness of motor functional MRI correlated to cortical mapping in Rolandic low-grade astrocytomas. Acta Neurochir (Wien). 1999;141:71–9.
6. Roux FE, Boulanouar K, Ranjeva JP, et al. Cortical intraoperative stimulation in brain tumors as a tool to evaluate spatial data from motor functional MRI. Invest Radiol. 1999;34:225–9.
7. Hirsch J, Ruge MI, Kim KH, et al. An integrated functional magnetic resonance imaging procedure for preoperative mapping of cortical areas associated with tactile, motor, language, and visual functions. Neurosurgery. 2000;47:711–21.
8. Roux FE, Ibarrola D, Tremoulet M, et al. Methodological and technical issues for integrating functional magnetic resonance imaging data in a neuronavigational system. Neurosurgery. 2001;9:1145–56. discussion 1156–1157.
9. Krings T, Schreckenberger M, Rohde V, et al. Functional MRI and 18F FDG-positron emission tomography for presurgical planning: comparison with electrical cortical stimulation. Acta Neurochir (Wien). 2002;144:889–99.
10. Wu JS, Zhou LF, Chen W, et al. Prospective comparison of functional magnetic resonance imaging and intraoperative motor evoked potential monitoring for cortical mapping of primary motor areas. Zhonghua Wai Ke Za Zhi. 2005;43:1141–5. in Chinese.
11. Petrella JR, Shah LM, Harris KM, et al. Preoperative functional mr imaging localization of language and motor areas: effect on therapeutic decision making in patients with potentially resectable brain tumors. Radiology. 2006;240:793–802.
12. Medina LS, Bernal B, Dunoyer C, et al. Seizure disorders: functional MR imaging for diagnostic evaluation and surgical treatment—prospective study. Radiology. 2005;236:247–53.
13. Holodny AI, Schulder M, Liu WC, et al. The effect of brain tumors on BOLD functional MR imaging activation in the adjacent motor cortex: Implications for image-guided neurosurgery. AJNR Am J Neuroradiol. 2000;21(8):1415–22.
14. Hou BL, Bradbury M, Peck KK, et al. Effect of brain tumor neovasculature defined by rCBV on BOLD fMRI activation volume in the primary motor cortex. Neuroimage. 2006;32(2):489–97.
15. Hsu YY, Chang CN, Jung SM, et al. Blood oxygenation level-dependent MRI of cerebral gliomas during breath holding. J Magn Reson Imaging. 2004;19(2):160–7.
16. Bandettini PA, Wong EC. A hypercapnia-based normalization method for improved spatial localization of human brain activation with fMRI. NMR Biomed. 1997;10:197–203.
17. Yetkin FZ, Swanson S, Fischer M, et al. Functional MR of frontal lobe activation: comparison with Wada language results. AJNR Am J Neuroradiol. 1998;19:1095–8.
18. Salvan CV, Ulmer JL, DeYoe EA, et al. Visual object agnosia and pure word alexia: correlation of functional magnetic resonance imaging and lesion localization. J Comput Assist Tomogr. 2004;28:63–7.
19. Holland SK, Plante E, Weber Byars A, et al. Normal fMRI brain activation patterns in children performing a verb generation task. Neuroimage. 2001;14:837–43.
20. Pillai JJ, Araque JM, Allison JD, et al. Functional MRI study of semantic and phonological language processing in bilingual subjects: preliminary findings. Neuroimage. 2003;19:565–76.
21. Pillai JJ, Zacà D. Relative utility for hemispheric lateralization of different clinical fMRI activation tasks within a comprehensive language paradigm battery in brain tumor patients as assessed by both threshold-dependent and threshold independent analysis methods. Neuroimage. 2011;54 Suppl 1: S136–45.
22. Just MA, Carpenter PA, Keller TA, et al. Brain activation modulated by sentence comprehension. Science. 1996;274(5284):114–6.
23. Phillips MD, Lowe MJ, Lurito JT, et al. Temporal lobe activation demonstrates sex-based differences during passive listening. Radiology. 2001;220:202–7.
24. Bookheimer SY, Zeffiro TA, Blaxton TA, et al. Regional cerebral blood flow during auditory responsive naming: evidence for cross-modality neural activation. Neuroreport. 1998;9:2409–13.

25. Desmond JE et al. Functional MRI measurement of language lateralization in Wada-tested patients. Brain. 1995;118:1411–9.
26. FitzGerald DB, Cosgrove GR, Ronner S, et al. Location of language in the cortex: a comparison between functional MR imaging and electrocortical stimulation. AJNR Am J Neuroradiol. 1997;18:1529–39.
27. Ojemann GA. Cortical organization of language. J Neurosci. 1991;11:2281–7.
28. Hickok G, Poeppel D. Dorsal and ventral streams: a framework for understanding aspects of the functional anatomy of language. Cognition. 2004;92(1–2): 67–99.
29. Saur D, Kreher BW, Schnell S, et al. Ventral and dorsal pathways for language. Proc Natl Acad Sci U S A. 2008;105:18035–40.
30. Binder JR, Swanson SJ, Hammeke TA, et al. Determination of language dominance using functional MRI: a comparison with the Wada test. Neurology. 1996;46:978–84.
31. Bahn MM, Lin W, Silbergeld DL, et al. Localization of language cortices by functional MR imaging compared with intracarotid amobarbital hemispheric sedation. AJR Am J Roentgenol. 1997;169:575–9.
32. Hertz-Pannier L, Gaillard WD, Mott SH, et al. Noninvasive assessment of language dominance in children and adolescents with functional MRI: a preliminary study. Neurology. 1997;48:1003–12.
33. Sabbah P, Chassoux F, Leveque C, et al. Functional MR imaging in assessment of language dominance in epileptic patients. Neuroimage. 2003;18:460–7.
34. Lurito JT, Lowe MJ, Sartorius C, Mathews VP. Comparison of fMRI and intraoperative direct cortical stimulation in localization of receptive language areas. J Comput Assist Tomogr. 2000;24:99–105.
35. Roux FE, Boulanouar K, Lotterie JA, et al. Language functional magnetic resonance imaging in preoperative assessment of language areas: correlation with direct cortical stimulation. Neurosurgery. 2003;52:1335–47.
36. Rutten GJ, Ramsey NF, van Rijen PC, et al. Development of a functional magnetic resonance imaging protocol for intraoperative localization of critical temporoparietal language areas. Ann Neurol. 2002;51:350–60.
37. Tomczak RJ, Wunderlich AP, Wang Y, et al. fMRI for preoperative neurosurgical mapping of motor cortex and language in a clinical setting. J Comput Assist Tomogr. 2000;24:927–34.
38. Yetkin FZ, Mueller WM, Morris GL, et al. Functional MR activation correlated with intraoperative cortical mapping. AJNR Am J Neuroradiol. 1997;18:1311–5.
39. Bizzi A, Blasi V, Falini A, et al. Presurgical functional MR imaging of language and motor functions: validation with intraoperative electrocortical mapping. Radiology. 2008;2:579–89.
40. Pouratian N, Bookheimer SY, Rex DE, et al. Utility of preoperative functional magnetic resonance imaging for identifying language cortices in patients with vascular malformations. J Neurosurg. 2002;97:21–32.
41. Signorelli F, Guyotat J, Schneider F, et al. Technical refinements for validating functional MRI-based neuronavigation data by electrical stimulation during cortical language mapping. Minim Invasive Neurosurg. 2003;46:265–8.
42. Giussani C, Roux FE, Ojemann J, et al. Is preoperative functional magnetic resonance imaging reliable for language areas mapping in brain tumor surgery? Review of language functional magnetic resonance imaging and direct cortical stimulation correlation studies. Neurosurgery. 2010;66(1):113–20.
43. Price CJ. The anatomy of language: a review of 100 fMRI studies published in 2009. Ann N Y Acad Sci. 2010;1191:62–88.
44. Han SD, Wible CG. Neuroimaging of semantic processing in schizophrenia: a parametric priming approach. Int J Psychophysiol. 2010;75(2):100–6.
45. Olichney JM, Taylor JR, Chan S, et al. fMRI responses to words repeated in a congruous semantic context are abnormal in mild Alzheimer's disease. Neuropsychologia. 2010;48(9):2476–87.
46. Kim N, Goel PK, Tivarus ME, et al. Independent component analysis of the effect of L-dopa on fMRI of language processing. PLoS One. 2010;5(8):e11933.
47. Vannest J, Karunanayaka PR, Schmithorst VJ, et al. Language networks in children: evidence from functional MRI studies. AJR Am J Roentgenol. 2009;192(5):1190–6.
48. Thulborn KR, Carpenter PA, Just MA. Plasticity of language-related brain function during recovery from stroke. Stroke. 1999;30(4):749–54.
49. Martin PI, Naeser MA, Ho M, et al. Overt naming fMRI pre- and post-TMS: two nonfluent aphasia patients, with and without improved naming post-TMS. Brain Lang. 2009;111(1):20–35.
50. Cousin E, Baciu M, Pichat C, et al. Functional MRI evidence for language plasticity in adult epileptic patients: preliminary results. Neuropsychiatr Dis Treat. 2008;4(1):235–46.
51. Hertz-Pannier L, Chiron C, Jambaqué I, et al. Late plasticity for language in a child's non-dominant hemisphere: a pre- and post-surgery fMRI study. Brain. 2002;125(Pt 2):361–72.
52. Pillai JJ. Insights into adult postlesional language cortical plasticity provided by cerebral blood oxygen level-dependent functional MR imaging. AJNR Am J Neuroradiol. 2010;31(6):990–6.
53. Duffau H, Capelle L, Denvil D, Sichez N, et al. Functional recovery after surgical resection of low grade gliomas in eloquent brain: hypothesis of brain compensation. J Neurol Neurosurg Psychiatry. 2003;74(7):901–7.
54. Turken AU, Dronkers NF. The neural architecture of the language comprehension network: converging evidence from lesion and connectivity analyses. Front Syst Neurosci. 2011;5:1.
55. Zhao J, Liu J, Li J, et al. Intrinsically organized network for word processing during the resting state. Neurosci Lett. 2011;487(1):27–31.

BOLD fMRI for Presurgical Planning: Part II

5

Meredith Gabriel, Nicole P. Brennan, Kyung K. Peck, and Andrei I. Holodny

Introduction

In the early 1990s, functional magnetic resonance imaging (fMRI) entered the field of neuroimaging as a unique resource in the arsenal of preoperative planning tools for brain tumor patients. fMRI is a technique that takes advantage of the differences in magnetic susceptibility between oxyhemoglobin and deoxyhemoglobin. It is a less invasive neuroimaging method than its positron emission tomography (PET) predecessor given that the contrast agent is endogenous [1]. fMRI is possible because oxyhemoglobin has a different magnetic resonance signal than deoxyhemoglobin. When a task is performed, oxygenated blood in excess of the amount needed (termed luxury perfusion) is delivered to the active area. The difference in magnetic susceptibility between deoxyhemoglobin concentrations and oxyhemoglobin concentrations creates the signal in functional imaging. This effect is termed the blood oxygen level-dependent signal (BOLD signal). fMRI provides good spatial localization (as low as 1 mm) and temporal acquisition resolution (as low as 1 s) though it is limited by the resolution of the hemodynamic response (8–30 s). The superior spatial resolution is particularly advantageous for mapping peri-tumoral eloquent areas for treatment planning [2].

fMRI can effectively map the sensory and motor areas. The motor gyrus is somatotopically organized, with all body parts represented in a way that is preserved across different people. fMRI can provide a multidimensional map in a single mapping session. fMRI maps of sensory/motor function help the surgeon assess the risks of surgery, as well as guide intraoperative mapping techniques [2, 3]. The primary motor and sensory areas are of particular interest in fMRI for surgical planning because iatrogenic damage to these areas can cause permanent neurological deficits. As a result, the precise localization of various motor and sensory areas is useful particularly in light of a space-occupying lesion.

Primary motor and sensory cortices are distinct in the functions they subserve. However, as a result of significant neuronal reciprocity in the region, injury to either can result in a mixed motor/sensory deficit. For example, injury to the primary motor gyrus usually leads to a permanent, largely irreversible paresis [4]. Injury to the sensory cortex, while producing the expected sensory perceptual deficits, can also lead to a similar type of paresis seen with injury to the motor strip as a result of the lack of proprioceptive information. There are a variety of other defi-

M. Gabriel • N.P. Brennan • K.K. Peck
Functional MRI Laboratory, Department of Radiology, Memorial Sloan-Kettering Cancer Center, New York, NY, USA

A.I. Holodny, M.D. (✉)
Department of Radiology, Division of Neuroradiology, Functional MRI Laboratory, Memorial Sloan-Kettering Cancer Center, Weill Medical College of Cornell University, 1275 York Avenue, New York, NY 10065, USA
e-mail: holodnya@mskcc.org

J.J. Pillai (ed.), *Functional Brain Tumor Imaging*, DOI 10.1007/978-1-4419-5858-7_5,

cits that are seen with injury to the postcentral gyrus depending upon whether the left or the right hemisphere is damaged. Some of these include two-point discrimination, astereognosis (inability to discern objects by feeling them) and agraphism (inability to write). In this chapter, the usefulness of BOLD fMRI in regard to preoperative motor mapping is discussed.

The Anatomical Organization of the Sensory Motor System

The four main regions that subserve motor control that are of interest to neurosurgeons are the primary motor cortex, the primary sensory cortex, the premotor cortex, and the supplementary motor area (SMA). The motor and sensory gyri taken together are often referred to as one larger area termed the primary sensory motor cortex [6].

The Primary Sensory/Motor Cortex

The primary motor cortex, located in the precentral gyrus, is responsible for executing movement (see Fig. 5.1). Its position delineates the frontal from the parietal lobes. The motor gyrus marks the posterior limit of the frontal lobe and the sensory gyrus marks the start of the parietal lobe. The motor gyrus is somatotopically mapped; different body regions are distinctly represented in cortical space in a common (but not steadfast) pattern medially to laterally. Historically, the motor gyrus has been localized using anatomical markers. The most salient anatomical marker of the motor gyrus is the reverse omega portion of the central sulcus (Fig. 5.1). This reverse omega typically demarcates the location of the hand motor region of the motor homunculus [5]. However, the presence of this marker is occasionally unreliable. Figure 5.2 shows a case where a reverse-omega sign would have incorrectly indicated the position of the motor gyrus. While cases like this are rare in our experience, they do occur. Further, lesions can obscure traditional anatomical markers making their identification based on visual inspection of MR images alone difficult. Figure 5.3 shows a case where anatomical markers have been obscured by tumor making anatomical prediction of the location of the motor gyrus impossible without a technique like fMRI.

The face/tongue region of the primary motor gyrus is located on the lateral/inferior aspect of the motor gyrus. This region is anatomically just posterior to Broca's area in the inferior frontal gyrus. Figure 5.4 shows an fMRI map of both hand and tongue motor movements acquired simultaneously in an intact patient. Of note, finding the tongue motor region by "pulling down" the sulcus, where one first locates the more cephald component of the central sulcus/reverse omega and follows the sulcus inferiorly, can be misleading and inaccurate. The inferior aspect of the central sulcus moves anteriorly as it is traced inferiorly and shortens making precise localization of the inferior aspect of the motor gyrus particularly difficult to discern anatomically alone. For this reason, fMRI is particularly useful for localizing the face/lips/tongue portion of the motor gyrus at its inferior aspect.

Another way in which fMRI contributes significantly to motor gyrus localization is in the foot motor region. The foot motor region is located most medially just over the interhemispheric fissure. This region is often localized medial and slightly posterior to the hand motor region in the axial plane (Fig. 5.5). Direct cortical stimulation (the surgeon's intraoperative gold standard for functional mapping) of this region is difficult because the sagittal sinus makes the cortex difficult to access. Therefore, fMRI localization of the foot motor region is valuable for presurgical planning.

fMRI typically maps these three main motor areas (foot, hand, and face/tongue) for neurosurgical planning. This is partly because these three areas span the gyrus medially to laterally and partly because tasks involving these areas are easily amenable to functional paradigms.

The primary sensory gyrus (also known as the postcentral gyrus) is located just posterior to the precentral gyrus from which it is divided by the central sulcus. Like the primary motor gyrus, the organization of the sensory gyrus is also somatotopically organized (Fig. 5.1).

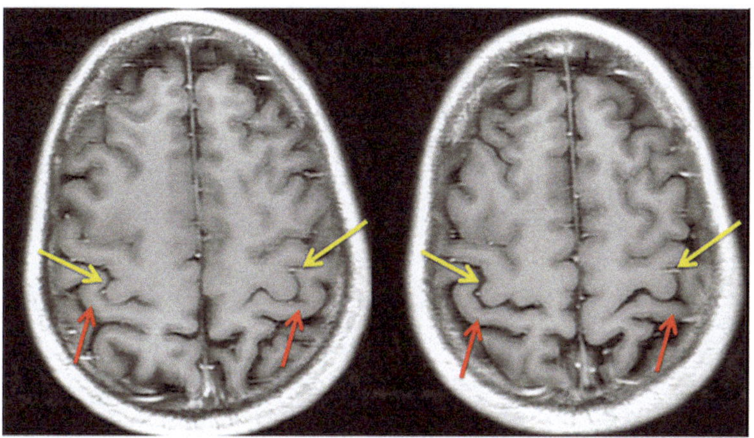

Fig. 5.1 The primary sensory/motor gyrus: The *yellow arrow* indicates the position of the reverse omega portion of the primary motor gyrus in the posterior frontal lobe. The *red arrow* shows the position of the sensory gyrus

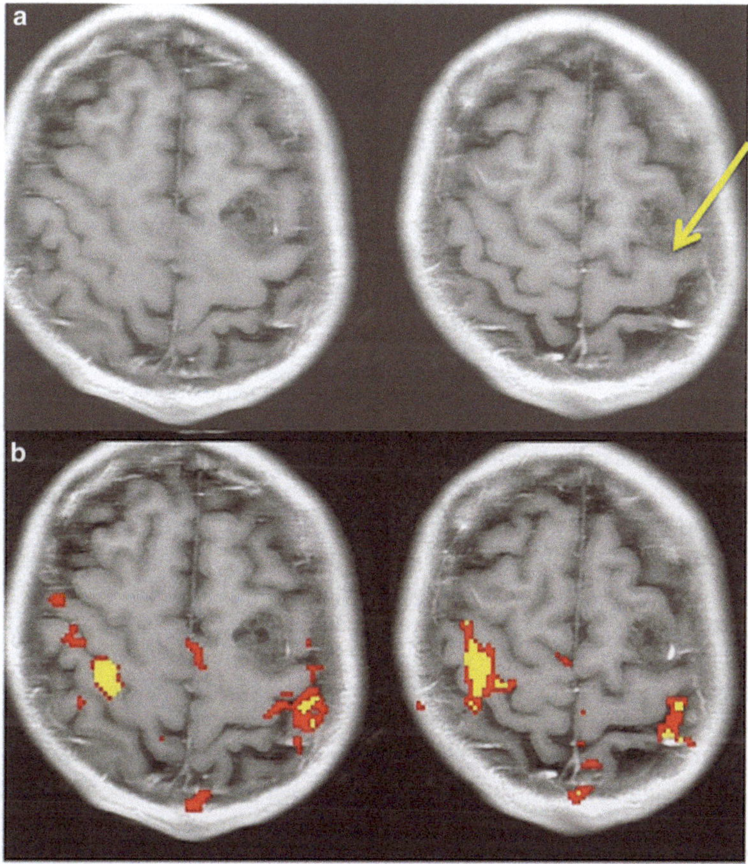

Fig. 5.2 Ambiguous anatomy. In rare instances the reverse omega (*yellow arrow*) does not indicate the position of the central sulcus. Without fMRI, this lesion would have been assumed to be in the motor gyrus

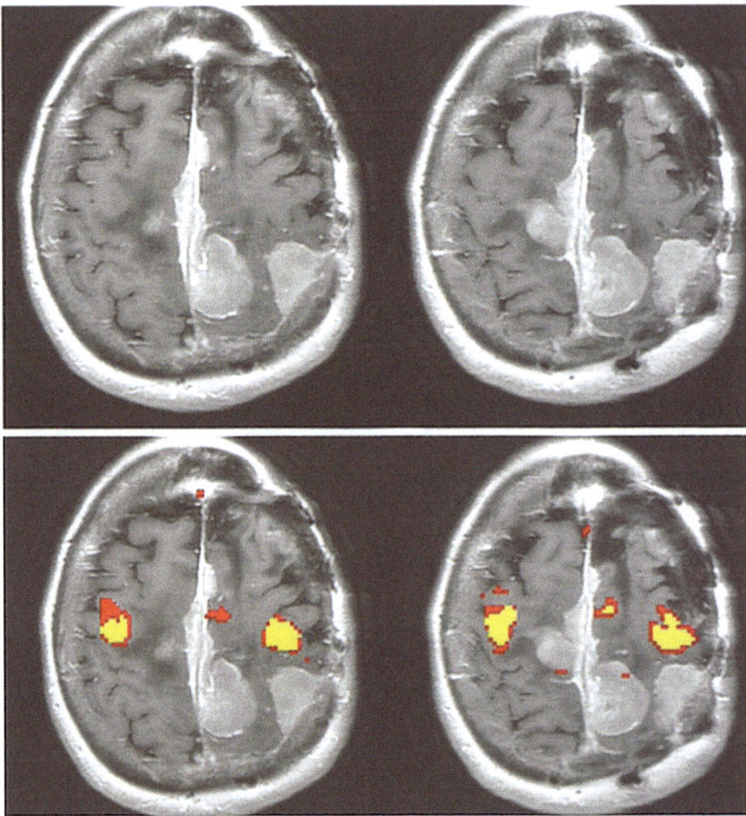

Fig. 5.3 Where is the motor gyrus? fMRI is particularly useful in cases where tumor has obscured normal anatomy. In this case multiple extra-axial lesions make the motor gyrus localization impossible without a technique like fMRI

Secondary Motor Areas

While the primary motor and sensory areas are the main focus of most neurosurgical planning targets, damage to secondary motor areas also carries a risk of morbidity [7–10]. As a result, their precise localization is becoming increasingly important during fMRI exams. The most common secondary motor areas of interest for neurosurgical planning are the supplementary motor area and the pre-motor area. To study the secondary areas, paradigms often focus on a unilateral volitional movement contrasted with rest [11].

Supplementary Motor Area

The SMA is located in the superior frontal gyrus just medial to the superior frontal sulcus (Fig. 5.6). While it is an expansive area with ill-defined anterior borders, the posterior border of the SMA is the foot motor region of the primary motor gyrus. The SMA is made up of an anterior portion (pre-SMA), more active on fMRI during language tasks and a posterior portion, more active on fMRI during motor tasks. The boundary between the pre-SMA and SMA proper has been delineated using a VCA line or a line drawn vertically from the AC/PC line [12].

Recent studies suggest that the motor portion of the SMA is, like the primary motor gyrus, also somatotopically arranged. In lower animals, it has been shown that the hind limb is located in caudal sites while the forelimb and facial movements are closer to the pre-SMA, the more anterior, language-related portion of the SMA, and are thus more rostral [13–17]. Although somatotopic organization is more commonly associated

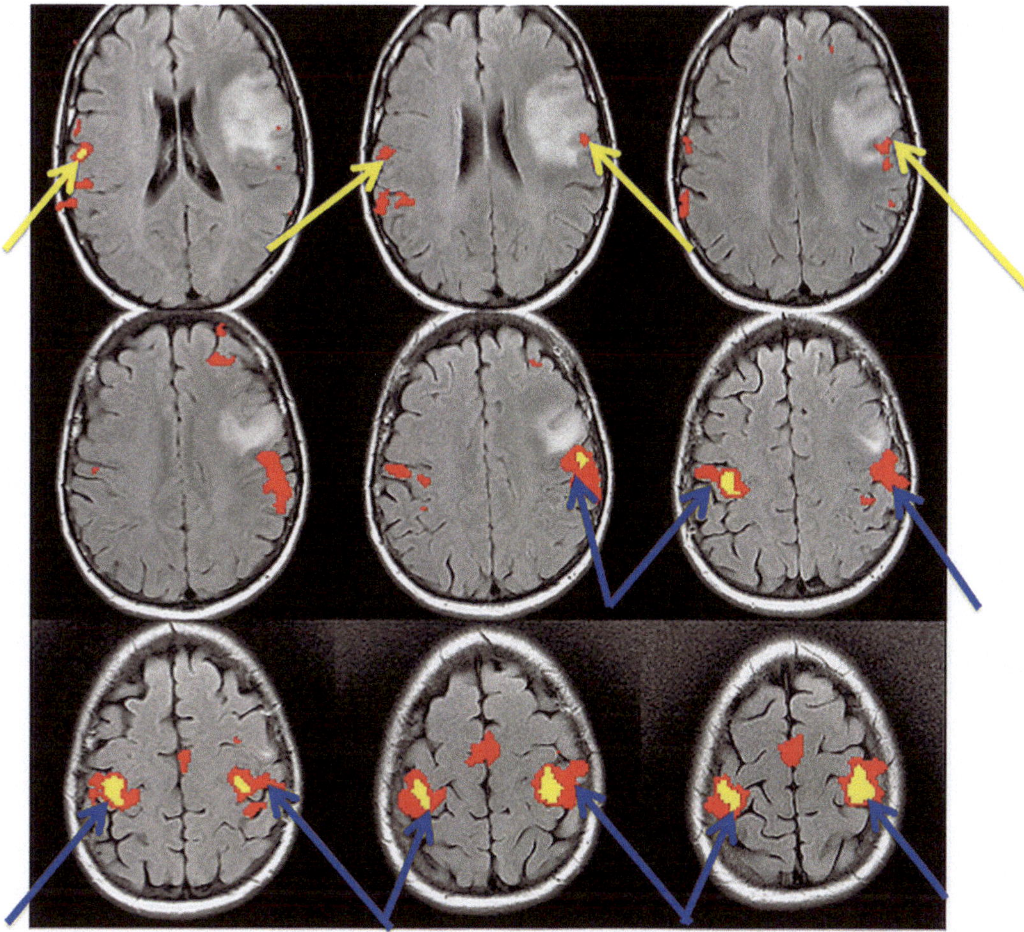

Fig. 5.4 Position of the hand (*blue arrow*) and tongue (*yellow arrow*). fMRI signals in the primary motor gyrus

with the primary motor cortex, the three main motor areas—hand, foot, and face/tongue—may also be somatotopically mapped along the more rostral axis of the SMA [18, 19].

The SMA is broadly responsible for motor planning and activates temporally before the primary motor gyrus [20–22]. Further, it is active when movements are both internally and externally cued [20]. The SMA is best known for being associated with voluntary movement but will also activate on fMRI during passive tasks [23]. The posterior portion of the SMA is more involved in finger movement tasks while the anterior part of the SMA is active during cognitive and language processing [24]. A centralized region of the SMA that is active during both language and motor tasks suggests a region that may be essential. Further investigation is needed to determine whether insult to this centralized region carries an increased incidence or degree of postoperative deficit.

More recent work suggests a role for the SMA in cortical compensation. BOLD fMRI can be used preoperatively to look at the patterns of activation as a tumor invades either the primary motor area or the SMA [25]. The SMA has been shown to be involved in temporal planning and organization of motor movements before execution, as well as sequencing of multiple movements [26]. Peck et al. characterized the role of the SMA in patients with high-grade gliomas and their role in cortical reorganization.

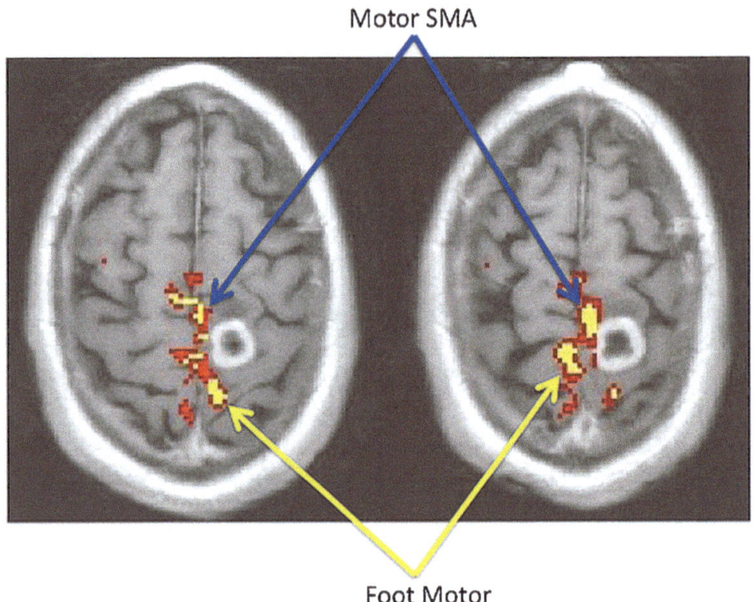

Fig. 5.5 Foot motor and supplementary motor (SMA) regions of the primary motor gyrus

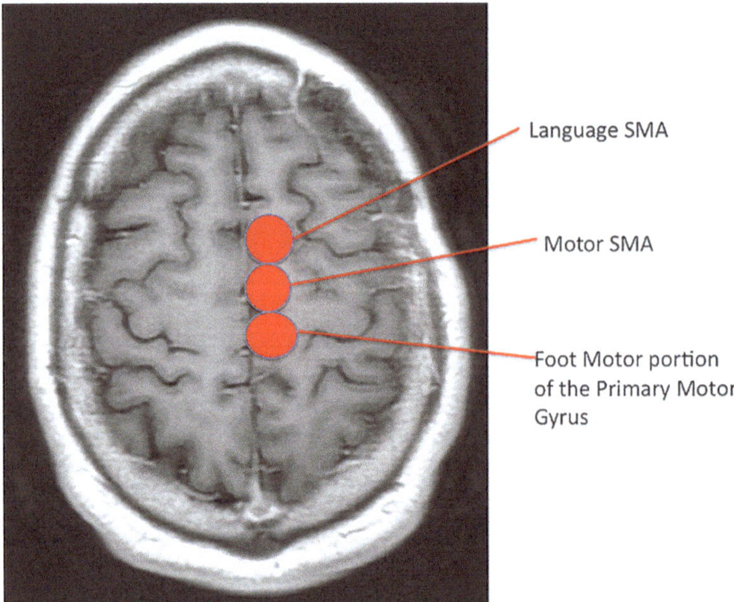

Fig. 5.6 Supplementary motor area: The supplementary motor area located in the superior frontal gyrus. The SMA is functionally segregated into motor (posterior) and speech (anterior) components

The study used fMRI to look at the BOLD hemodynamic responses in the primary motor and SMA of tumor patients. Here, block paradigms were used to assess latency differences so that the more sensitive hemodynamic response would be isolated. This work concluded that patients with glial tumors located within the primary motor cortex experienced lesion-induced compensation in the BOLD magnitude and firing pattern in both the primary motor cortex and the SMA. Cortical reorganization was visibly demonstrated with the SMA's role assuming functions for which the PMC was likely previously responsible [25, 27].

Why fMRI?

FMRI is especially useful for the purpose of locating the primary sensory motor cortex if normal sulci and/or gyral patterns are distorted or in rare cases when reorganization has occurred secondary to an invasive tumor [28]. fMRI, as a preoperative neuroimaging tool to localize the sensory/motor system, is popular for a variety of reasons. This method is minimally invasive and easily repeatable. Further, given that patients with brain tumors are often impaired, fMRI of sensory motor regions can be acquired with a variety of paradigms that are both volitional and passive. Patients undergo preoperative motor mapping for a multitude of reasons, the majority of which are when anatomical landmarks cannot be identified with certainty by traditional anatomical means. fMRI is also being investigated as a tool to predict deficits [5]. Lastly, fMRI can be used to interrogate cortical reorganization in the motor system, the clinical utility of which is still under investigation [25].

Several studies within the past decade provide evidence for the usefulness of fMRI preoperative sensory motor mapping. In a 2007 study by Pujol et al., patients were examined to identify the sensory motor cortex over a 5-year period. They performed a hand motion paradigm (opening and closing). The fMRI map correctly identified the location of the sensory motor cortex in 96 % of the cases—141 patients out of 147 examined. The 4 % that could not be identified displayed head motion greater than 2 mm. Although both conventional MRI and fMRI were used and compared in this study, fMRI significantly increased the confidence of the motor gyrus identification [29].

Studies investigating the outcomes of fMRI for preoperative identification of eloquent areas are ongoing. An important step in this direction was published by Petrella et al. The study investigated presurgical fMRI in 39 patients who were candidates for tumor resection. Two paradigms were used to map sensory motor areas. Treatment plans following inspection of the fMRI results were altered in 49 % of patients. In this study, fMRI sufficiently changed treatment options offering patients who would have otherwise been deemed inoperable the chance for surgical resection. Additionally, in nine patients for whom surgery was not originally offered, five were reconsidered for a craniotomy with intraoperative mapping. In cases where the course of treatment continued as planned, fMRI provided the neurosurgeons with further confidence in their surgical decision-making [30]. In a 2003 study by Wilkinson et al. [2], preoperative maps created through fMRI data were essential for safe resection by way of allowing for gross total resections and no postoperative deficits in 17 patients mapped with fMRI. Identifying the eloquent areas to prevent damage during tumor removal is of the utmost importance during mapping [31]. Tumors initially believed to be of too high risk for safe resections were now possible to resect since anatomical locations were available through preoperative fMRI scanning. In this study, no patients displayed permanent neurological damage after surgery.

Paradigms

fMRI localization is dependent upon the paradigm used to elicit the activation. In the motor system, these paradigms are relatively straightforward. Common paradigms for the motor area are finger tapping, tongue motion, and foot motion. Finger tapping most commonly involves having patients tap their fingers whilst in the scanner while simultaneously avoiding movement of the arms or the shoulders. During the tongue motion paradigm, patients are asked to keep teeth closed to avoid head motion artifacts and sweep their tongue against the back of their teeth. Motor foot localization consists of repetitive flexion and extension of the toes without moving the ankles. In most cases, small movements of the foot, hand, or tongue provide a significant signal, particularly when head motion is absent [11].

There are a variety of ways to perform motor paradigms with patients. Some are designed to localize the motor gyrus in both hemispheres simultaneously with bilateral finger tapping (to asses motor gyrus displacement) and in some cases patients can be asked to both move their tongue while tapping their fingers to localize both hand and tongue in a single experimental run. Yet another design involves no rest; that is, instead of alternating between a single motor task and rest, patients are instead asked to alternate between finger tapping and tongue motion. In all cases, careful attention should be paid to minimizing head motion. Short scanning time and clear instruction help to minimize artifacts.

fMRI exams of motor function, like any fMRI exam, can be performed using a block design or an event-related design. In many fMRI exams there are two states that are statistically contrasted in post-processing analysis. In an event-related design the patient performs one event (a finger tap for example), which is followed by rest. This type of paradigm allows for detailed estimation of the hemodynamic response [32]. Event-related designs, while possible in patient populations, are arguably preferred in basic science fMRI as more precise neuroanatomic parameters can be extracted from single events. However, this type of design requires many repetitions because the change from baseline for any one event is small (on the order of about 2–6 %). Accordingly, event-related designs tend to be longer than block designs given the need for many repetitions for adequate statistical power. This can be problematic for brain tumor patients who, in our experience, can have trouble keeping still and following complicated instructions with rapid alternations in task demand.

Block designs, by contrast, average the signal from many of the same types of events over a single epoch [23]. For example, a typical block-designed motor task would have the patient resting for five images and finger tapping for five images. This alternating cycle of rest and task would repeat five or six times and last approximately 5 min depending on the time to repeat (TR) of the images [31, 33–35]. The advantage to the block design is that the task-related images and the rest-related images are signal averaged. Therefore, the block design maximizes detection of the signal while the event-related design maximizes estimation of the signal [32, 36]. However, with this said, there is a role for event-related motor paradigms. Work done by Marquart et al. indicated that for finger movement tasks, where head motion artifacts are less likely to occur, a block trial is preferred for greater activation seen within the sensory motor cortex and/or the SMA. However, for toe and tongue movement tasks that are more susceptible to movement artifacts, event related or "single-event" paradigms adequately localized the foot motor areas [37].

There are also many special considerations when using fMRI maps for clinical use. For example, in brain tumor patients it is helpful to have a shorter task or "paradigm" duration as patients have a harder time than normal controls in keeping their head still. While fMRI data is often acquired using an event-related design in healthy control subjects, brain tumor patients as a result often benefit from the signal averaging afforded by block designs. Further, areas can be activated that are associated with the task being investigated but not essential for the task. This of course is an important consideration for BOLD fMRI mapping for neurosurgical planning where the goal is to isolate essential eloquent areas. With this said, fMRI is commonly used to map eloquent areas pre-surgically and has been shown to be sufficiently accurate, particularly in motor areas, for neurosurgical planning in a multitude of studies [2, 23].

Paresis

Paresis or weakness occurs often when the primary motor gyrus is injured or infiltrated by tumor or edema [6]. Paradigms for patients with paresis or weakness should be altered on a case-by-case basis. For example, sequential finger tapping can be modified to hand clenching for patients with partial hand paralysis [6]. In patients with complete paralysis, sensory stimulation of the hand (such as brushing, stroking, or rubbing) often elicits motor activation as well as sensory

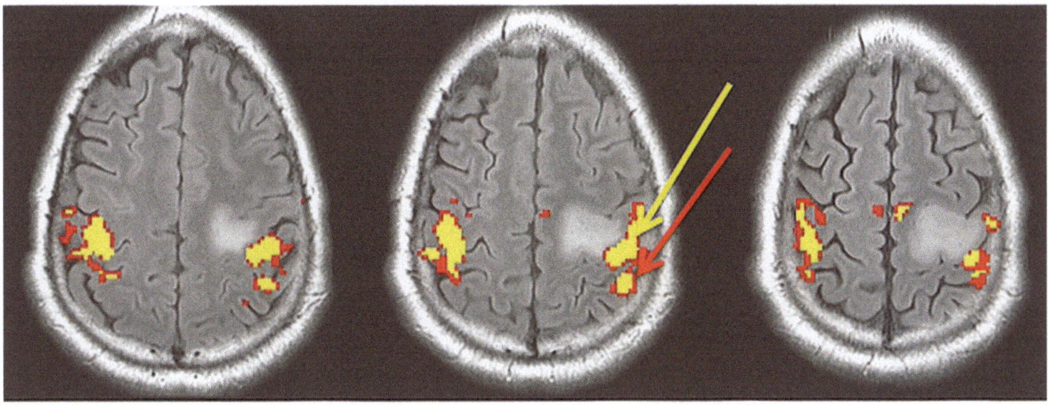

Fig. 5.7 Sensory fMRI paradigms often activate the motor gyrus as well. Bilateral hand scrubbing paradigm activates both primary motor (*yellow arrow*) and sensory (*red arrow*)

activation as a result of significant reciprocity between the sensory motor systems [6] (Fig. 5.7). The same can be done for the face and foot. Instead of asking the patient to move the affected area, the examiner strokes or scrubs the paretic region. While this fMRI map is biased toward the sensory gyrus, often strong motor signals are still seen [6, 11]. Extra caution in interpretation must be taken when dealing with preoperative scanning of patients with paresis. Scans on paretic patients tend to, in our experience, have more head motion as they struggle to move the affected limb during the fMRI exam [38].

Artifacts

Artifacts during fMRI scanning are common in patients with brain tumors [39]. Artifacts can be motion related or can result from anything that disrupts the T2* signal (i.e., susceptibility artifact). Motion-related artifacts can be periodic (arising from heartbeat, breathing) or random as is often the case with head motion. It is important to note that modern statistical analyses can easily remove periodic artifacts as long as they vary with a different frequency than the stimulus presentation. Trend (motion that occurs in a linear fashion) is also fairly straightforward to correct for because it looks different from the cycling BOLD signal. Stimulus-correlated motion (for example, nodding the head concurrently while performing a finger-tapping paradigm) however can look so similar to real oscillating signal that it can be difficult to remove with standard motion correction algorithms and may in turn adversely affect the study. Other artifacts like signal dropout can be caused by dental work, blood products, hemosiderin from a previous surgery, or infarct and can also be a source of false-negative function (Fig. 5.8). Dropout artifacts from the air tissue interface at the base of the brain are also common in the brain tumor patient population [23]. As a result, T2* source images should be routinely inspected.

Effect of Tumor on fMRI

Presence of a tumor can affect the BOLD fMRI signal. The BOLD signal is dependent upon a predictable vascular response, which can be affected by a tumor's abnormal neovasculature. The BOLD contrast is a measure of the proportional changes in the amount of oxygenated blood that replaces deoxygenated blood during a task. Tissue that is negative in and around a tumor on fMRI can become active after surgery when mass effect associated with tumor is removed and normal perfusion is restored [40]. This false negative phenomenon is referred to as tumor-induced neurovascular uncoupling and was first described by

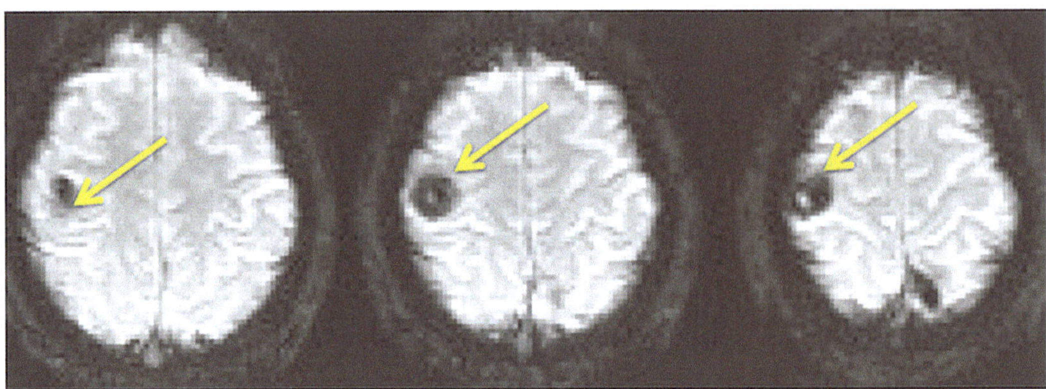

Fig. 5.8 Dropout artifact. T2* signal loss can cause false-negative determinations of function in fMRI. In this case the artifact was caused by hemorrhage

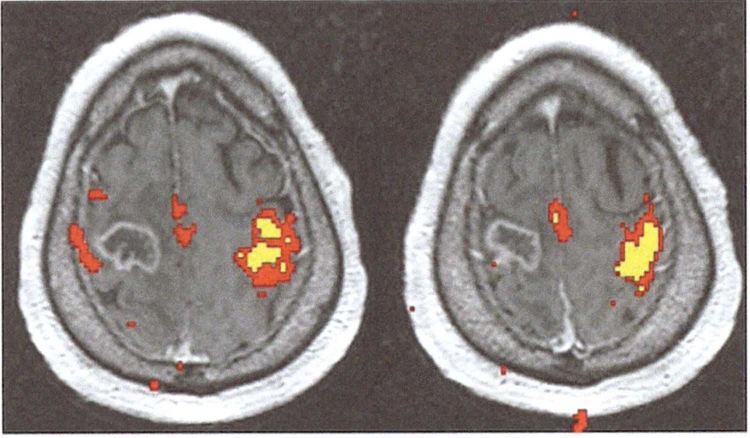

Fig. 5.9 Diminished BOLD response adjacent to a tumor. fMRI signal magnitude during a bilateral finger-tapping task is diminished adjacent to a glioblastoma multiforme. The exact mechanism which accounts for this phenomenon is unknown; caution in interpretation should be exercised in and around lesions

Holodny et al. [41]. The authors showed that the fMRI activation volume on the tumor side of the brain was diminished in relation to the healthy contralateral side. This effect is hypothesized to be caused by a loss of autoregulation in the tumor vasculature. Figure 5.9 shows an example of this commonly seen phenomenon during a finger-tapping fMRI paradigm. The study by Krings et al. in 2002 supported the decoupling theory. The patients in this study suffering from moderate paresis had tumors affecting the motor cortex and reduced signal magnitude within the primary motor cortex. In cases where patients were completely paretic, the fMRI signal was even further diminished. However, in these patients, the signal from the supplementary motor cortex and the contralateral hemisphere increased. This effect is most likely explained by compensation [42]. In Ludemann et al.'s work the BOLD signal of patients with larger highly vascularized tumors tended to be smaller than the signals of patients with smaller less vascularized gliomas. Lastly, it has been suggested that bilateral motor paradigms be used in fMRI preoperative mapping so that the contralateral hemisphere BOLD activation acts as a control reference [43]. In this way it is easier to make determinations about displaced anatomy and reduced BOLD magnitudes.

The effects of BOLD decoupling on the interpretation of fMRI maps vary. In motor mapping, where the main goal is often localization of a single gyrus, a diminished fMRI signal is irrelevant as long as it correctly identifies the gyrus in question. For example, Holodny et al. [44] found that there was a significant difference in the volume of activation in the primary motor cortex on the tumor side of the brain versus the non-tumor side. This effect was most seen in glioblastoma multiformes. Despite decoupling effects on the BOLD fMRI signal, the motor cortex was still correctly identified [44]. However, caution should still be exercised in the case where tumor and other factors associated with the tumor completely eliminate the fMRI signal as these maps are at risk of errors in interpretation. Holodny et al. [41] have shown that BOLD fMRI activation can be not only diminished but also eliminated.

Combination of Methods

There are a variety of other mapping techniques that can be complementary to fMRI for presurgical planning. These techniques vary in aspects such as resolution (both spatial and temporal), or their ability to preferentially localize or lateralize function. The methods also vary in invasiveness. Common methods used in place of or in addition to fMRI are magnetoencephalography (MEG), electroencephalography (EEG), PET, and diffusion tractography (DTI).

Magnetoencephalography

In Korvenoja et al.'s 2006 work, both MEG, described in Chap. XX of this book, and fMRI were used to locate the primary sensory motor cortex. Their study showed that MEG predicated a more accurate and specific location of the gyrus of interest in comparison to fMRI. In all 15 patients, the localization of the central sulcus with MEG was correct. Since fMRI activation activates the entire network of structures required for a motor task (essential as well as secondary areas) it can be difficult to interpret the localization of the motor gyrus where the pre-motor, primary motor, and sensory gyri may activate on fMRI simultaneously compromising specificity. This is not an issue with MEG. The spatial resolution for these two methods also varies; MEG can achieve 5 mm while fMRI can be as low as 1 mm [45].

Other studies, such as the one performed by Kober et al. in 2001, indicated comparable identification of the primary motor gyrus using either MEG or fMRI and thus showed a strong degree of clinical usefulness for identifying the sensory/motor region of the brain [46]. Both of these techniques allow for much more precise preoperative planning for surgery than traditional anatomical MR markers. However, of the two, MRI scanners are much more readily available than MEG scanners and is thus a more popular method.

Electroencephalography

A method similar to MEG is EEG, which directly measures the cortical electrical activity of the brain through potentials. Both of these techniques have superb temporal resolution. Using somatosensory evoked potentials (SSEPs) as measured by EEG and fMRI together, the central sulcus is often identified, particularly in the operating room just preceding direct cortical stimulation [33]. EEG is, however, a much more invasive methodology than fMRI. Further, SSEPs as a result of their electrical sensitivity often fail to identify the rolandic region making fMRI integration into the neurosurgical navigation system helpful in these cases [47].

Positron Emission Tomography

PET, a neuroimaging technique described in Chap. XX, is a brain mapping technique that preceded fMRI historically. It is based on blood glucose metabolism. When performing a paradigm, the cerebral metabolism is measured and statistical operations similar to those used for fMRI are used to create a map of function [23]. A 1999 study performed by Ritter et al. showed that there was good concordance between PET and fMR imaging in regard to locating the primary motor and somatosensory cortex. Their work showed that the distance of peak PET and fMRI activation centroids averaged 7.9 mm (range 1–18 mm; $p>0.05$) [28]. Unlike PET, fMRI has the added benefit of not requiring an invasive radioactive tracer.

Diffusion Tractography

Diffusion tractography, an MR method that measures water diffusivity in the brain, is used to map the white matter tracts. This topic is considered more thoroughly in Chap. XX. Combining DTI with grey matter fMRI localizations provides a more complete picture of the functional anatomy around a tumor. Once the precentral gyrus is localized, there is further consideration given to the descending white matter tracts [38, 39, 48–51]. The corticospinal tract, the major tract leading from the primary motor cortex to the spinal cord, if violated, can lead to irreversible paresis [52]. Further, in regard to brain tumors, this combination of fMRI and DTI allows for the presurgical evaluation of the effects of rolandic brain tumors on the pyramidal (corticospinal) tract [49]. fMRI has also been used to enhance the ability to identify tracts of interest within a brain where deformed anatomy is present by providing a seed-point for DTI post-processing [52].

Intraoperative Mapping

fMRI is often integrated into the intraoperative mapping environment. Figure 5.10 shows a motor map integrated into the Brainlab Neuronavigation System (Feldkirchen, Germany). Intraoperative direct cortical stimulation is considered the gold standard for functional localization in the operating room. It entails stimulating the exposed cortex with electrical current in order to localize the motor gyrus [53]. It is this gold standard that fMRI and any other functional technique is compared against. BOLD fMRI commonly guides intraoperative mapping. When the motor gyrus is localized using fMRI preoperatively, these maps can guide direct cortical stimulation and save time assaying the rolandic anatomy in some cases. Further, direct cortical stimulation can only measure the gyral surfaces and does not always elicit a motor response. Therefore, fMRI has proven valuable and can act as a significant addition to the neuronavigational toolbox [2, 3, 54].

Coregistered fMRI images can be formatted to a surgical microscope and functional areas can be projected directly onto the surface of the exposed brain. Work done by Krishnan et al. used neuronavigation around the motor strip during surgery superimposing motor localizations for foot, hand, and tongue [55]. Visualizing fiber tracks and connections within the navigational system also helps minimize the risk of iatrogenic injury by acting as a functional reference point during surgery. Intraoperative mapping using direct cortical stimulation has the advantage of assaying cortex essential for a function whereas fMRI shows all areas both essential and supportive for a task [55].

There are small subsets of centers performing intraoperative BOLD fMRI in surgical units that include an MRI. Feigl et al. concluded that intraoperative fMRI mapping safely guided the neurosurgeons avoiding damage to functional areas during surgery. Real-time data from a 3-T MRI scanner can be efficiently used—especially since no offline post-processing is needed [56]. Work done by Nabavi et al. yielded similar results. Their work looked at patients undergoing awake craniotomies with cortical stimulation in an MRI-assisted operating room. Intraoperative imaging added about 20–60 min to the procedure. 94 % of the patients in the study stated that they would undergo the procedure again if needed.

Real-Time fMRI

Real-time functional magnetic resonance imaging (rtfMRI) allows live evaluation of brain activation. Trials that are contaminated with head motion can be detected and corrected during the scanning session rather than rendering a study not usable in post-processing after the scan.

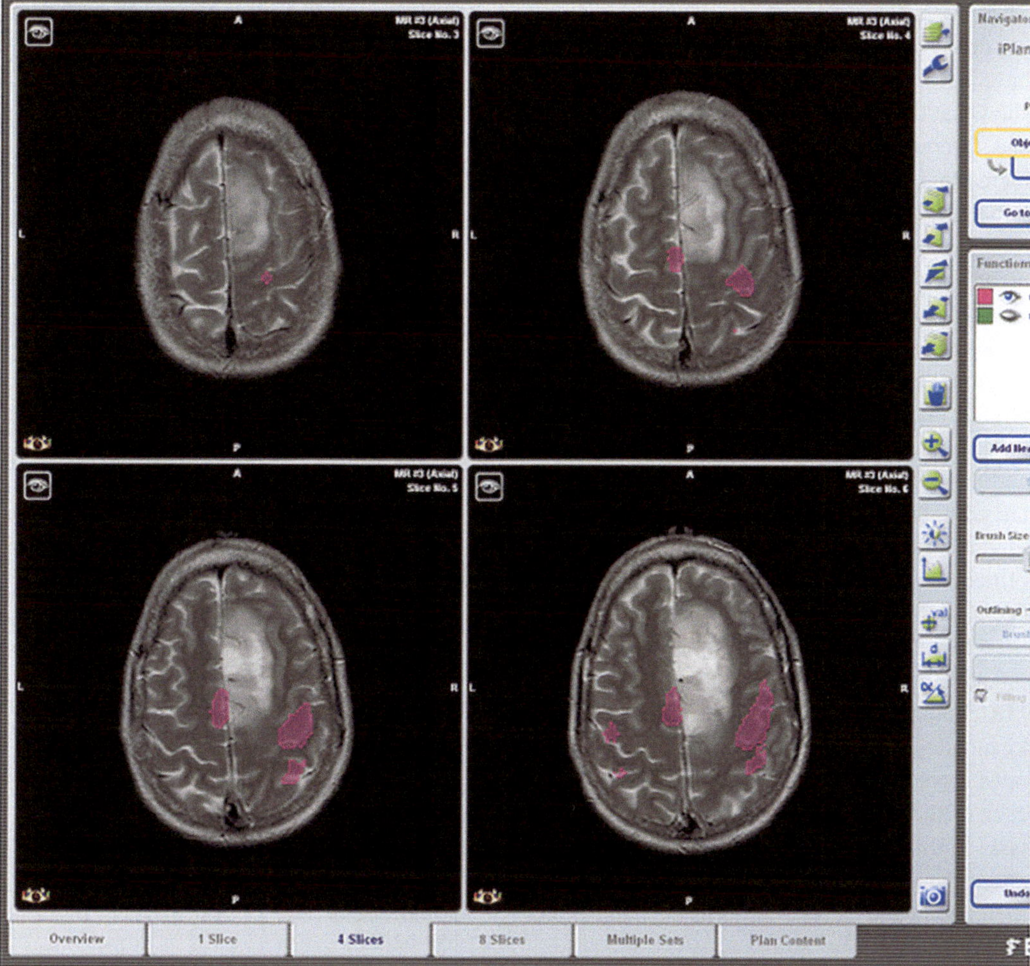

Fig. 5.10 Intraoperative figure integrating motor fMRI. A bilateral finger-tapping fMRI paradigm can easily be integrated into a neurosurgical navigation system and may decrease time required for invasive mapping procedures (Brainlab, Feldkirchen, Germany)

More widespread implementation of real time may shorten procedures and yield a higher proportion of usable fMRI data [1, 57].

Conclusions/Future Directions

Within the past decade, fMRI has become a common tool for presurgical sensory motor mapping. fMRI is a significant preoperative asset for tumors located within the central region [33]. Using various motor paradigms, fMRI has significantly improved the neurosurgeon's confidence in functional localization during resection and also has changed surgical options for many patients. This noninvasive tool allows for easy display and integration with other neuroimaging techniques. Although fMRI is a useful preoperative tool, it is not a perfect tool. Tumors that affect the normal vascular coupling of neuronal activity will affect the fMRI measurement.

fMRI continues to be developed in novel fields, such as digit mapping, a more specified mapping of the hand motor area. Work done by Sanchez-Panchuelo et al. used a 7T scanner to make high-resolution maps of digit representation.

Thus, high-field scanners are providing increasing detail of motor representations. Robust maps have been made using high-field magnets that show that the thumb (digit 1) as the most inferior and lateral while digits 2–5 are represented increasingly superior. The higher spatial resolution and high-field mapping provides a promising tool for increased precision of the functional organization and specificity of different areas within the central region [58].

Visual inspection of a patient performing a bilateral finger-tapping paradigm common in the clinical mapping environment does not allow for an accurate correlation between a precise task and the fMRI BOLD response. This is particularly an issue when analyzing the effects of tumor on the motor gyrus. fMRI maps can be difficult to interpret in the context of increased or decreased magnitude and the pattern of activation. Some groups have tried to enhance interpretative power in these cases by developing MR-compatible devices that measure finger kinematics. For example, Schaechter et al. developed a system to measure angular velocity from each of the ten digits while performing a motor task. In this way, more inferences can be drawn about the differences between tumor-infiltrated motor gyri and normal patterns of hand motor activation [59].

fMRI, while advancing in the preoperative neurosurgical planning, continues to make strides.

References

1. Decharms RC. Applications of real-time fMRI. Nat Rev Neurosci. 2008;9(9):720–9.
2. Wilkinson ID, Romanowski CAJ, Jellinek DA, Morris J, Griffiths PD. Motor functional MRI for pre-operative and intraoperative neurosurgical guidance. Br J Radiol. 2003;76(902):98–103.
3. Paleologos TS, Wadley JP, Kitchen ND, Thomas DG. Clinical utility and cost-effectiveness of interactive image-guided craniotomy: clinical comparison between conventional and image-guided meningioma surgery. Neurosurgery. 2000;47(1):40–7. discussion 47–8.
4. Kasahara M, Menon DK, Salmond CH, et al. Altered functional connectivity in the motor network after traumatic brain injury. Neurology. 2010;75(2):168–76.
5. Stippich C, Blatow M. Clinical functional MRI : presurgical functional neuroimaging. Berlin; New York: Springer; 2007.
6. Tieleman A, Deblaere K, Van Roost D, Van Damme O, Achten E. Preoperative fMRI in tumour surgery. Eur Radiol. 2009;19(10):2523–34.
7. Zentner J, Hufnagel A, Pechstein U, Wolf HK, Schramm J. Functional results after resective procedures involving the supplementary motor area. J Neurosurg. 1996;85(4):542–9.
8. Fontaine D, Capelle L, Duffau H. Somatotopy of the supplementary motor area: evidence from correlation of the extent of surgical resection with the clinical patterns of deficit. Neurosurgery. 2002;50(2):297–303. discussion 303–5.
9. Krainik A, Lehericy S, Duffau H, et al. Postoperative speech disorder after medial frontal surgery: role of the supplementary motor area. Neurology. 2003;60(4): 587–94.
10. Bannur U, Rajshekhar V. Post operative supplementary motor area syndrome: clinical features and outcome. Br J Neurosurg. 2000;14(3):204–10.
11. Brennan NP. Preparing the paitent for the fMRI study and optimization of paradigm selection and delivery. In: Holodny AI, editor. Functional neuroimaging. New York: Informia Healthcare; 2008. p. 13–21.
12. Dassonville P, Zhu XH, Ugurbil K, Kim SG, Ashe J. Functional activation in motor cortex reflects the direction and the degree of handedness (vol 94, pg 14015, 1997). Proc Natl Acad Sci U S A. 1998;95(19): 11499.
13. Matsuzaka Y, Aizawa H, Tanji J. A motor area rostral to the supplementary motor area (presupplementary motor area) in the monkey: neuronal activity during a learned motor task. J Neurophysiol. 1992;68(3): 653–62.
14. Luppino G, Matelli M, Camarda RM, Gallese V, Rizzolatti G. Multiple representations of body movements in mesial area 6 and the adjacent cingulate cortex: an intracortical microstimulation study in the macaque monkey. J Comp Neurol. 1991;311(4): 463–82.
15. Fried I, Katz A, McCarthy G, et al. Functional organization of human supplementary motor cortex studied by electrical stimulation. J Neurosci. 1991;11(11): 3656–66.
16. Mitz AR, Wise SP. The somatotopic organization of the supplementary motor area: intracortical microstimulation mapping. J Neurosci. 1987;7(4): 1010–21.
17. Arienzo D, Babiloni C, Ferretti A, et al. Somatotopy of anterior cingulate cortex (ACC) and supplementary motor area (SMA) for electric stimulation of the median and tibial nerves: an fMRI study. Neuroimage. 2006;33(2):700–5.
18. Chainay H, Krainik A, Tanguy ML, Gerardin E, Le Bihan D, Lehericy S. Foot, face and hand representation in the human supplementary motor area. Neuroreport. 2004;15(5):765–9.

19. Rijntjes M, Dettmers C, Buchel C, Kiebel S, Frackowiak RSJ, Weiller C. A blueprint for movement: functional and anatomical representations in the human motor system. J Neurosci. 1999;19(18): 8043–8.
20. Nachev P, Kennard C, Husain M. Functional role of the supplementary and pre-supplementary motor areas. Nat Rev Neurosci. 2008;9(11):856–69.
21. Tanji J, Kurata K. Comparison of movement-related activity in 2 cortical motor areas of primates. J Neurophysiol. 1982;48(3):633–53.
22. Brinkman C, Porter R. Supplementary motor area in the monkey: activity of neurons during performance of a learned motor task. J Neurophysiol. 1979;42(3): 681–709.
23. Tharin S, Golby A. Functional brain mapping and its applications to neurosurgery. Neurosurgery. 2007;60(4):185–201.
24. VanOostende S, VanHecke P, Sunaert S, Nuttin B, Marchal G. FMRI studies of the supplementary motor area and the premotor cortex. Neuroimage. 1997;6(3):181–90.
25. Peck KK, Bradbury M, Hou BL, Brennan NP, Holodny AI. The role of the supplementary motor area (SMA) in the execution of primary motor activities in brain tumor patients: functional MRI detection of time-resolved differences in the hemodynamic response. Med Sci Monit. 2009;15(4):Mt55–62.
26. Tanji J. The supplementary motor area in the cerebral-cortex. Neurosci Res. 1994;19(3):251–68.
27. Peck KK, Bradbury M, Psaty EL, Brennan NR, Holodny AI. Joint activation of the supplementary motor area and presupplementary motor area during simultaneous motor and language functional MRI. Neuroreport. 2009;20(5):487–91.
28. Bittar RG, Olivier A, Sadikot AF, Andermann F, Pike GB, Reutens DC. Presurgical motor and somatosensory cortex mapping with functional magnetic resonance imaging and positron emission tomography. J Neurosurg. 1999;91(6):915–21.
29. Pujol J, Deus J, Acebes JJ, et al. Identification of the sensorimotor cortex with functional MRI: frequency and actual contribution in a neurosurgical context. J Neuroimaging. 2008;18(1):28–33.
30. Petrella JR, Shah LM, Harris KM, et al. Preoperative functional MR imaging localization of language and motor areas: effect on therapeutic decision making in patients with potentially resectable brain tumors. Radiology. 2006;240(3):793–802.
31. Kim PE, Singh M. Functional magnetic resonance imaging for brain mapping in neurosurgery. Neurosurg Focus. 2003;15(1):E1.
32. Birn RM, Cox RW, Bandettini PA. Detection versus estimation in event-related fMRI: choosing the optimal stimulus timing. Neuroimage. 2002;15(1): 252–64.
33. Rombouts SARB, Barkhof F, Scheltens P. Clinical applications of functional brain MRI. Oxford: Oxford University Press; 2007.
34. Zarahn E, Aguirre G, DEsposito M. A trial-based experimental design for fMRI. Neuroimage. 1997; 6(2):122–38.
35. Aguirre G, D'Esposito M. Experimental design for brain fMRI. In: Moonen CTW, Bandettini PA, editors. Functional MRI. Berlin: Springer; 2000. p. 369–80.
36. Liu TT, Frank LR, Wong EC, Buxton RB. Detection power, estimation efficiency, and predictability in event-related fMRI. Neuroimage. 2001;13(4):759–73.
37. Marquart M, Birn R, Haughton V. Single- and multiple-event paradigms for identification of motor cortex activation. AJNR Am J Neuroradiol. 2000;21(1): 94–8.
38. Stippich C. Presurgical functional magnetic resonance imaging (fMRI). Clin Neuroradiol. 2007;2: 69–87.
39. Krings T, Reinges MHT, Erberich S, et al. Functional MRI for presurgical planning: problems, artefacts, and solution strategies. J Neurol Neurosurg Psychiatry. 2001;70(6):749–60.
40. Roux FE, Boulanouar K, Ibarrola D, Tremoulet M, Chollet F, Berry I. Functional MRI and intraoperative brain mapping to evaluate brain plasticity in patients with brain tumours and hemiparesis. J Neurol Neurosurg Psychiatry. 2000;69(4):453–63.
41. Holodny AI, Schulder M, Liu WC, Maldjian JA, Kalnin AJ. Decreased BOLD functional MR activation of the motor and sensory cortices adjacent to a glioblastoma multiforme: implications for image-guided neurosurgery. AJNR Am J Neuroradiol. 1999; 20(4):609–12.
42. Krings T, Topper R, Willmes K, Reinges MHT, Gilsbach JM, Thron A. Activation in primary and secondary motor areas in patients with CNS neoplasms and weakness. Neurology. 2002;58(3):381–90.
43. Schreiber A, Hubbe U, Ziyeh S, Henning J. The influence of gliomas and nonglial space-occupying lesions on blood-oxygen-level-dependent contrast enhancement. AJNR Am J Neuroradiol. 2000;21:1055–63.
44. Holodny AI, Schulder M, Liu WC, Wolko J, Maldjian JA, Kalnin AJ. The effect of brain tumors on BOLD functional MR imaging activation in the adjacent motor cortex: implications for image-guided neurosurgery. AJNR Am J Neuroradiol. 2000;21(8):1415–22.
45. Korvenoja A, Kirveskari E, Aronen HJ, et al. Sensorimotor cortex localization: comparison of magnetoencephalography, functional MR imaging, and intraoperative cortical mapping. Radiology. 2006; 241(1):213–22.
46. Kober H, Nimsky C, Moller M, Hastreiter P, Fahlbush R, Ganslandt O. Correlation of sensorimotor activation with functional magnetic resonance imaging and magnetoencephalography in presurgical functional imaging: a spatial analysis. Neuroimage. 2001;14(5): 1214–28.
47. Petrovich N, Holodny AI, Tabar V, et al. Discordance between functional magnetic resonance imaging during silent speech tasks and intraoperative speech arrest. J Neurosurg. 2005;103(2):267–74.

48. Parmar H, Sitoh YY, Yeo TT. Combined magnetic resonance tractography and functional magnetic resonance imaging in evaluation of brain tumors involving the motor system. J Comput Assist Tomogr. 2004; 28(4):551–6.
49. Stippich C, Kress B, Ochmann H, Tronnier V, Sartor K. Preoperative functional magnetic resonance tomography (FMRI) in patients with rolandic brain tumors: indication, investigation strategy, possibilities and limitations of clinical application. Rofo. 2003;175(8):1042–50.
50. Ulmer JL, Salvan CV, Mueller WM, et al. The role of diffusion tensor imaging in establishing the proximity of tumor borders to functional brain systems: implications for preoperative risk assessments and postoperative outcomes. Technol Cancer Res Treat. 2004;3(6): 567–76.
51. Holodny AI, Schwartz TH, Ollenschleger M, Liu WC, Schulder M. Tumor involvement of the corticospinal tract: diffusion magnetic resonance tractography with intraoperative correlation - case illustration. J Neurosurg. 2001;95(6):1082.
52. Schonberg T, Pianka P, Hendler T, Pasternak O, Assaf Y. Characterization of displaced white matter by brain tumors using combined DTI and fMRI. Neuroimage. 2006;30(4):1100–11.
53. Xie J, Chen XZ, Jiang T, et al. Preoperative blood oxygen level-dependent functional magnetic resonance imaging in patients with gliomas involving the motor cortical areas. Chin Med J (Engl). 2008;121(7): 631–5.
54. Gasser T, Ganslandt O, Sandalcioglu E, Stolke D, Fahlbusch R, Nimsky C. Intraoperative functional MRI: implementation and preliminary experience. Neuroimage. 2005;26(3):685–93.
55. Krishnan R, Raabe A, Hattingen E, et al. Functional magnetic resonance imaging integrated neuronavigation: correlation between lesion-to-motor cortex distance and outcome. Neurosurgery. 2004;55(4): 904–14.
56. Feigl GC, Safavi-Abbasi S, Gharabaghi A, et al. Real-time 3 T fMRI data of brain tumour patients for intra-operative localization of primary motor areas. Eur J Surg Oncol. 2008;34(6):708–15.
57. Schwindack C, Siminotto E, Meyer M, et al. Real-time functional magnetic resonance imaging (rt-fMRI) in patients with brain tumours: preliminary findings using motor and language paradigms. Br J Neurosurg. 2005;19(1):25–32.
58. Sanchez-Panchuelo RM, Francis S, Bowtell R, Schluppeck D. Mapping human somatosensory cortex in individual subjects with 7T functional MRI. J Neurophysiol. 2010;103(5):2544–56.
59. Schaechter JD, Stokes C, Connell BD, Perdue K, Bonmassar G. Finger motion sensors for fMRI motor studies. Neuroimage. 2006;31(4):1549–59.

DTI for Presurgical Mapping

6

Andrew P. Klein, John L. Ulmer, Wade M. Mueller, Flavius D. Raslau, Wolfgang Gaggl, and Mohit Maheshwari

Introduction

The most clinically advanced application of diffusion tensor imaging (DTI) currently is white matter mapping prior to surgical resection of brain tumors. The potential and realized successes of DTI in this setting have propelled the clinical translation of the technology. It has quickly become an invaluable tool for neurosurgeons and neurosurgery patients, not only at academic centers but within many community practices as well. Presurgical DTI can provide prognostic information, help create a patient-specific neurosurgical plan by defining spatial relationships between the lesion and functional white matter networks, and guide intraoperative assessments. Combined with four other preoperative and perioperative localization techniques (including functional MRI), DTI becomes an asset that maximizes the extent of tumor resection and minimizes postsurgical neurological deficits. Understanding the DTI technique, data visualization methods, effect of pathological processes, and limitations is essential for accurate interpretation and optimal utilization of the technology. In this chapter, we focus on the emerging and powerful clinical application of presurgical DTI.

DTI Translation

DTI's rapid transition from the research realm to daily clinical practice is the result of its high translatability for presurgical planning and operative decision-making. The relationship of the determinants of technology translation is conceptualized by the formula

$$\boldsymbol{T} = (\boldsymbol{A} - \boldsymbol{I}) + \boldsymbol{S} + \boldsymbol{C} + \boldsymbol{R} \tag{6.1}$$

T represents the translatability of the technology in changing the existing clinical algorithm. ***A*** represents the magnitude of the application's clinical impact, which considers individual impact, volume of patients affected, and societal impact. ***I*** represents the relative invasiveness of the application compared to alternative clinical strategies. ***S*** represents the rate of development and clinical translation of a technology. ***C*** represents the comfort level of practicing physicians in adopting the technology. Finally, ***R*** represents the relative resource impact perceived by decision-makers

A.P. Klein, M.D. (✉) • J.L. Ulmer, M.D.
• F.D. Raslau, M.D. • W. Gaggl, M.S.E., Ph.D.
Department of Radiology, Medical College of Wisconsin, 8701 Watertown Plank Road, Milwaukee, WI 53226, USA
e-mail: aklein@mcw.edu

W.M. Mueller, M.D.
Department of Neurosurgery, Medical College of Wisconsin, Milwaukee, WI, USA

M. Maheshwari, M.D.
Children's Hospital and Health System, Medical College of Wisconsin, 9000 W. Wisconsin Avenue, Wauwatosa, WI 53226, USA

J.J. Pillai (ed.), *Functional Brain Tumor Imaging*, DOI 10.1007/978-1-4419-5858-7_6,

involved in implementing the technology. As such, a positive ***R*** represents resource gain while a negative value represents expenditure. Decision-makers generally include more than one entity, and the weighted interests and influence of the involved entities determine the value of the ***R*** term.

Using this formula helps explain why DTI has a high translatability. DTI has a high positive ***A*** value, or a superior clinical impact, because it is the most effective way to preoperatively visualize the relationships of white matter tracts to the resectable brain lesion. Details of this concept are covered later in the chapter. Because DTI is non-invasive, (***A–I***) is positive. Sequences are readily available on new MR systems and commercially available software makes workflow efficient and intuitive. Therefore, ***S*** is also positive. Although ***R*** may have a negative value in certain situations because of costs related to hardware or software upgrades to existing MRI scanners, this is easily overcome by the strongly positive clinical impact, ***A***, and the increasing realization that DTI for presurgical white matter mapping is becoming the standard of care. Institutions without DTI capability will eventually be vulnerable to the perception of inferior clinical care and undesirable medicolegal scenarios.

The ***C*** value, comfort level of practicing physicians in adopting the technology, is critical. The practicing physicians are primarily the neuroradiologists and neurosurgeons. White matter functional anatomy is becoming an integral component of neuroradiology fellowship programs. Thus, for the newly trained neuroradiologist, ***C*** is actually positive. For the practicing neuroradiologist trained before the era of presurgical brain mapping, additional training in white matter functional anatomy is not insurmountable. In fact, the momentum from the high translatability of DTI will necessitate training in these individuals, propelling a mildly negative ***C*** value to neutral or positive. The ***C*** value as it relates to the neurosurgeon is perhaps even more integral to the translation of DTI. It is the neurosurgeon who directly puts this technology to use. Neurosurgeons who have recently trained at academic centers with clinical DTI and functional MRI (fMRI) demand this technology. They bear witness to the positive results of presurgical brain mapping and rely on it. The ***C*** value as it relates to the neurosurgeon is becoming increasingly positive. Neurosurgeons trained before the era of presurgical brain mapping may continue to perform tumor resections without this technology. However, it is at the patient's disadvantage because DTI and presurgical brain mapping are the standard of care at many institutions.

Neurosurgery: Goals and Risks

The primary goals for neurosurgical resection of brain tumors are to establish a histological diagnosis and achieve maximal cyto-reduction. Because of the notorious histologic heterogeneity in gliomas, gross total resections are preferable to subtotal resections or biopsies for accurate diagnosis. With an accurate histologic diagnosis, the patient's prognosis as well as the optimal treatment algorithm can be established. Treatment algorithms may include adjuvant radiotherapy and/or chemotherapy. Maximal cyto-reduction has been theorized to decrease cell populations that could convert to higher grades [1, 2] and improve the effectiveness of adjuvant therapies by altering cell kinetics and reducing cell populations resistant to chemoradiation. In point of fact, resection extent of high-grade and low-grade gliomas has been shown to correlate with survival [1, 3–6]. In terms of quality of life, up to 53 % of glioma patients may show improved neurologic function after resection [7]. Surgical excision of primary brain tumors can also decrease steroid dependence and seizure activity.

These benefits of histological characterization and cyto-reduction must be weighed against the risks. Brain tumor resections do not carry an insignificant risk to the patient. Prior to the era of modern presurgical brain mapping, neurological complication rates for brain tumor resections ranged from 7 to 26 % [7–15]. The most feared complications include both impairments to elementary functions such as motor and vision, as well as higher cognitive functions such as speech, language, and memory. DTI and presurgical brain mapping have had a profound impact on this risk–benefit analysis.

During initial internal translation of presurgical DTI at the Medical College of Wisconsin (MCW) in 2004, a pilot study included 33 left dominant high-risk posterior frontal lobe tumors that were resected [16]. Eighteen patients had tumors resected prior to DTI implementation while 15 had their tumor resections after preoperative DTI was available. New speech and motor deficits occurred in 44 % of the former group and 47 % of the latter group. However, as is often the case in the immediate postoperative setting, transient deficits were seen and there was varying recovery of these functions for both groups. In the group without presurgical DTI, 39 % of patients had *persistent* speech and motor deficits at 1 month after surgery. This contrasts with persistent speech and motor deficits at 1 month in only 7 % of the presurgical DTI patients. It follows that presurgical DTI resulted in significantly better recovery of neurological function ($p<0.05$) following *high-risk* left frontal lobe tumor resections in age-, gender-, histology-, tumor size-, and location-matched controls performed by the same neurosurgeon with identical technique. The profound impact of DTI during this initial translation cemented its future at MCW for high-risk tumor cases with proximity to eloquent white matter structures. Since then, overall complication rates have fallen well below this 7 % benchmark [17].

Presurgical Mapping Process

Establishing an efficient workflow is necessary to create a reliable presurgical brain mapping service. Upon referral, usually by a neurosurgeon, neuropsychologist, or neurologist, the patient arrives for the DTI/fMRI exam. At this time, an outside MRI exam has already been loaded into the PACS or the patient hand carries a disc for the neuroradiologist to review. Upon review of the imaging, review of the electronic medical record, and direct patient interaction, the neuroradiologist selects specific mapping parameters including underlay anatomical sequences, the need for contrast, DTI protocol, and fMRI paradigms. The patient is then trained in the subselected fMRI paradigms, with any combination of language, motor, pre-motor, and vision categories. Patient experience for DTI is similar to conventional MR imaging and requires no special instructions. After the mapping data have been acquired, analyzed, and optimized for viewing, the neuroradiologist reviews the findings with the referring clinician(s). The mapping images are sent to the institutional PACS and then a decision is made whether or not to import the data into the intraoperative neuronavigation system. The presurgical mapping data then complement and guide intraoperative strategies, including white matter functional testing and electrocortical mapping.

Localization Sources

DTI is only one critical component of the presurgical and perioperative mapping process. There are five complementary preoperative and perioperative localization sources that establish functional network proximity risks necessary to preserve neurological function. These sources are clinical presentation, functional anatomy at standard imaging, presurgical functional mapping techniques (which include DTI), intraoperative functional white matter testing, and intraoperative electrocortical mapping. Each of these sources is imperfect alone, but can prove to be critical when combined with the others. Let us take a closer look.

Clinical presentation often yields valuable information regarding at-risk functional networks. Sources are available for detailed discussion of functional systems and lesion localization [18, 19]. The presenting neurologic deficit (sometimes associated with seizure) often indicates direct involvement or mass effect by tumor and/or edema upon a structure that is normally vital for carrying out that particular function. For example, a brain tumor patient presenting with a persistent or a transient seizure-induced language deficit indicates with a fairly high positive predictive value (PPV) that the lesion has proximity to eloquent structures. However, because of propagation of epileptogenic activity, the PPV is not 100 %. Assessments regarding the negative predictive value (NPV) in this capacity should not be made as seizures and deficits may be absent even though a lesion has proximity to eloquent structures.

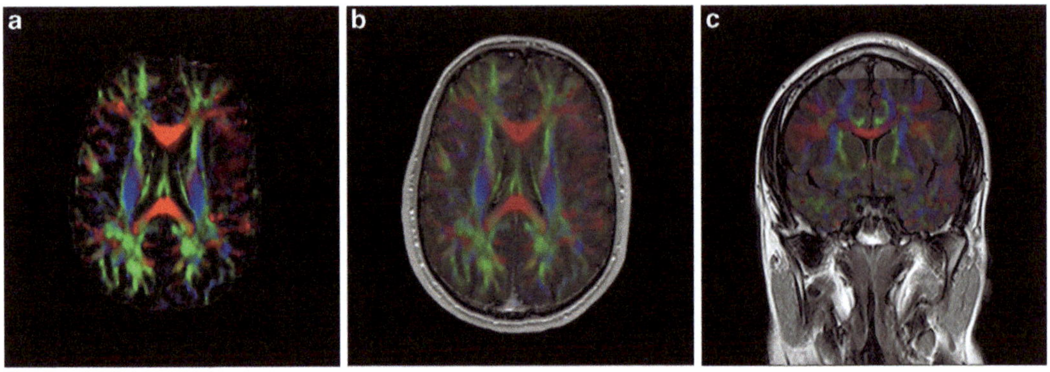

Fig. 6.1 (a) High-resolution axial color-coded FA map. (b) High-resolution axial color-coded FA map faded to 50 % and superimposed on an anatomic axial post-contrast SPGR image at the same slice location. (c) High-resolution coronal color-coded FA map superimposed on an anatomic coronal FLAIR image at the same slice location

Additionally, handedness determines the likelihood of left hemisphere language dominance [19, 20]. Right-handed individuals have a 98 % chance of being left hemisphere dominant for language function while left-handed individuals have a 67 % chance of being left dominant. The other 33 % of left-handers either are right hemisphere dominant for language or have shared hemisphere function. In the vast majority of patients, presenting neurologic deficit and handedness will accurately predict hemispheric language dominance. However, the importance of fMRI as a confirmatory test cannot be stressed enough. Consider that while 98 % of right-handed individuals are left hemisphere dominant for speech and language function, 2 % are not. That means for every 100 mapping cases performed on right-handers, two of them will have significant language function in the right hemisphere. Ignoring or not adequately scrutinizing language fMRI data could lead to significant postoperative speech and language impairment.

Knowledge of *functional anatomy at standard imaging* is critical in the interpretation of presurgical DTI data. In clinical practice, the color-coded FA maps are superimposed on anatomic imaging sequences to optimally characterize relationships of white matter structures to pathologic processes (Fig. 6.1a–c). For further discussion of color-coded FA maps see below. DTI by itself can be limited in establishing functional network proximity because of pathophysiologic constraints. For example, anatomic distortion of perilesional white matter from edema/infiltrating tumor may obscure and/or reorient tracts, making them difficult to discern at color-coded DTI (Fig. 6.2a, b). This is a frequent occurrence with high-grade gliomas. With the use of standard imaging, expected relationships of tracts to each other and to gyral and sulcal landmarks can help problem-solve and successfully predict functional network proximity when tract directions are altered or fractional anisotropy is nearly lost. In addition to aiding DTI interpretation, functional anatomy at standard imaging is key in the interpretation of fMRI, particularly in cases of decreased or absent cortical activation due to neurovascular uncoupling [21]. As mentioned previously, review of the pertinent functional anatomy on a patient's standard diagnostic MR exam can aid in the selection of specific fMRI paradigms.

Presurgical mapping anatomy techniques include DTI, fMRI, magnetoencephalography (MEG), WADA testing, positron emission tomography (PET), MRI, MR spectroscopy, and computed tomography (CT). The goal of these techniques is to preoperatively define spatial relationships between a lesion's borders and functional brain networks. At the heart of this lies the complementary duo of DTI and fMRI. DTI evaluates the white matter and fMRI evaluates the functional cortex. Value of DTI and fMRI data in a particular case usually depends upon the

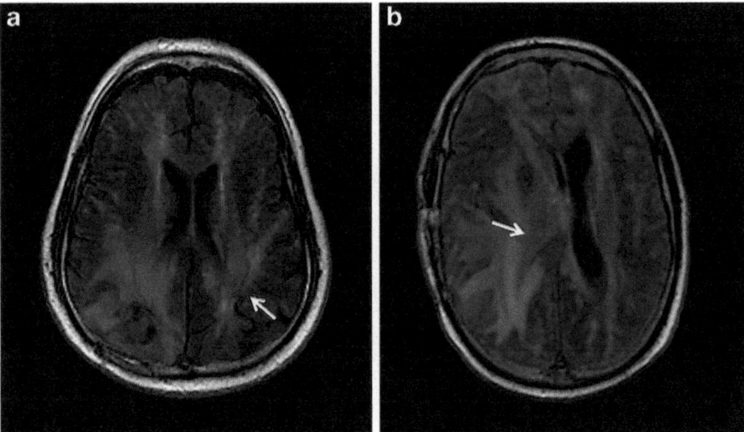

Fig. 6.2 Axial FLAIR images with superimposed, faded DTI data in two different patients with right-sided high-grade gliomas. In (**a**) perilesional tumor infiltration and/or edema results in markedly reduced white matter fractional aniosotropy. The right arcuate fasciculus cannot be confidently identified, unlike the preserved contralateral arcuate fasciculus (*white arrow*). In (**b**) a large right posterior temporal lobe lesion (not shown) creates marked mass effect on adjacent structures. Portions of the right corona radiata expected to contain corticospinal motor fibers are displaced transversely and appear *red* instead of *blue* (*white arrow*)

location of the lesion. Scenarios exist where cortical lesions have little proximity to functional white matter and deep lesions are remote to functional cortex. Most often, however, DTI and fMRI will provide useful and complementary information. Investigators found that the combined use of DTI, anatomic imaging, and fMRI was superior to anatomic imaging than fMRI alone for pre-operative functional system risk-proximity designations [22]. Optimal use of these techniques for presurgical brain mapping requires an understanding of the functional and dysfunctional anatomy. While there are good resources available for functional and dysfunctional anatomy reviews [18, 19], our understanding continues to evolve. Motor and vision functional networks are fairly well understood and have been deliberately avoided during neurosurgical procedures for many years. Primary motor cortex, SMA, corticospinal tracts, and corticobulbar tracts for motor function and visual cortex (especially occipital poles for central vision) and optic radiations (not Meyer's loop) for visual function constitute identifiable structures at presurgical mapping. Conversely, identifying speech/language cortical regions and white matter tracts is complicated by the fact that our understanding of these functional networks is much less concrete. fMRI can give us indirect evidence of cortical language areas, though it is complicated by a combination of factors including temporal resolution limits, paradigm contrast, lesion-induced neurovascular uncoupling, and other artifacts. Autoradiographic tract tracing and DTI studies in nonhuman primates have revealed a tremendous amount of detail regarding white matter tract organization [23, 24]. Much of this information is presumed to be transferable to the human brain. Unfortunately, the lack of speech and language capabilities in nonhuman primates remains a major obstacle in applying these data to the human language system. Emerging theories of ventral and dorsal language streams [25–27] may aid in establishing which association tracts are necessary and thus to be avoided during surgery. At our institution, components of the dominant superior longitudinal fasciculus (SLF) including the arcuate fasciculus (AF) are considered eloquent structures and are intentionally preserved at the time of neurosurgical resections.

Intraoperative localization techniques include *functional white matter testing* and *electrocortical mapping*. When used in conjunction with lesion border-risk designations derived from

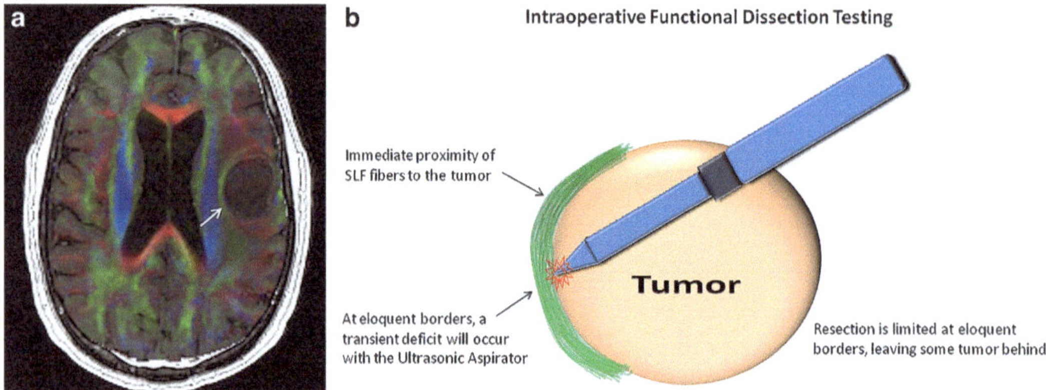

Fig. 6.3 In (**a**) there is a cystic lesion within the left frontal white matter. Horizontal fibers of the SLF (*white arrow*) are displaced and have immediate proximity to the medial border of the lesion. In a *left* hemisphere language dominant patient, this is considered a high-risk surgical resection. (**b**) illustrates the method of intraoperative functional dissection testing for this high-risk medial tumor border. Using lesion border-risk information derived from presurgical DTI, language function is tested while the neurosurgeon dissects with the ultrasonic aspirator. If a transient language deficit occurs, an impending permanent deficit is likely if dissection is continued along that plane. Therefore, functional *white* fibers along this border are spared and some tumor is left behind

presurgical mapping, these techniques can be utilized most efficiently. The neurosurgeon can tailor the use of these intraoperative localization techniques based upon the presurgical mapping data and thus reduce operation times. For example, the neurosurgeon can specifically test language and motor functions while dissecting along a lesion's high-risk borders. Intraoperative electrical stimulation is one method used for functional white matter testing [28, 29]. At MCW, intraoperative functional dissection testing is performed. In conjunction with lesion border-risk designations derived from presurgical DTI, an ultrasonic aspirator is used that not only provides tissue fragmentation, irrigation, aspiration, and coagulation but also has a close-distance nonlethal and transient effect on neuronal tissue (Fig. 6.3a, b). If the patient develops a transient speech or language deficit upon dissection, impending functional white matter injury is predicted only millimeters beyond the dissection plane. A transient deficit limits resection along that tumor border. However, if a tumor border is deemed to be free of eloquent white matter at preoperative DTI, a grossly clean margin will be dissected using the ultrasonic aspirator. Intraoperative electrocortical mapping has its own advantages and disadvantages. This technique is not susceptible to the effects of neurovascular uncoupling and is especially valuable in cases where lack of cortical activation due to neurovascular uncoupling is suspected on presurgical fMRI [21, 30]. However, electrocortical mapping is limited in reaching eloquent cortex due to pial barriers and can be compromised by perilesional seizure induction. Electrocortical mapping and functional white matter testing are powerful tools, made more powerful by presurgical mapping data.

DTI Protocols, Acquisition

For CC-FA maps, a dual-refocused spin echo technique is used to minimize distortions and maximize signal-to-noise ratio (SNR). DTI resolution is determined by readout time and gradient strength. Diffusion weighting and higher resolution reduce SNR. Greater diffusion gradient encoding directions lengthen the duration of the DTI scan. At least 6 orthogonal gradient encoding directions are required to construct a diffusion ellipsoid, but 12 or more are preferred to minimize directional under-sampling at fiber crossings and at acute angulations. However, some venders only allow odd numbers of encoding directions for reasons of colinearity. The

CC-FA sequence protocols at MCW were designed by *Wolfgang Gaggl* in his capacity as research engineer. At 1.5T, 3 separate data sets with 3 mm slice thickness, 13 gradient encoding directions, *b* value of 900, NEX of 2, TE of 70 ms, and TR min of 11 s are used to acquire a total of 40 contiguous slices. Typically, 128 × 128 matrix and an FOV = 20–24 cm will be acquired, with in-plane resolution generally at 1.8 × 1.8 mm. Some vendors will automatically interpolate the DTI data to 256 × 256, which has a smoothing effect. Acquisition time is 5.5 min for each data set, with a total time of 16.5 min for all three data sets. The *Gaggl* modular approach provides the latitude to modify the slice thickness and gain necessary for adequate SNR simply by changing the number of runs. Three averaged data sets at 1.5T provide an SNR equivalent to a single run with an NEX = 6, with SNR to spare. If a patient can only withstand one or two 5.5-min acquisitions, the data are aesthetically compromised, but still diagnostic. For 2.5 and 2 mm slice thicknesses, however, four and six averaged 5.5-min data sets, respectively, are required to achieve diagnostic SNR. Movement between data acquisitions can be corrected in post-processing. The DTI data are suitable, though not optimal, for fiber tracking if needed (see fiber tracking section below).

At 3T MRI sequence parameters are similar, though slice thickness is typically reduced, higher TR may be needed, *b* value = 1,000 or greater, and up to 50 slices are acquired. For 3 mm slice thickness, two data sets are averaged, but we generally acquire data at 2 mm slice thickness requiring three acquisitions to achieve nearly isotropic voxels of 1.87 × 1.87 × 2 mm with sufficient signal. DTI data at 1.5T or 3T are acquired in the axial plane and reconstructed in coronal and sagittal planes and superimposed onto desired underlay images for all cases. Because DTI is acquired with other mapping data, including fMRI, patients with prior surgeries or biopsies are scanned at 1.5T to reduce susceptibility. Sequence parameters are customized to optimize patient compliance and minimize motion effects, depending on the length of time required to acquire DTI and other mapping data. Generally though, three runs at 3 mm (1.5T) or 2 mm (3T) slice thicknesses suffice.

DTI Data Visualization

DTI is rooted in the concept that white matter microstructure, primarily axons, provides a barrier for random diffusion of water molecules. By acquiring data along at least six different gradient directions, ellipsoids representing relative directional movements of water can be calculated. Each ellipsoid is defined by one major and two minor eigenvectors based on the major and minor directions of water movement. The ellipsoid, or diffusion tensor, is the basis by which relative directional information of white matter can be displayed on a voxel-by-voxel basis.

Information from the three components of the diffusion tensor vector can be displayed in color-coded FA maps. These maps enable one to visualize the anatomic organization of white matter tracts with the added value of directionality. At any one voxel on the image, one of the three colors is assigned according to the eigenvector with the greatest eigenvalue. By convention, green represents the anteroposterior (or posteroanterior) direction, red the transverse (right to left or left to right) direction, and blue the craniocaudal (or caudocranial) direction [31]. Color intensities are scaled in relation to the magnitude of the FA value. A benefit of color-coded FA maps is the ability to visualize global white matter architecture by the same method conventional MR images are displayed, i.e., in the axial, coronal, and sagittal planes. With a thorough understanding of white matter anatomy, a tremendous amount of valuable information can be garnered prior to surgery. DTI atlases are available for a detailed illustration of white matter anatomy [32]. At our institution, the color-coded FA map is the primary method by which DTI data are utilized in the presurgical mapping process.

Fiber tracking, or tractography, is an additional means of displaying DTI data. A three-dimensional representation of a white matter tract is constructed based on the directionality information derived from FA values. Using mathematical algorithms, fiber tract trajectories are estimated based on the major eigenvector at sampled locations, propagating from a "seed point." Numerous different DTI tractography algorithms have been proposed in the literature, either deterministic or probabilistic [33–37]. The former method only uses the best estimate of the major eigenvector to propagate the fiber trajectories, while the latter includes a method for estimating and displaying the uncertainty in propagation between two points. Most commercially available fiber tracking software packages coupled with scanners have a deterministic mathematical algorithm.

A unique characteristic of fiber tracking is the capability of distinguishing specific functional white matter tracts [38–40]. For example, fiber tracking can help display the relative position of the corticospinal motor fibers within the corona radiata, distinguishing it from adjacent functionally distinct sensory and thalamocortical fibers [41]. All of these fibers demonstrate a blue appearance on color-coded FA maps. Although the relative position of corticospinal motor fibers can be estimated on color-coded FA maps with a knowledge of white matter anatomical organization, fiber tracking enables a more explicit visual demonstration. In a clinical setting, fiber tracking has been shown to distinguish specific white matter tracts adjacent to brain tumors [42–44]. One could argue that the more information the neurosurgeon has prior to surgery regarding spatial relationships of specific functional white matter tracts to the resectable lesion, the more confident and efficient he/she can be with intraoperative subcortical white matter testing. This could lead to shorter operation times and better outcomes.

There are limitations of DTI which affect interpretation of both color-coded FA maps and tractography. Crossing fiber tracts present a challenge for current DTI algorithms. Because tract orientation information for a single voxel is based on the major eigenvector, the DTI model fails to accommodate complex intra-voxel heterogeneity resulting from multiple fiber populations within each voxel. For example, the compact horizontal portion of the superior longitudinal fasciculus hinders identification of cortico-bulbar fiber as they originate from the lower precentral gyrus, traverse the superior longitudinal fasciculus, and emerge as part of the corona radiata. Therefore, an understanding of white matter anatomy is critical in the interpretation of DTI, knowing what information can and cannot be depicted. Newer diffusion imaging techniques such as high angular diffusion imaging (HARDI) show promise in better resolving crossing tracts and could be on the horizon for clinical translation [45–48]. However, these techniques also have limitations, namely, long imaging times and complex post-processing. Acute fiber angulations at the interface between cortex and white matter also pose a challenge for current DTI techniques. This limits the ability to determine exact fiber origins and terminations, a critical component of fiber tracking. Pathophysiologic factors including tumor and edema can reduce anisotropy and hinder depiction of white matter tracts while mass effect from either of these can cause regional changes in tract orientation [40, 49]. The fact that DTI data are influenced by the underlying pathology makes understanding the technical aspects so critical in interpretation. Finally, DTI with echoplanar imaging is exquisitely sensitive to regional field distortions at bone– or air–tissue interfaces and susceptibility artifact from hemorrhage, surgical hardware, and metal (Fig. 6.4a). This has important implications in presurgical brain mapping when determining lesion border-risk assessments. Superimposing DTI data onto anatomical MR images is critical in evaluating the magnitude of geometric distortions. While higher order shimming may help minimize these distortions (Figs. 6.4b, c), overlay nudge functions may be used to realign DTI data to their corresponding white matter structures on MRI when these distortions exist in the vicinity of a lesion. Optimized re-registration of the two data sets should be centered at the surgical lesion. New acquisition and post-processing techniques addressing the issue of DTI geometric distortions have been proposed [50, 51].

A few points of caution specifically regarding fiber tracking need to be addressed. It is important to remember that the 3-D depictions of fiber trajectories at tractography do not correspond to individual axons. They are merely indirect visual representations of the major eigenvector within

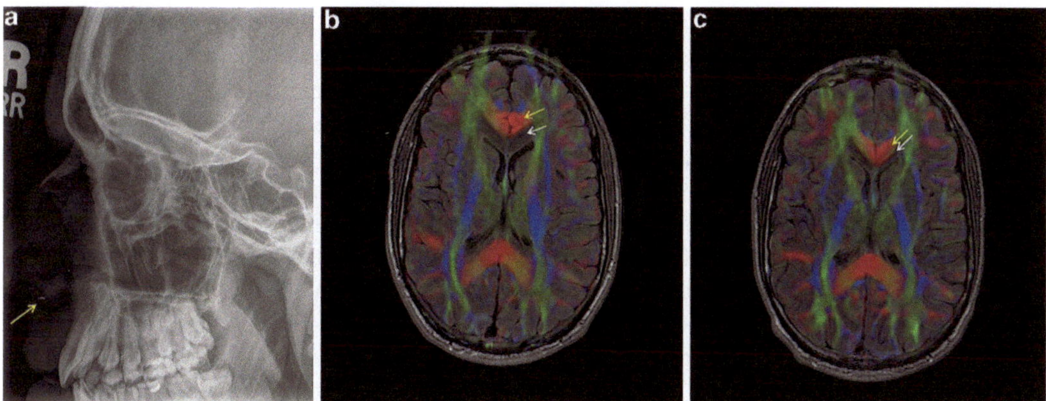

Fig. 6.4 (**a**) Plain X-ray of the face shows a small metallic foreign body in the inferior nasal soft tissues. Axial FLAIR images with superimposed color-coded FA maps obtained without (**b**) and with (**c**) higher order shimming. Regional frontal field distortions in (**b**) are minimized in (**c**). Notice how the distortions result in the *red* corpus callosum genu fibers (*yellow arrow*) on DTI to be located anterior to its corresponding anatomic structure (*white arrow*) on FLAIR imaging. The DTI technique is exquisitely sensitive to metallic susceptibility artifact, even when the object is extracranial. Higher order shimming can reduce distortions

voxels propagated along the course of the white matter tract. Due to limitations in spatial resolution at MR imaging, the 3-D tract components are much larger than the actual size of the axons. Additionally, relying disproportionately on fiber tracking results can lead to false-negative judgments about lesion border-risk assessments. For example, peri-tumoral edema or tumor infiltration of white matter may reduce the anisotropy below the designated threshold for the tractography algorithm. This leads to erroneous termination of fibers at tractography when in fact the fibers may still exist. Lowering the anisotropy threshold to enable propagation of the tract through low-anisotropy regions does not optimally solve this problem because it results in reduced accuracy of the major eigenvector [52]. Further, image noise, crossing fiber populations, and diverging/converging trajectories all can alter the orientation of the major eigenvector and cause falsely premature termination of a fiber tract [53, 54].

The importance of a high NPV for lesion border-risk assessments cannot be overstated. Because of intraoperative white matter stimulation techniques, presurgical DTI does not need to have a high PPV of critical functional network proximity to resectable brain lesions. In other words, a false-positive prediction of functional white matter proximity to the lesion at DTI will not cause harm to the patient. The lesion border in question can be further evaluated by intraoperative stimulation and functional testing. However, presurgical DTI does need a high NPV. A false-negative prediction at DTI could lead to failure to test functions along a dissection border and consequent injury to critical white matter structures. In a recent study of ten patients with low-grade gliomas or malformations near language tracts, 17 of 21 (81 %) intraoperative subcortical stimulations were concordant with presurgical fiber tracking results [55]. Negative fiber tracking does not rule out the presence of a fiber tract, especially when invaded by tumor. This underscores a crucial advantage of color-coded FA maps over fiber tracking. With the former, there is no loss of data, minimizing the chance for a false-negative prediction. Global white matter anatomic visualization with color-coded FA maps remains an important feature of presurgical brain mapping. An understanding of the limitations of DTI and fiber tracking is necessary to prevent postsurgical functional deficits. As a complementary technique, DTI can help intraoperative assessments strive for an NPV of 100 %.

DTI Interpretation

Neurosurgeons are interested in identifying sensorimotor, premotor, vision, and language functional networks and their relationships to the resectable lesion. Attempts have been made to estimate "safe" distances between a lesion border and functional cortex or white matter on fMRI and DTI studies, respectively. However, there is no accepted "safe" distance. In fact, with the phenomenon of brain shifting at the time of surgery, it is dangerous to quantify preoperative distances and apply them to the intraoperative setting. DTI and fMRI are best used for qualitative assessment of spatial relationships.

When interpreting DTI preoperatively, it is important to describe the relationships of white matter tracts to the lesion. If there are enhancing and nonenhancing components to the lesion, white matter relationships are described relative to each of these components. The term "immediate proximity" is used to describe a tract contacting or within a few millimeters to a lesion border. This relationship conveys to the neurosurgeon that there is a high likelihood of tract injury along this dissection border if caution is not exercised, caution perhaps in the form of functional white matter testing. "Relative proximity" is used to describe a relationship with the tract/lesion border distance somewhere between "immediate" and "remote." Precisely defining these qualitative assessments in terms of distance is fraught with error, as reasoned above. If the procedure is to be performed awake, and a tract with lesion border proximity is amenable to intraoperative functional testing, the neurosurgeon can test this function as he/she dissects along that lesion border.

In an effort to establish consistent terminology with description of pathologically altered white matter tracts at DTI, five terms have been proposed with their corresponding appearances [56]. "Deviation" refers to a tract with altered course secondary to bulk mass effect. "Infiltration" refers to any portion of the tract with reduced anisotropy, but otherwise preserved order and morphology. Both tumor infiltration and edema infiltration can have a similar appearance, and often coexist. "Interruption" describes discontinuity of a tract on tractography or color-coded FA maps. "Interruption" is preferred over the term "destruction" as this latter term can have a misleading presumption of loss of white matter function. "Degeneration" is used to describe a tract with significantly reduced size and/or anisotropy remote from a lesion affecting the same neural pathway. This is the same concept as Wallerian degeneration. Finally, "splaying" refers to a tract separated by a lesion into distinct fiber components, deviated from the expected trajectory.

Often times in the case of high-grade gliomas, it can be difficult to distinguish non-enhancing tumor from edema and treatment change (if applicable). All three of these entities appear hyperintense on FLAIR imaging. In cases of a highly aggressive lesion with proximity to critical functional white matter structures, debulking the enhancing component of the lesion with preservation of adjacent functional tracts becomes the primary goal. Establishing border relationships to the enhancing component at DTI is critical. For optimal visualization, color-coded FA maps are faded to 50 % and superimposed on anatomic FLAIR images and post-contrast SPGR images (if the lesion enhances).

Case Illustration: 64-year-old right-handed man with progressive right visual field difficulties, word finding problems, and headache. MRI of the brain was performed that demonstrates a heterogeneous rim-enhancing left parieto-occipital mass with extensive mass effect and surrounding abnormal signal (Fig. 6.5a). The patient was presumed to be left hemisphere dominant for speech and language given his symptoms and right-handedness. Speech and language fMRI confirmed this. Prior to surgery, DTI was performed to better characterize relationships of white matter tracts to the lesion. DTI data faded and superimposed on post-contrast SPGR images show that the anterior border of the enhancing mass has immediate proximity to the vertical fibers of the arcuate fasciculus (white arrow), the bundle of fibers containing FOF, ILF, and optic radiations (yellow arrow), and the tapetum (dashed white arrow) (Fig. 6.5b). The medial border of the mass has immediate proximity to forceps major, which is deviated slightly mesially (dashed yellow arrow). DTI data faded and super-

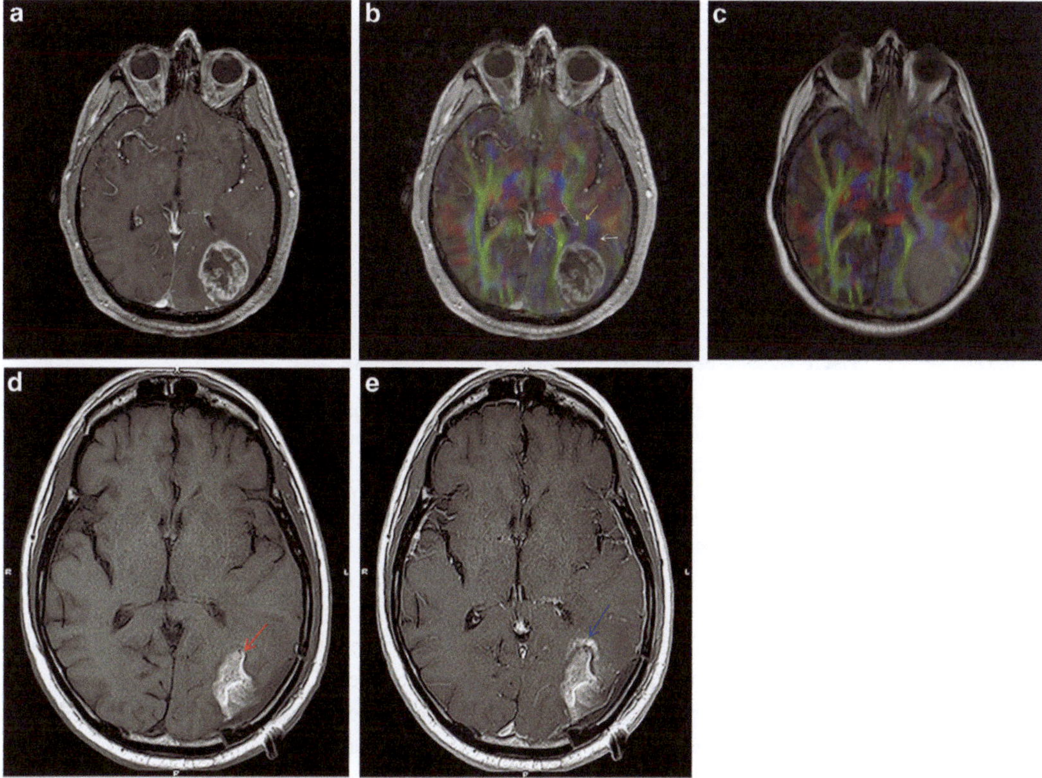

Fig. 6.5 DTI case illustration (**a**–**e**)

imposed on FLAIR imaging best show infiltration of these bordering tracts manifested by FLAIR hyperintensity and asymmetrically reduced anisotropy (Fig. 6.5c). These border assessments have implications for language (arcuate fasciculus), semantic language function (FOF), visual memory (ILF), and vision (optic radiations).

Surgery was performed under general anesthesia as the patient was not able to tolerate an awake procedure. Axial pre-contrast T1-weighted image of the brain following surgery reveals a blood-filled resection cavity with T1 shortening (red arrow) (Fig. 6.5d). Axial post-contrast image at the same level demonstrates a small amount of residual enhancing neoplasm along the anterior margin of the cavity (blue arrow), at the known interface of vertical fibers of the arcuate fasciculus, bundle of fibers containing the FOF, ILF, and optic radiations, and the tapetum (Fig. 6.5e). Frozen sections of the tumor during the operation were consistent with high-grade glioma. The neurosurgeon opted for a subtotal tumor resection with preservation of language (arcuate fasciculus) and central vision (optic radiations) functions, especially considering that cure was not possible with this aggressive lesion and intraoperative functional testing could not be utilized. Subsequent final histopathological diagnosis was glioblastoma multiforme.

Case illustration: 38-year-old male presented to an outside emergency department with left foot weakness. An MRI was performed revealing an enhancing intra-axial mass centered within the subcortical white matter of the right paracentral lobule. The patient was referred for presurgical brain mapping, including DTI and fMRI. Evaluation of the DTI data faded and superimposed on anatomic axial (Fig. 6.6a) and coronal (Fig. 6.6b) post-contrast images reveals a ball-in-glove configuration (Fig. 6.6c). Right-sided corticospinal motor fibers are displaced about the mass and have immediate proximity to the lesion's borders, making this a high-risk surgical lesion. The superior precentral gyrus (with

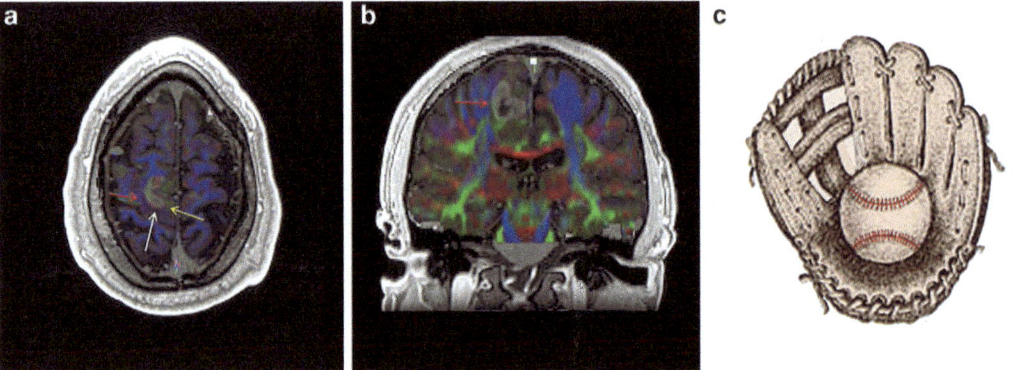

Fig. 6.6 (**a**, **b**) High-risk "ball-in-glove" case illustration. (**c**) Ball-in-glove drawing. A commonly encountered phenomenon in presurgical mapping of white matter for glioma patients (and often other tumors) is the "ball-in-glove" configuration. Because gliomas are white matter-based lesions, and often round, they displace tracts about their periphery. The configuration is similar to a "ball-in-glove" with the lesion mimicking a baseball and the white matter tracts mimicking the palm and finger extensions of a baseball glove. This visualization can help the neurosurgeon, especially if specific tract border designations are described

corticospinal fibers) wraps around the posteromedial (yellow arrow), posterior (white arrow), and posterolateral (red arrow) borders of the mass. Upon scrolling through the images, the corticospinal fibers continue to course along the posterior-inferior border of the mass (not shown). An awake neurosurgical resection with functional white matter testing was performed to best address these high-risk lesion border designations. Transient intraoperative left leg paresis occurred during dissection along the posteromedial tumor border. Consequently, the neurosurgeon opted to leave a small amount of residual tumor at this location. The neurosurgeon was able to use a priori knowledge of lesion border designations from DTI in conjunction with intraoperative functional white matter dissection testing to avoid injury to the corticospinal fibers, avoiding hemiparesis in this high-risk surgical patient. Final histopathologic diagnosis was anaplastic astrocytoma.

Recent and Future Directions

One of the more recent advances with DTI and fMRI is the ability to import mapping data into neuronavigation systems. This allows the neurosurgeon real-time and interactive access to spatial relationships between the lesion and functional systems. Some of the neuronavigation systems incorporate their own basic DTI and fMRI processing software. However, lack of compatibility between other commercially available DTI/fMRI software and the select few neuronavigation platforms has proven to be an obstacle for the widespread use of this powerful technology. Some headway has been made in overcoming this proprietary hitch, but not without temporary concession (Fig. 6.7). Forging ahead is the only reasonable solution as intraoperative use of presurgical mapping data has already displayed its strengths. Not only is there is a high correlation (but not perfect) between results of preoperative DTI data used intraoperatively with intraoperative subcortical mapping [57], but also use of preoperative DTI in neuronavigation has been shown to significantly improve postsurgical outcome and survival in glioma patients [58]. Further, subcentimeter spatial agreement (8.7 ± 3.1 mm) between neuronavigational DTI and subcortical white matter stimulation has been demonstrated, though it will be compromised by brain shift at craniotomy and throughout the resection [59]. It is clear that going forward, neuronavigation represents an important element in the evolution of clinical functional imaging [60].

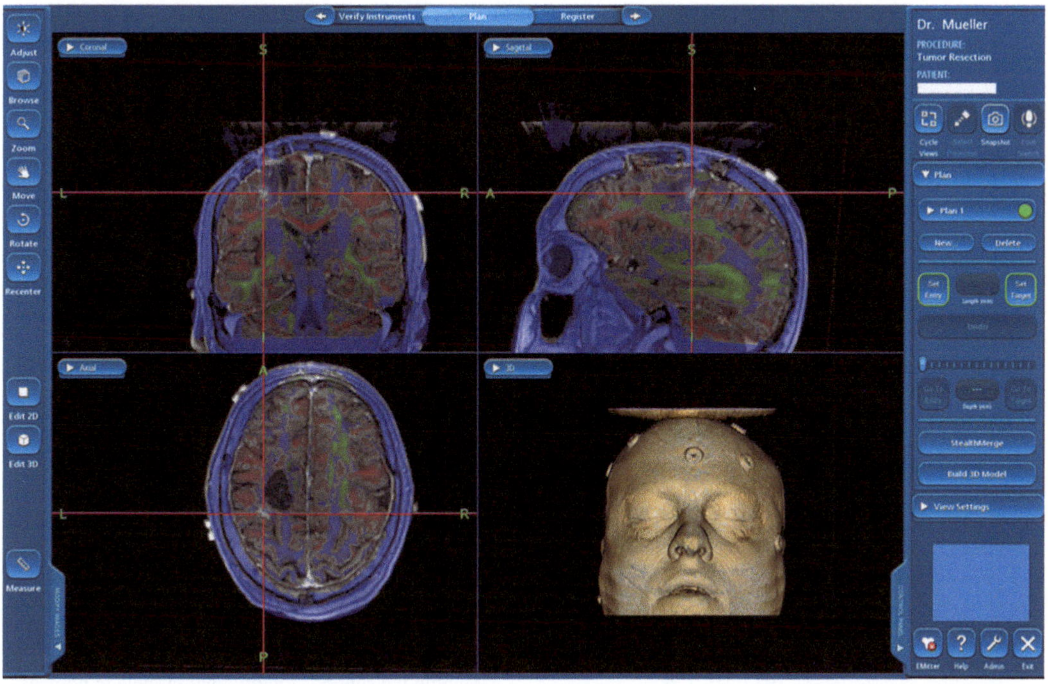

Fig. 6.7 Screen capture from a neuronavigation system with imported commercially distinct brain mapping software data. Color-coded DTI data are superimposed on conventional post-contrast MR images. Notice how there are numerous scattered areas throughout the white matter without the expected *red*, *blue*, or *green* FA designation. The neuronavigation system does not permit the import of full 24-bit color (RGB) information, and as a result the reduced-resolution imagery permitted appears crude (*dark*). The interpolation methods utilized to reconstruct 3D information in the neuronavigation system do not handle color-coded information correctly, resulting in artifactual (interpolated) values (colors). Work-arounds for this problem include using lower resolution imagery, avoiding interpolation by "burning in" the functional information onto anatomical background imagery, and utilizing somewhat shifted color schemes to minimize the appearance of interpolated artifacts. Unfortunately, there is little incentive for the relatively few neuronavigation companies to resolve compatibility issues with the more numerous commercially available DTI/fMRI software packages, especially considering that the neuronavigation systems have some form of proprietary packaged DTI/fMRI processing software (courtesy of J. Reuss and R. Pyritz)

Summary

Successful clinical translation of DTI is evidence of its vital role in presurgical brain mapping and positive effect on neurosurgical outcomes. By helping establish spatial relationships between specific lesion borders and functional networks prior to and during surgery, DTI is cementing its role in high-risk neurosurgical resections and becoming the standard of care. Future improvements may include intraoperative functional MR imaging data acquisition with the use of high-field intraoperative systems, possibly with real-time brain-shift correction. Quantification of DTI data, further use of additional DTI parameters such as radial and axial diffusivity, and improved fiber tracking algorithms are likely on the horizon as well. In the meantime, the application of presurgical brain mapping will continue to be the anchor for the technology and revolutionize the way we care for neurosurgical patients.

References

1. Smith JS, Chang EF, Lamborn KR, et al. Role of extent of resection in the long-term outcome of low-grade hemispheric gliomas. J Clin Oncol. 2008;26: 1338–45.
2. Bernstein M, Berger M. Neurooncology: the essentials. 2nd ed. New York, NY: Thieme; 2008.

3. Lacroix M, Abi-Said D, Fourney DR, et al. A multivariate analysis of 416 patients with glioblastoma multiforme: prognosis, extent of resection, and survival. J Neurosurg. 2001;95:190–8.
4. Stummer W, Pichlmeier U, Meinel T, ALA-Glioma Study Group, et al. Fluorescence-guided surgery with 5-aminolevulinic acid for resection of malignant glioma: a randomized controlled multicentre phase III trial. Lancet Oncol. 2006;7:392–401.
5. Ryken TC, Frankel B, Julien T, et al. Surgical management of newly diagnosed glioblastoma in adults: role of cytoreductive surgery. J Neurooncol. 2008;89: 271–86.
6. Claus EB, Horlacher A, Hsu L, et al. Survival rates in patients with low-grade glioma after intraoperative magnetic resonance image guidance. Cancer. 2005;103:1227–33.
7. Chang S, Parney IF, McDermott M, et al. Perioperative complications and neurological outcome of first versus second craniotomy among patients enrolled in the Glioma Outcomes Project. J Neurosurg. 2003;98: 1175–81.
8. Ciric I, Ammirati M, Vick N, et al. Supratentorial gliomas: surgical considerations and immediate postoperative results. Gross total resection versus partial resection. Neurosurgery. 1987;21:21–6.
9. Fadul C, Wood J, Thaler H, et al. Morbidity and mortality for excision of supratentorial gliomas. Neurology. 1988;38:1374–9.
10. Sawaya R, Hammoud M, Schoppa D, et al. Neurosurgical outcomes in a modern series of 400 craniotomies for treatment parenchymal tumors. Neurosurgery. 1998;42:1044–55.
11. Brell M, Ibanez J, Caral L, et al. Factors influencing surgical complications of intra-axial brain tumors. Acta Neurochir (Wien). 2000;142:739–50.
12. Deveaux BC, O'Fallon JR, Kelly PR. Resection, biopsy, and survival in malignant glial neoplasms: a retrospective study of clinical parameters, therapy, and outcome. J Neurosurg. 1993;78(5):767–75.
13. Vorster SJ, Barnett GH. A proposed preoperative grading scheme to assess risk for surgical resection of primary and secondary intraaxial brain tumors. Neurosurg. 1998 Focus 4, article 2.
14. Taylor MD, Berstein M. Awake craniotomy with brain mapping as the routine surgical approach to treating patients with supratentorial intraaxial tumors: a prospective trial of 200 cases. J Neurosurg. 1999;90:35–41.
15. Bohinski RJ, Kokkino AK, Warnick RE, et al. Glioma resection in a shared resource operating room after optimal image-guided frameless stereotactic resection. Neurosurgery. 2001;48:731–42.
16. Mueller W. DTI for neurosurgeons: cases and concepts. 2010 International brain mapping and intraoperative surgical planning society (IBMISPS) brain, spinal cord mapping and image guided therapy conference, 27 May 2010, Bethesda, MN; 2010
17. Ulmer JL, Berman JI, Mueller, WM, et al. Issues in translating imaging technology and presurgical diffusion tensor imaging. In: Faro SH, Mohamed FB, Law M, Ulmer JL, editors. Functional neuroradiology: principles and clinical applications. 1st ed. Springer; 2011.
18. Aralasmak A, Ulmer JL, Kocak M, et al. Association commissural, and projection pathways and their functional deficit reported in literature. J Comput Assist Tomogr. 2006;30(5):695–716.
19. Brazos PW, Masdeu JC, Biller J. Localization in clinical neurology. 5th ed. Philadelphia: Lippincott Williams & Wilkins; 2007.
20. Oldfield RC. The assessment and analysis of handedness: the Edinburgh inventory. Neuropsychologia. 1971;9:97–113.
21. Ulmer JL, Hacein-Bey L, Mathews VP, et al. Lesion-induced pseudo-dominance at fMRI: implications for pre-operative assessments. Neurosurgery. 2004;55:569–81.
22. Ulmer JL, Salvan CV, Mueller WM, et al. The role of diffusion tensor imaging in establishing the proximity of tumor borders to functional brain systems: implications for preoperative risk assessments and postoperative outcomes. Technol Cancer Res Treat. 2004;3:567–76.
23. Schmahmann JD, Pandya DN. Fiber pathways of the brain. New York: Oxford University Press; 2006.
24. Makris N, et al. Segmentation of subcomponents within the superior longitudinal fascicle in humans: a quantitative, in vivo, DT-MRI study. Cereb Cortex. 2005;15(6):854–69.
25. Price CJ. The anatomy of language: contributions from functional neuroimaging. J Anat. 2000;197(Pt 3):335–59.
26. Hickok G, Poeppel D. Dorsal and ventral streams: a framework for understanding aspects of the functional anatomy of language. Cognition. 2004;92:67–99.
27. Duffau H. New insights into the anatomo-functional connectivity of the semantic system: a study using cortico-subcortical electrostimulations. Brain. 2005;128:797–810.
28. Berger M. Minimalism through intraoperative functional mapping. Clin Neurosurg. 1996;43:324–37.
29. Duffau H, et al. Intraoperative mapping of the subcortical language pathways using direct stimulations. Brain. 2002;125(1):199–214.
30. Ulmer JL, Krouwer HG, Mueller WM, et al. Pseudo-reorganization of language cortical function at FMR Imaging: a consequence of tumor-induced neurovascular uncoupling. AJNR Am J Neuroradiol. 2003;24:213–7.
31. Pajevic S, Pierpaoli C. Color schemes to represent the orientation of anisotropic tissues from diffusion tensor data: application to white matter fiber tract mapping of the human brain. Magn Reson Med. 1999;42:526–40.
32. Klein AP. Diffusion tensor imaging atlas of the brain. In: Faro SH, Mohamed FB, Law M, Ulmer JL, editors. Functional neuroradiology: principles and clinical applications. 1st ed. Springer; 2011.
33. Mori S, Crain BJ, Chacko VP, et al. Three dimensional tracking of axonal projections in the brain by magnetic resonance imaging. Ann Neurol. 1999;45:265–9.

34. Conturo TE, Lori NF, Cull TS, et al. Tracking neuronal fiber pathways in the living human brain. Proc Natl Acad Sci U S A. 1999;96:10422–7.
35. Basser P, Pajevic S, Pierpaoli C. In vivo fiber tractography using DT-MRI data. Magn Reson Med. 2000;44:625–32.
36. Lazar M, Alexander A. Bootstrap white matter tractography (BOOT-TRAC). Neuroimage. 2005;24:524–32.
37. Parker G, Haroon H, Wheelr-Kingshott C. A framework for a streamline-based probabilistic index of connectivity (PICo) using a structural interpretation of MRI diffusion measurements. J Magn Reson Imaging. 2003;18:242–54.
38. Mori S, Kaufmann WE, Davatzikos C, et al. Imaging cortical association tracts in the human brain using diffusion-tensor-based axonal tracking. Magn Reson Med. 2002;47:215–23.
39. Catani M, Howard RJ, Pajevic S, Jones DK. Virtual in vivo interactive dissection of white matter fasciculi in the human brain. Neuroimage. 2002;17:77–94.
40. Jellison BJ, Field AS, Medow J, Lazar M, Salamat MS, Alexander AL. Diffusion tensor imaging of cerebral white matter: a pictorial review of physics, fiber tract anatomy, and tumor imaging patterns. AJNR Am J Neuroradiol. 2004;25:356–69.
41. Han BS, Hong JH, Hong C, et al. Location of the corticospinal tract at the corona radiata in human brain. Brain Res. 2010;1326:75–80.
42. Holodny A, Schwartz T, Ollenschleger M, et al. Tumor involvement of the corticospinal tract: diffusion magnetic resonance tractography with intraoperative correlation. J Neurosurg. 2001;95:1082.
43. Clark C, Barrick T, Murphy M, et al. White matter fiber tracking in patients with space-occupying lesions of the brain: a new technique for neurosurgical planning? Neuroimage. 2003;20:1601–8.
44. Berman J, Berger M, Mukherjee P, et al. Diffusion-tensor imaging-guided tracking of fibers of the pyramidal tract combined with intraoperative cortical stimulation mapping in patients with gliomas. J Neurosurg. 2004;101:66–72.
45. Tuch D. Q-ball imaging. Magn Reson Med. 2004;52: 1358–72.
46. Frank LR. Characterization of anisotropy in high angular resolution diffusion-weighted MRI. Magn Reson Med. 2002;47:1083–99.
47. Tournier J, Calamante F, Gadian D, et al. Direct estimation of the fiber orientation density function from diffusion-weighted MRI data using spherical deconvolution. Neuroimage. 2004;23:1176–85.
48. Wedeen VJ, Hagmann P, Tseng W, et al. Mapping comlex tissue architecture with diffusion spectrum magnetic resonance imaging. Magn Reson Med. 2005;54:1377–86.
49. Tropine A, Vucurevic G, Delani P, et al. Contribution of diffusion tensor imaging to delineation of gliomas and glioblastomas. J Magn Reson Imaging. 2004;6:905–12.
50. Wang FN, Huang TY, Lin FH, et al. PROPELLER EPI: an MRI technique suitable for diffusion tensor imaging at high field strength with reduced geometric distortions. Magn Reson Med. 2005;54(5):1232–40.
51. Gaggl W, Jesmanowicz A, Prost RW. *Eddy Current correction in diffusion tensor imaging using phase-correction in k-space*. Annual meeting of the organization for human brain mapping, 18–23 June 2009, San Francisco, USA; 2009.
52. Basser PJ, Pajevic S. Statistical artifacts in diffusion tensor MRI (DT-MRI) caused by background noise. Magn Reson Med. 2000;44:41–50.
53. Anderson A. Theoretical analysis of the effects of noise on diffusion tensor imaging. Magn Reson Med. 2001;46:1174–88.
54. Lazar M, Alexander A. Divergence/convergence effects on the accuracy of white matter tractography algorithms. ISMRM 2003; Toronto, Canada p. 2160.
55. Leclercq D, Duffau H, et al. Comparison of diffusion tensor imaging tractography of language tracts and intraoperative subcortical stimulations. J Neurosurg. 2010;112:503–11.
56. Field AS, Alexander AL. Diffusion tensor tractography around brain tumors: concepts and applications. "Imaging Brain Tumors: From Physiology to Therapy" (Clinical categorical course), International society for magnetic resonance in medicine (ISMRM) 16th scientific meeting and exhibition; 2008 May 5; Toronto, Canada; Syllabus.
57. Coenen VA, Krings T, Axer H, et al. Intraoperative three-dimensional visualization of the pyramidal tract in a neuronavigation system (PTV) reliably predicts true position of principal motor pathways. Surg Neurol. 2003;60:381–90.
58. Wu JS, Zhou LF, Tang WJ, et al. Clinical evaluation and follow-up outcome of diffusion tensor imaging-based functional neuronavigation: a prospective, controlled study in patients with gliomas involving pyramidal tracts. Neurosurgery. 2007;61:935–48. discussion 948–49.
59. Berman JI, Berger MS, Chung SW, et al. Accuracy of diffusion tensor magnetic resonance imaging tractography assessed using intraoperative subcortical stimulation mapping and magnetic source imaging. J Neurosurg. 2007;107:488–94.
60. Pillai JJ. The evolution of clinical functional imaging during the past 2 decades and its current impact on neurosurgical planning. AJNR Am J Neuroradiol. 2010;31(2):219–25.

Magnetoencephalographic Imaging for Neurosurgery

7

Phiroz E. Tarapore, Edward F. Chang, Rodney Gabriel, Mitchel S. Berger, and Srikantan S. Nagarajan

Introduction to Magnetoencephalography

Multiple modalities of noninvasive functional brain imaging have made a tremendous impact on preoperative mapping of neurosurgery patients. Since its advent in 1991, functional magnetic resonance imaging (fMRI) has emerged as the dominant modality for imaging of the functioning brain for several reasons. fMRI uses MRI to measure changes in blood oxygenation level-dependent (BOLD) signals due to neuronal activation. It is a safe, noninvasive method that allows for whole-brain coverage, including the ability to examine activity in deep brain structures. Importantly, the widespread availability of commercial and open-source tools for analysis of fMRI data has enabled many researchers to embrace this technology easily. However, since the BOLD signal is an indirect measure of neural activity and is fundamentally limited by the rate of oxygen consumption and subsequent blood flow mechanism, fMRI lacks the temporal resolution required to image the dynamic and oscillatory spatiotemporal patterns that are associated with cognitive processes. Furthermore, it might not accurately reflect true neuronal processes, especially in regions of altered vasculature. In fact, the exact frequency band of neuronal processes that corresponds to the BOLD signal is still being actively debated [1, 2]. Finally, in the context of speech and language studies, because fMRI measurements involve loud scans caused by fast forces on MR gradient coils, the scans themselves invoke auditory responses that have to be deconvolved from the signals in order to examine other stimulus-related activity. Hence, to image brain activity noninvasively on a neurophysiologically relevant timescale and to observe neurophysiological processes more directly, silent imaging techniques that have high temporal and spatial resolution are needed.

Temporal changes in cortical function can be noninvasively measured using methods with high (e.g., millisecond) temporal resolution, namely magnetoencephalography (MEG) and electroencephalography (EEG). MEG measures tiny magnetic fields outside of the head that are generated by neural activity. EEG is the measurement of electric potentials generated by neural activity using an electrode array placed directly on the scalp. In contrast to fMRI, both MEG and EEG directly measure electromagnetic (EM) fields emanating from the brain with excellent temporal resolution (<1 ms) and allow the study of neural oscillatory processes over a wide frequency range (at least 1–600 Hz). MEG and EEG also provide

P.E. Tarapore, M.D. • E.F. Chang, M.D.
M.S. Berger, M.D.
Department of Neurological Surgery, University of California, San Francisco, CA, USA

R. Gabriel, B.S. • S.S. Nagarajan, Ph.D. (✉)
Department of Radiology and Biomedical Imaging, University of California, San Francisco, 513 Parnassus Avenue, S362, San Francisco, CA 94143, USA
e-mail: sri@ucsf.edu

J.J. Pillai (ed.), *Functional Brain Tumor Imaging*, DOI 10.1007/978-1-4419-5858-7_7,

complementary information about brain activity because of their differing sensitivity to sources of current within the brain [3]. MEG is primarily sensitive to tangential currents in the brain closer to the surface and unaffected by the poor conductive properties of the skull [4]. EEG, on the other hand, is primarily sensitive to radial EM sources, and significantly affected by the conductive properties of intervening tissues including the brain, skull, and scalp. This problem of variable conductivity is further compounded in the case of brain tumors, where the conductivity of the perilesional tissues are largely unknown. Since the bioelectric currents produced by neurons also generate magnetic fields which are not subject to environmental distortions, measurements of these magnetic fields using MEG offer an undistorted signature of underlying cortical activity. Therefore, MEG and EEG have complementary profiles in their sensitivity to underlying neural activity [3].

In this chapter, a review is initially presented on how brain activity can be reconstructed from MEG measurements. We also discuss the implications of such reconstructions on spatial and temporal resolution. Subsequently, we review the clinical applications of MEG in neurosurgery patients.

Sensing the Brain's Magnetic Fields

Biomagnetic fields detected by MEG are extremely small, in the tens-to-hundreds of femto-Tesla (fT) range—seven orders of magnitude smaller than the earth's magnetic field. As a result, appropriate data collection necessitates a magnetically shielded room and highly sensitive detectors called Superconducting quantum interference devices (SQUIDs) [5]. The fortuitous anatomical arrangement of cortical pyramidal cells allows the noninvasive detection of their activity by MEG. The long apical dendrites of these cells are arranged parallel to each other and often perpendicular to the cortical surface, and their EM fields sum up to magnitudes large enough to be detected at the scalp. Synchronously fluctuating dendritic currents result in electric and magnetic dipoles that produce these electromagnetic fields [6, 7]. These dendritic currents from the brain are typically sensed using detection coils called flux transformers or magnetometers, which are positioned closely to the scalp and connected to SQUIDs. SQUIDs act as magnetic-field-to-voltage converters, and their typically nonlinear response is linearized by flux-locked loop electronic circuits. SQUIDs have a sensitivity of ~10 fT per square root of Hz which is adequate for detection of the brain's magnetic fields [5, 8].

Modern MEG systems often consist of simultaneous recordings from many differential sensors that cover the whole head, with the total number of SQUIDs varying from 100 to 300. Typical MEG systems have sensors that are spaced approximately 2.2–3.6 cm apart. Although the maximum sampling rate is approximately 12 kHz, most MEG data is usually recorded at about 1 kHz, thereby maintaining excellent temporal resolution for measuring the dynamics of cortical neuronal activity at the millisecond level.

From Sensing to Imaging

MEG sensor data analysis provides qualitative information about the activity of brain regions underlying the sensor array. This analysis largely relies on the intuition of experienced users regarding the sensitivity profile of the sensors. To quantify underlying brain activity from observed sensor data, it must be reconstructed. This reconstruction of brain activity from MEG data typically involves two major components—a forward model and an inverse model.

The forward model consists of three subcomponents—a source model, a volume conductor, and a measurement model. Typical source models assume that the MEG measurements outside the head are generated primarily by electric current dipoles located in the brain. This model is consistent with available measurements of coherent synaptic and intracellular currents in cortical columns that are thought to be major contributors to MEG and EEG signals. Although several more complex source models have been proposed recently, the equivalent current dipole is still the dominant source model in the literature [9]. Given the distance between the sources in the brain and the sensors outside the head, the dipole is still a reasonable approximation of the sources [10].

Volume conductor models refer to the equations that govern the relationship between the source model and the sensor measurements—i.e., the electric potentials or the magnetic fields. These surface integral equations, obtained by solving Maxwell's equations under quasi-static conditions, can be solved analytically for special geometries of the volume conductor, such as a sphere or ellipsoid. For realistic volume conductors, various numerical techniques such as finite-element and boundary-element methods are employed. These methods are very time consuming and their use may appear impractical in many settings because of the lack of knowledge about specific parameters used in these models [9].

Measurement models refer to the specific measurement systems used in EEG and MEG including the position of the sensors relative to the head. For instance, different MEG systems measure different types of gradients of the magnetic fields with differential configuration of reference sensors. The measurement model incorporates information about the type of measurement and the geometry of the reference sensors. Since MEG sensor arrays are fixed relative to the head of a subject, it is necessary to measure the position of the head relative to the sensor array. Typically, this is accomplished by attaching head-localization coils to fiducial markers on the scalp, passing current through these coils, measuring the magnetic field created by the currents, and triangulating to locate the head-position relative to the sensor array. In many MEG systems, head localization is accomplished every 5–10 min because it disrupts normal data collection. Within a block of 10 min, with subjects in a supine position with their heads securely positioned in the array, typically head movements are found to be less than 5 mm. However, more modern systems are sometimes equipped with continuous head-localization procedures that enable constant updating of the sensor locations relative to the head, thereby correcting for head movement [8].

Coregistration is an integral part of forward-model construction. It involves defining three fiducial points on an individual subject's head surface, thereby creating the landmarks for a three-dimensional Cartesian coordinate system that includes the brain and the position of the MEG sensors relative to it. Based on these fiducial landmarks, a transformation matrix is obtained that enables coregistration with the subjects MRI. This process allows the source locations and sensors to be defined in MRI coordinates and enables interpretation of inverse model reconstructions in terms of the underlying brain anatomy provided by MRI.

The source, volume conductor, and measurement models are typically incorporated in the "forward-field matrix," which describes a linear relationship between sources and measurements. Usually, the forward-field matrix is known or can be easily calculated. Most commonly, in MEG, the forward field is calculated for equivalent electric current dipoles assuming that they are in a spherical volume conductor model [9].

Inverse algorithms are used to solve the bio-electromagnetic inverse problem, i.e., estimating neural sources from MEG and EEG measurements obtained outside the human head. Because the source distributions are inherently five-dimensional (three in space, one in time, and one for power fluctuations in different frequency bands) and only a few measurements are made outside the head, estimation is ill-posed; in other words, there are no unique solutions for a given set of measurements. To circumvent this problem of nonuniqueness, various estimation procedures incorporate prior knowledge and constraints about source characteristics such as possible source locations, the source spatial extent, the total number of sources or the source time, and source frequency characteristics.

Inverse algorithms can be broadly classified into two categories—parametric dipole fitting and tomographic imaging methods. Parametric dipole fitting methods assume that a small set of current dipoles (usually 2–5) can adequately represent some unknown source distribution. In this case, the dipole locations and moments form a set of unknown parameters which are typically found

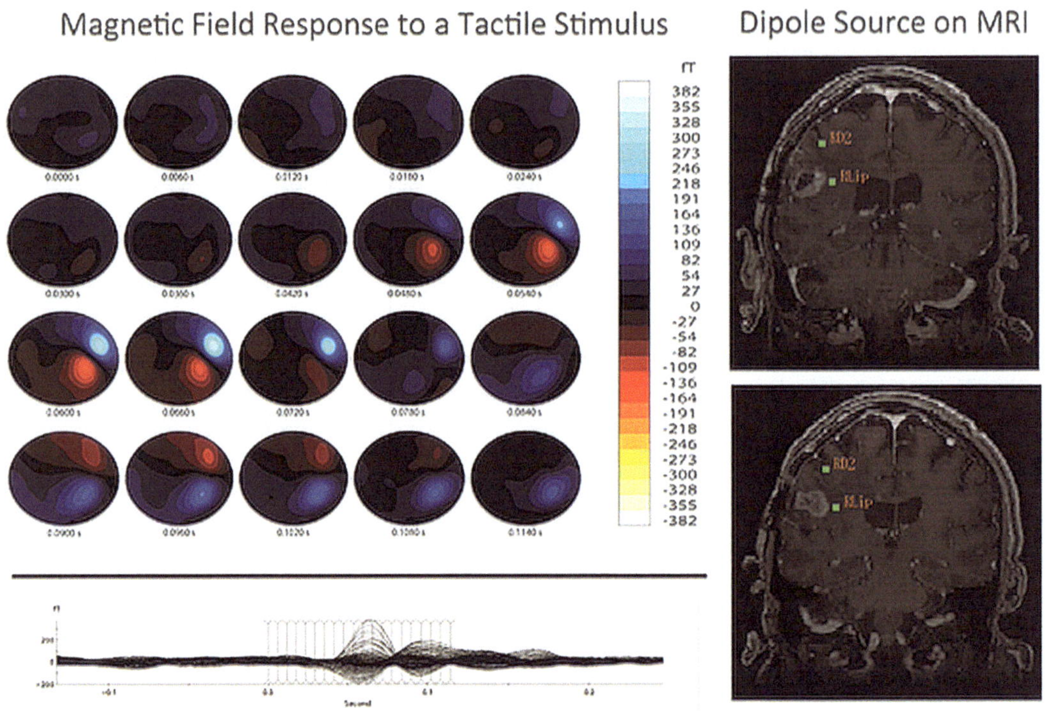

Fig. 7.1 Example case of parametric dipole localization of somatosensory stimuli to the right lip (RLip) and right index finger (RD2). Multiple stimulus trials are performed for each site and cortical magnetic fields are recorded. The trials are averaged and a single dipole is reconstructed for each site using the least-square fit method. The resulting dipoles are then displayed on a coregistered, T1-weighted post-gadolinium coronal MR slice

using either a nonlinear least-square fit or search procedures. Parametric dipole fitting has been successfully used clinically for localization of early sensory responses in somatosensory and auditory cortices. Figure 7.1 shows an example of parametric dipole localization in the context of a somatosensory-evoked response, and shows that responses to vibrotactile stimuli can often be localized to activity arising from primary somatosensory cortex in the contralateral hemisphere.

Two major problems exist in dipole-fitting procedures. First, due to nonlinear optimization, there are problems of local minima when more than two dipole parameters are estimated. This problem is usually manifested by sensitivity to initialization and some subjectivity is involved in evaluating the validity of solutions. A second, more difficult problem in parametric methods is that these methods often require a priori knowledge of the number of dipoles. This information about model order is not known, especially in complex brain mapping conditions. While parametric dipole methods are ideal for point or focal sources, they perform poorly for distributed clusters of sources. Nevertheless, many studies to date using MEG have used dipole-fitting procedures to make inferences about cortical activity, especially those arising from primary cortical regions (e.g., visual, auditory, and somatosensory cortex).

Tomographic imaging is an alternative approach to the inverse problem. These methods impose constraints on source locations based on anatomical and physiological information that can be derived from information obtained with other imaging modalities. Anatomical MRI provides excellent spatial resolution of head and brain anatomy, and fMRI techniques provide ameasure of summated neural activation based on associated hemodynamic changes. This information can be used to improve solutions to the inverse problem. If we assume that the dominant sources in an MEG recording are the transmembrane and intracellular currents in the apical dendrites of the cortical pyramidal cells, then source image can be constrained to the cortex, which can be extracted from a coregistered volume MRI of the subject's head. By tessellating the cortex into disjoint regions and representing sources in each region by an equivalent current dipole, the forward model relating the sources and the measurements can be written as a linear model with additive noise. Such a formulation transforms the inverse problem into a linear imaging method since it now involves the estimation of electrical activity at discrete locations over a finely sampled reconstruction grid based on discrete measurements. Nevertheless, this imaging problem, although linear, is also highly ill-posed because of the limited number of sensor measurements available in comparison to the number of elements used in the tesselation grid. Various solutions have been proposed for solving the tomographic imaging problem, but because there are many more unknowns to estimate simultaneously (source amplitude and time-courses) than there is sensor data, this problem also remains underdetermined.

Instead of simultaneous estimation of all sources, a popular alternative is to scan the brain and estimate source amplitude at each source location independently. It can be shown that such scanning methods are closely related to whole-brain tomographic methods, and the most popular scanning algorithms are adaptive spatial filtering techniques, more commonly referred to as "adaptive beamformers" or just "beamformers" [11]. Adaptive beamformers have been shown to be quite simple to implement and are powerful techniques for characterizing cortical oscillations. Although they are robust in dealing with moderately correlated sources, one major problem with adaptive beamformers is that they are extremely sensitive to the presence of strongly correlated sources. In the case of auditory and language studies, since auditory cortices are largely synchronous in their activity across the two hemisphere, these algorithms tend to perform poorly for auditory evoked datasets. Many modifications have been proposed for reducing the influence of correlated sources 12–14].

Adaptive spatial filters are particularly suited for time–frequency analyses of oscillatory activity, where coherent activity is assumed to be less of a problem across multiple frequency bands. Time–frequency analysis enables examination of the location, timing, and frequency band of induced oscillatory activity. Research tools such as NUTMEG (http://nutmeg.berkeley.edu) or Fieldtrip (fieldtrip.fcdonders.nl) can be used to perform five-dimensional imaging from MEG data. One may then observe the spatiotemporal patterns of oscillatory power fluctuations across the entire cortical mantle in relation to specific stimuli such as visual stimuli or speech production or motor tasks (see Fig. 7.2 below) [12, 15].

Algorithms have also been proposed for simultaneous estimation of all source amplitudes. These solutions require that brain sources be specified either implicitly or explicitly in the form of probability distributions. In these cases the solutions often require a Bayesian inference procedure for estimating some aspect of the posterior distribution given the data and the priors. Recently, we showed that the many seemingly disparate algorithms for tomographic source imaging can be unified. Using a hierarchical Bayesian modeling framework with a general form of prior distribution (called Gaussian scale mixture) and two different types of inferential procedures, we also found that these algorithms are in some cases equivalent [16]. These insights allow the development of novel algorithms to incorporate and improve upon prior efforts in this enterprise.

Recent algorithms have shown that significant improvements in performance can be achieved by modern Bayesian inference methods that allow for accurate reconstructions of a large number of sources from typical configurations of MEG sensors [16–18]. Figure 7.3 shows source reconstructions of auditory evoked responses using one such novel algorithm, as well as reconstructions from popular benchmark algorithms for comparisons that highlight their poorer spatial resolution and sensitivity to correlated sources and noise.

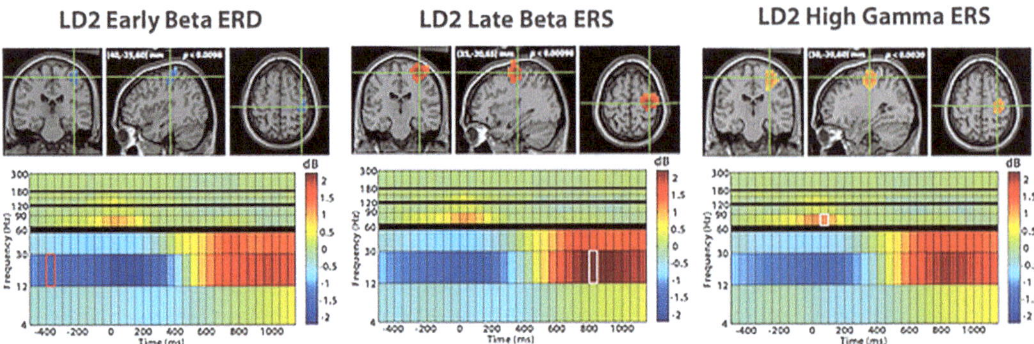

Fig. 7.2 Shown above are the grand average reconstruction results for left index finger movement. The functional maps are superimposed on the MNI template brain and are statistically thresholded at $p < 0.05$ (corrected for multiple comparisons). In each panel, the crosshairs mark the spatiotemporal peak for the reconstructed source, with the corresponding spectrogram shown below it. The functional map plotted on the MRI corresponds to the time–frequency window *highlighted* on the spectrogram

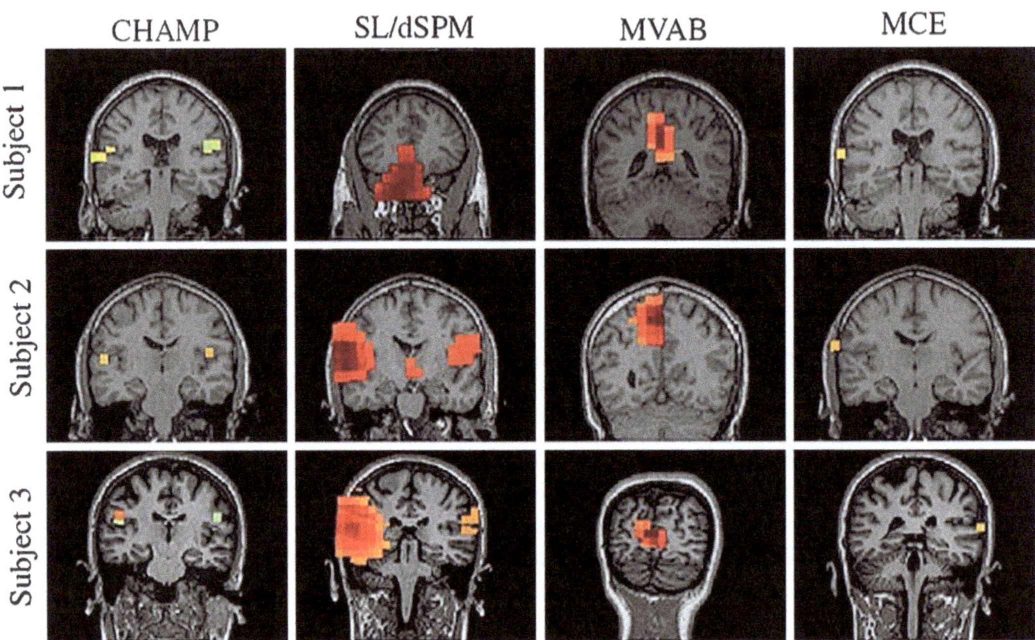

Fig. 7.3 Source reconstructions of auditory responses for three patients using four different algorithms. Champagne (CHAMP) is designed to estimate the number and location of a sparse set of flexible dipoles that adequately explain sensor data while also successfully reconstructing highly correlated sources. Standardized low-resolution brain electromagnetic tomography (SL) and dynamic statistical parametric mapping (dSPM) can localize the dipole but their area of activation is much more diffuse. Minimum variance adaptive beamforming (MVAB) is dependent on prior assumptions about source distribution and has difficulty reconstructing correlated brain activity such as bilateral auditory inputs. Minimum current estimation (MCE) produces focal estimates of dipoles, but with additional spurious peaks and bilateral activations outside of auditory cortical areas

Even though significant breakthroughs have occurred in the source reconstruction algorithm development effort, an enduring problem in MEG- and EEG-based imaging is that the brain's response to sensory or cognitive events is small when compared to the numerous sources of noise, artifact (biological and nonbiological), and interference from spontaneous brain activity.

Other sources of noise include Gaussian thermal noise and Gaussian electrical noise, both of which originate from the MEG or EEG sensors themselves. Background room interference from power lines and electronic equipment can also be problematic, as can biological noise such as heartbeat, eye blink, or other muscle artifact. Ongoing brain activity itself, including the drowsy-state alpha (~10 Hz) rhythm can drown out evoked brain sources.

All existing methods for brain source localization in MEG and EEG are hampered by these sources of noise. For example, the magnitude of the stimulus-evoked auditory cortical sources are on the same order as the noise on a single trial, so 75–200 averaged trials are typically needed to clearly resolve the sources. This requirement for repetition limits the type of research questions that can be asked and is prohibitive for examining processes such as learning that can occur over fewer trials. On a practical level, the multiple trials are time consuming, and it is difficult for a subject to hold still or pay attention throughout the experiment.

Noise in MEG and EEG data is typically reduced by a variety of preprocessing algorithms before being fed into source localization algorithms. One simple form of preprocessing is to filter out frequency bands not containing a brain signal of interest. Additionally and more recently, independent component analysis (ICA) has been used to remove artifactual components such as eye blinks [19, 20]. More sophisticated techniques have also recently been developed using graphical models [19]. Consequently, algorithms for source localization from MEG and EEG data typically use a two stage procedure—the first for noise/interference removal and the second for source localization. More recently algorithms that integrate interference suppression with source reconstructions have also been proposed and allow for robust source reconstruction [17, 18, 21].

Temporal and Spatial Resolution of MEG Imaging

Since MEG data can be acquired at a submillisecond timescale, temporal resolution of MEG imaging is only limited by the sampling rate (typically ~1 kHz). In principle, cortical oscillations can be observed up to 500 Hz. In contrast, determining the spatial resolution of MEG imaging is challenging because it is highly dependent on the reconstruction algorithm chosen, as well as variety of factors such as signal-to-noise and interference ratio, model formulation, forward-model accuracy, coregistration errors, and accuracy of priors. In general, the spatial resolution of MEG reconstruction is not limited by sensor spacing, because many adaptive methods can perform better than estimated based on spatial sampling criteria. For instance, while sensor spacing in many axial gradiometer systems is 2.2 cm, reconstruction accuracy can in some cases be as small as 3 mm. In general, coregistration errors alone can account for 3 mm of error in localization information for dipole-fitting procedures. While tomographic imaging algorithms, such as minimum-norm methods, have poor spatial resolution (on the order of a few centimeters), the spatial resolution of adaptive spatial filtering methods and tomographic reconstruction methods based on machine learning techniques are difficult to compute because these estimates depend on the data itself, as well as other factors such as data quality. As a rule of thumb, for typical datasets, these newer methods can reconstruct tens-to-hundreds of sources at about 5 mm distances (assuming time–frequency separation and detectability). This estimate can be considered an approximate spatial resolution for MEG, keeping in mind that under certain circumstances the spatial resolution can be even greater.

A common myth, related to the spatial resolution of MEG, is its lack of sensitivity to gyral crown activity and relative insensitivity to deep sources. While it is a fact that for single spherical volume conductor models MEG sensors are insensitive to radially pointing dipoles, this does not necessarily translate to gyral sources. It has been shown that, using realistic volume conductor models (such as boundary-element methods or multiple local-sphere models), some sensitivity to radial sources can be recovered, and that there is no predominant loss of sensitivity to gyral sources [22]. Furthermore, while there is a significant drop in sensitivity to deeper sources because their contributions will fall by approximately the square of the distance to the sensors. However, mid-brain sources present two additional problems. First, they may not have dipolar organization due to their architecture, although dipole approximation may not be inaccurate given the distance to the sensors. Second, the uncertainties in the lead-field increase for deep brain sources, making them more difficult to reconstruct. In general, recovery of deep sources is an issue of the signal-to-noise ratio. If high signal-to-noise ratio data are recorded, there is no inherent problem in recovery of deep sources with some of the newer Bayesian reconstruction methods.

Current Applications in Preoperative Neurosurgery

Epilepsy Surgery

Epileptic foci in patients with intractable epilepsy often lack obvious anatomic correlates. Accurate localization of the epileptogenic zone is essential for seizure-free outcomes after resection. Precise localization of normal functional areas is also critical when the surgical corridor is adjacent to eloquent cortices. The decision on the extent and location of cortical resection for epileptic foci can be difficult and therefore a multimodal approach is preferred. Decisions on the extent of resection outside of the actual lesion must take into account the balance between preventing postoperative neurological deficits and minimizing the volume of residual epileptogenic tissue. MEG is particularly useful for both patients with non-lesional epilepsy and those with large lesions [23–26], including mesial temporal lobe epilepsy [27].

Single epileptic spikes are defined as having duration of less than 70 ms. Localization of the epileptogenic zone involves manual identification of real interictal spikes from the averaged sensor data and subsequent calculation of the location and orientation of the associated ECD [8, 28–30]. One study with 455 patients demonstrated a sensitivity of 70 % for identifying abnormal interictal activity [28] and several studies have also shown MEG localization of interictal spikes can lead to favorable surgical outcomes [27, 31–33]. One disadvantage of this interictal spike localization approach is that it introduces a large amount of subjectivity from the manual visual inspection for interictal spikes (whether it is a real spike or non-epileptic origin).

Using an adaptive spatial filtering method, power changes in frequency bands associated with epileptic activity may be investigated and possibly provide a more accurate and objective methodology for preoperative evaluation with MEG. Epileptic spikes are primarily evident in the alpha, beta, and gamma frequency bands of MEG recordings (Fig. 7.4). Guggisberg et al. describe a unique algorithm using an adaptive spatial filtering method that isolates real epileptiform activity from these high frequency bands [34]. This technique initially involves manual identification of interictal spikes for MEG recordings followed by automated localization of the sources of the spike-locked power changes in the beta and gamma bands using an adaptive spatial filtering method. Transient increases seen in the beta and gamma power bands that were time-locked to interictal epileptic spikes may be used to reliably localize epileptogenic foci. While still subjective, the average power changes in the frequency bands offer an alternative localization method more robust than ECD models of single spikes. Furthermore, patients need to have a sufficient amount of interictal spikes in their recordings for effective preoperative evaluation.

Distinguishing whether generalized epileptiform discharges are from primary or secondary bilateral sources is an important decision-making factor for epilepsy surgery. Secondary bilateral synchrony is described as the rapid bilateral spread of epileptic activity from a focal cortical area of electrical abnormality. We demonstrated the usefulness of MSI in the evaluation of 16 patients with suspected secondary bilateral synchrony [35]. In this approach, interictal spikes were manually identified from MEG sensor recordings and the corresponding dipoles were fitted and visualized by MSI. This analysis revealed a unilateral, focal area of inter-

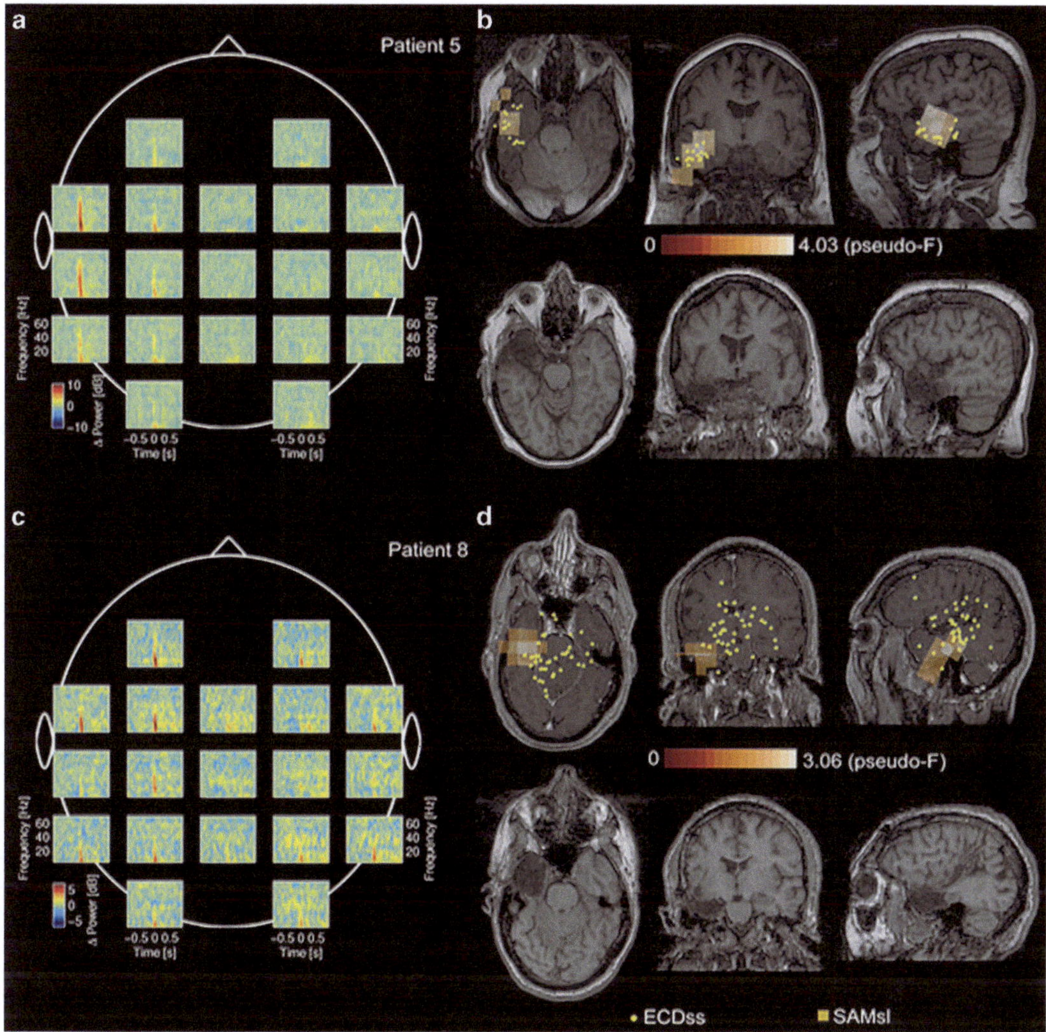

Fig. 7.4 MEG results in two typical patients. (**a**, **c**) Short-time Fourier transforms reveal transient power increases time-locked to the peak of interictal epileptic spikes at 0 s in a broad frequency band ranging from delta to gamma rhythms, with high-frequency changes being more focal than low-frequency changes. (**b**, **d**) An adaptive spatial filter localizes spike-locked beta and gamma power increases (*squares* in *upper row*) to the zone that was later surgically resected (*lower row*), and, in case of patient 5, to the area of clusters of corresponding ECD (*yellow dots*). *ECDs* refers to equivalent current dipoles of single spikes; *SpkFilt*, spike-locked dual-state synthetic aperture magnetometry

ictal spiking in the majority of patients and supported the decision to pursue resection in half of the patients.

While solitary anatomic lesions are highly prognostic of favorable seizure-free outcomes, the presence of multiple lesions can make decision-making highly complicated especially when scalp EEG is not well localizing. MSI has been applied successfully for localization in patients with multiple cerebral cavernous malformations [36]. One report found that MEG was useful in guiding the extended lesionectomy of surrounding abnormal cortex in cavernous malformations [37]. Similar results have been described for seizure localization in tuberous sclerosis patients with multiple tubers [38]. Overall, MSI is an important adjunct in presurgical decision-making for epilepsy surgery, especially when there was discordance between scalp EEG and anatomic findings on MRI.

Functional Mapping for Preoperative Planning for Tumors

Gliomas often infiltrate eloquent brain areas, and it is essential to consider their proximity in the presurgical planning for patients with brain tumors. Mass lesions can frequently distort normal neuroanatomy, which makes the identification of eloquent cortices inaccurate with normal neuroanatomical landmarks. MEG offers an added dimension for functional mapping in these patients [39–41]. This modality has been used for localization of the sensorimotor cortex along the central sulcus [42–45] as well as mapping the primary auditory [46, 47] and visual cortices [48].

The primary motor cortex and the sensory cortex are located on the anterior and posterior wall of the central sulcus, respectively. Identifying the hand region [42, 43, 49–51] and the mouth region [51, 52] of the primary sensorimotor cortex has been useful for presurgical evaluation, and also confirmed with intracranial direct cortical stimulation mapping.

Motor-evoked fields can be recorded by time-locking the MEG signal corresponding to movement [53], and single ECD fitting of the corresponding evoked field generated from the average sensor data [43, 49, 51, 52, 54]. Using this approach, Schiffbauer et al. compared MSI to intraoperative mapping in tumor patients receiving painless tactile somatosensory stimulation to the lip, hand, and foot and found that both approaches had a favorable degree of quantitative correlation [51]. Similarly, a favorable degree of quantitative correlation was also seen from utilizing dipole fitting with MEG versus fMRI [54]. Confirmed with ECOG, dipole fitting of evoked magnetic fields to median nerve stimulation proved to be superior to fMRI for 15 patients in identifying the sensorimotor cortex [43]. Following dipole fitting of the mouth motor cortex, ECS sites were usually anterior and lateral to MEG localization of the lip somatosensory cortex [52].

The use of MEG spatial filtering holds promise for a more robust method for mapping the motor cortex in presurgical patients [42, 50, 55]. The use of a spatial filter beamformer while subjects performed a self-paced index finger movement can generate high resolution imaging of the spatiotemporal patterns of premotor and motor cortex activity [55]. Peaks of the tomographic distribution of beta-band event-related desynchronization sources reliably localized the hand motor cortex in a group of 66 patients, which was confirmed with ECS [50] (Fig. 7.5).

In pediatric patients as well, the pre-movement motor field component in average brain response was localized. In this case, motor field time-locked to electromyography onset was successfully localized to areas corresponding to the hand region in 95 % of cases ($n=10$), which was confirmed with ECOG [42]. Furthermore, displacement of the sensorimotor cortex by space-occupying brain lesions does not seem to interfere with localization of the hand motor cortex [42, 50].

Future Applications

Lateralization of Language Function

Identification of a patient's dominant hemisphere is crucial when the surgical site is located near presumed language cortex. Traditionally, hemispheric language dominance is evaluated by the Wada test, which is an invasive procedure. Furthermore, crossflow of amobarbital to the contralateral hemisphere through the circle of Willis can make results inaccurate. MEG offers a noninvasive and potentially a more accurate alternative for determining hemispheric dominance.

Using MEG, language laterality can be measured by determining the asymmetry of equivalent dipole sources between both hemispheres [56]. Using this approach, MSI and Wada tests were concordant in determining dominant hemisphere

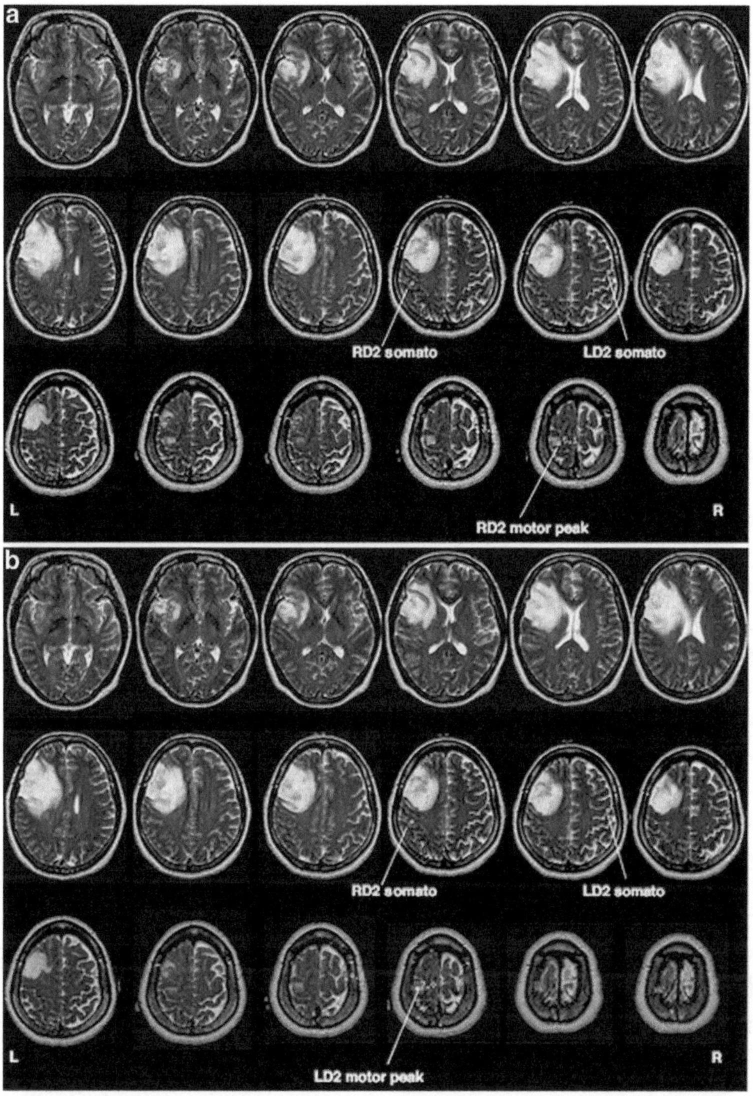

Fig. 7.5 (**a**) Localization of **β**-band desynchronization preceding right index finger flexion for a subject with a frontal tumor. The location of hand motor cortex relative to a single dipole localization of hand somatosensory cortex is also shown. (**b**) Localization of **β**-band desynchronization due to left index finger flexion in the same subject, showing contralateral hand motor cortical activation in the right hemisphere

in 86 % of a group of 35 patients with high sensitivity and specificity [57]. Dipole sources of the late auditory evoked field components in both hemispheres can be determined while subjects undergo a recognition task for spoken words or listening to synthesized vowel sounds [56, 58]. The laterality of increased suppression of MEG activity in the 8–50 Hz range in the inferior frontal gyrus regions corresponded to the dominant hemisphere and was consistent with the Wada test among 95 % of the patients [59].

Location of the language cortex (i.e., Broca's area and Wernicke's area) also holds clinical value as mass lesions can distort the anatomy and also because of interindividual anatomic variation among patients. The m100 of auditory evoked fields reside in the supratemporal auditory cortex [60], which is often surrounded by language-related cortex [61]. Grummich et al. compared MEG to fMRI in locating Wernicke and Broca's area among 172 patients [62]. These language areas were localized in all patients, however 4 % of cases differed in MEG and fMRI and in 19 % one modality showed activation while the other did not. Similarly, Kober et al. located Wernicke area in the posterior part of the left superior temporal gyrus and motor speech area in the left inferior frontal gyrus using spatially filtered MEG [63]. Most recently, Hirata et al. used synthetic aperture magnetometry (an improvement over MEG dipole methods) to prospectively determine language lateralization, and found high concordance with Wada testing and intraoperative cortical stimulation results [64]. In a recent study, we have extended the approach of Hirata et al. and are able to accurately characterize dynamics of language dominance using MEG.

Recordings were conducted during a verb-generation task on 21 subjects who were referred for a variety of neurological pathology. Using the MEG data, we were able to detect decreases in power in the beta-frequency band during the process of verb generation. With these data, we were able to calculate a laterality index (LI), which quantified the "leftness" or "rightness" of the subject's language function (Fig. 7.6). These data were then validated against Wada test results. In this cohort, we were able to predict with 100 % certainty the lateralization of language in each patient.

We then tested our model prospectively to evaluate its robustness. In a second group of 14 patients, we applied our model and confirmed findings with Wada testing. Overall, we found that our estimation of language lateralization based on this examination also correlates very highly with WADA results.

Assessing Functional Connectivity

The term functional connectivity essentially defines the complex functional interaction between local and more remote brain areas. This concept should be considered clinically as disturbances in these networks as abnormalities in functional connecting during resting state are observed primarily in brain tumor patients when compared to healthy controls [65, 66]. Furthermore, neurocognitive effects are correlated with functional connectivity changes in brain tumor patients, especially in patients with low-grade gliomas [67, 68]. Therefore, the mapping of functional connectivity may be an important component in surgical planning [69].

Utilizing MEG, Guggisberg et al. describe the changes in the time–frequency space of functional connectivity in 15 brain tumor patients compared to healthy controls [69] (See Figs. 7.7 and 7.8). Mean imaginary coherence between brain voxels was calculated as an index for functional connectivity. When compared with healthy controls, all patients with brain tumors had diffuse brain areas with decreased alpha coherence. Decreased connectivity was seen around the lesion area in patients with lesion-induced neurological deficits. In the resting connectivity in the delta and gamma frequency bands in patients with brain tumors, functional connectivity was decreased in patients with brain tumors and further decreased in left-sided versus right-sided tumors [51, 66]. Specifically, there is a decrease in high frequency bands for long-distance connections and an increase in slower frequency bands for more local connections [65].

In a recent follow-up study, we have found that these measures of functional connectivity can potentially be used to guide intraoperative electro-cortical stimulation (ECS) mapping. Prospectively, we compared MEG functional connectivity maps with ECS maps of eloquent cortex in 57 brain tumor patients over a 9-month period. Maps of functional connectivity were generated from preoperative MEG recordings (Fig. 7.9a). By comparing peri-tumoral regions against the corresponding regions in the contralateral hemisphere, we identified regions of altered connectivity. These maps were then compared with ECS-generated maps of language and motor function (Fig. 7.9b–d). Based upon these comparisons, we determined the predictive value

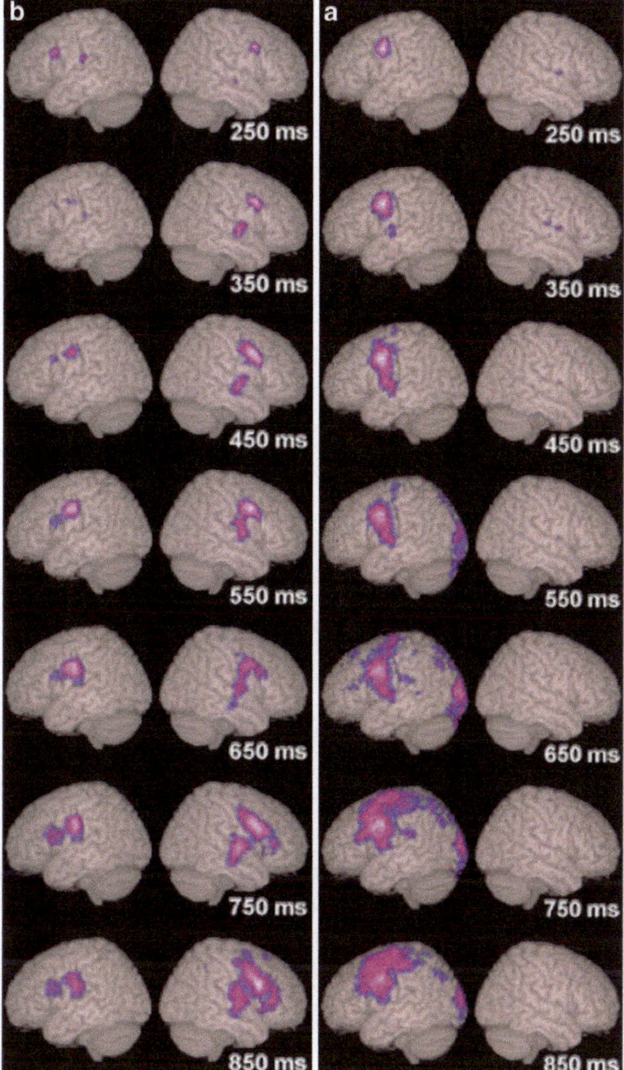

Fig. 7.6 Time course of average verb-generation activations for left-IAP patients (**a**) and right-IAP patients (**b**) for the stimulus-locked condition. Activations were thresholded at half of the absolute maximum power value over the shown time course. Time windows of 650 ms through 850 ms for superior temporal and supramarginal gyrus were used in determining language laterality

of the functional connectivity map. The negative predictive value of decreased connectivity was 87 %, while the positive predictive value of increased connectivity was 64 %. These results are encouraging and demonstrate that MSI can be a useful adjunct to preoperative mapping in this patient population.

Another study by Bosma et al. showed that patients with low-grade gliomas had higher long-distance synchronization in the delta, theta, and lower gamma frequency bands than healthy controls [67]. The increase of relative power in the theta and alpha band correlated with impaired executive function, information

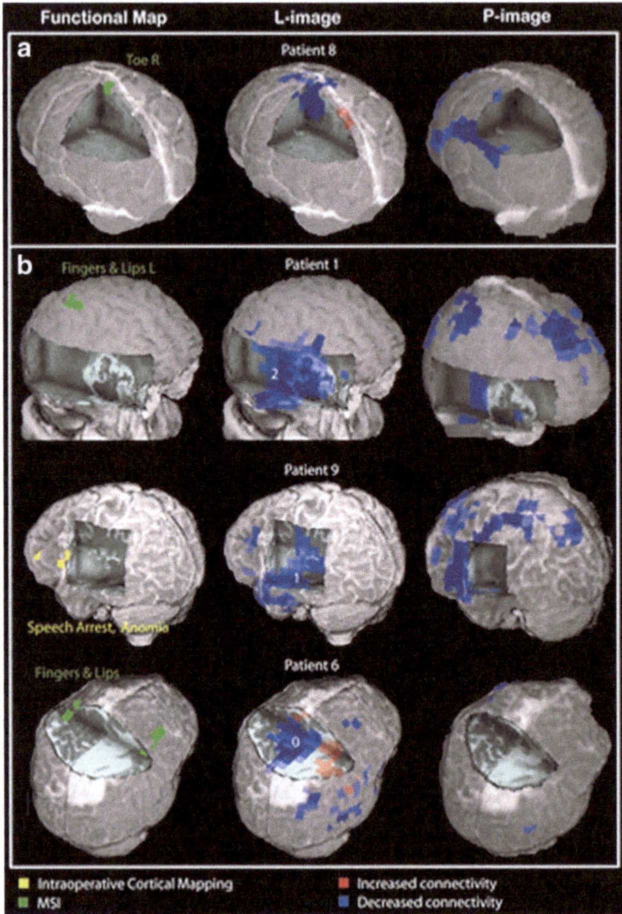

Fig. 7.7 Functional maps obtained with magnetoencephalographic imaging or intraoperative cortical mapping as well as two different kinds (L- and P-) images of functional connectivity in four patients with brain tumors superimposed over their 3D-rendered individual brain. The L-image is a lesion-specific image of connectivity and the P-image is a patient-specific image of connectivity. (**a**) Twenty-five-year-old woman *with* a central paresis of the right foot due to an astrocytoma WHO grade III that infiltrated the left medial sensorimotor cortex. Note that the L-image displays a corresponding decrease in functional connectivity in the sensorimotor cortex of the right foot. (**b**) The L-images of three tumor patients *without* presurgical functional deficits indicate functional disconnection (in *blue*) of different proportions of the corresponding tumor tissue (graded 0–2, with 0 indicating smallest proportion with disconnection). In agreement with the L-images and the clinical status, functional cortex was mapped outside of disconnected (*blue*) areas by MSI and cortical mapping in all patients. In addition, L-images predicted the functional status after radical surgery: whereas patient 6 suffered from postsurgical sensible deficits in the left arm and leg, no deficits were observed in patient 1 and 9. P-images show diffuse or scattered areas with significantly lower connectivity estimates than a healthy control population, but these areas are unrelated to tumor location and brain regions with functional deficits

processing, and working memory [67]. The delta and theta band activities were more intense in the cortex proximal to the tumor and the surrounding edematous tissues, and patients with increased volume of enhanced delta activity exhibited poor recovery of function in the early postoperative period [70].

Summary

MEG is rapidly becoming an ideal method for preoperative evaluation of patients undergoing intracranial neurosurgery. The noninvasive ability to derive high resolution spatial and

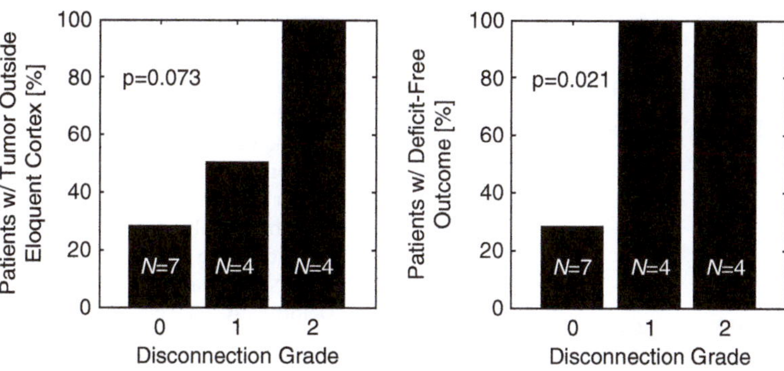

Fig. 7.8 Bar plots illustrating the percentage of patients without critical tissue within the tumor area and without functional deficits after tumor resection, in relation with the functional disconnection score derived from L-images

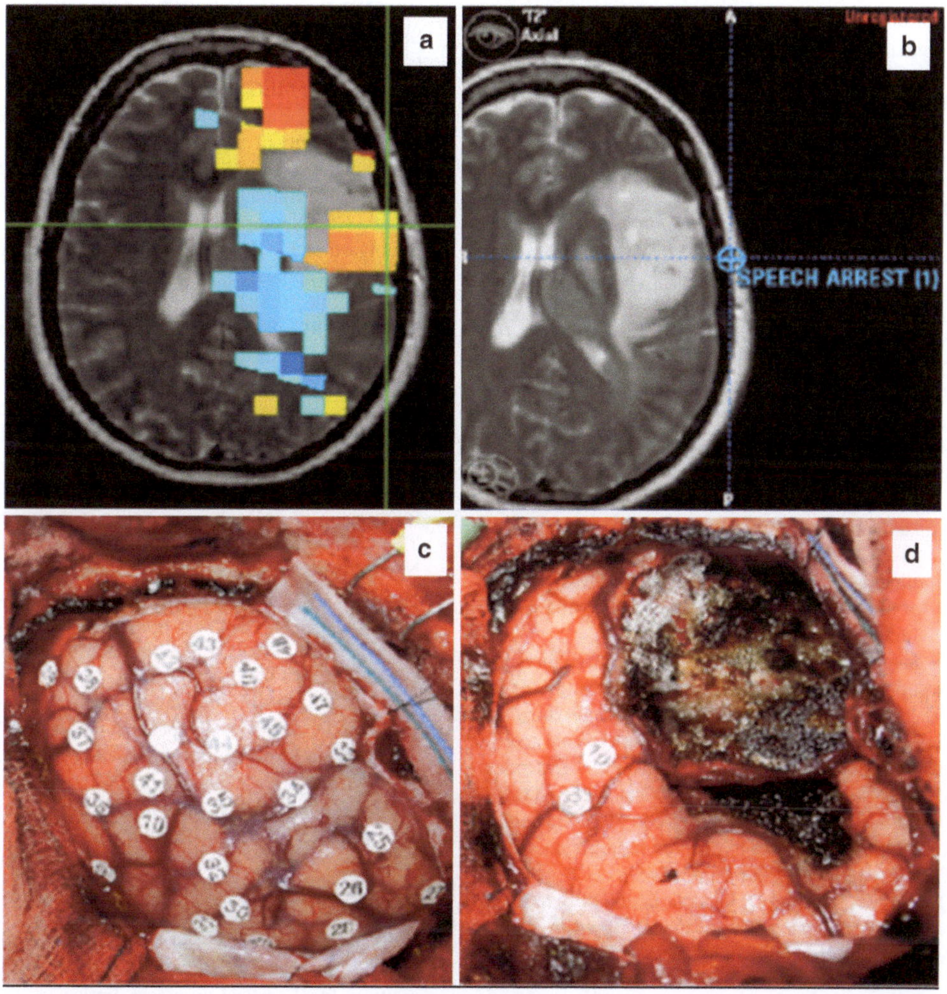

Fig. 7.9 Example case of a 46 year-old right-handed woman with a left fronto-temporo-insular low-grade glioma. (**a**) MEG connectivity analysis, showing increased cortical connectivity values posterior to the tumor in the posterior frontal operculum (indicated by the *orange* and *yellow* voxels marked by the *green cross*). (**b**) Intraoperative neuronavigation image indicating the area where speech arrest was elicited during ECS mapping, marked by the *blue cross*. Comparison of images (**a**) and (**b**) revealed good correlation between the area of speech arrest and an area of increased cortical connectivity. (**c**) Intraoperative photograph taken before tumor resection; #9 and #10 mark the area of speech arrest. (**d**) Intraoperative picture after tumor resection. The temporal and insular component of the tumor has been removed; the functional language points identified (marked with the numbers *9* and *10*) have been preserved

temporal cortical activity will play an increasingly important role in clinical decision-making for neurosurgery.

References

1. Logothetis N, Merkle H, Augath M, Trinath T, Ugurbil K. Ultra high-resolution fMRI in monkeys with implanted RF coils. Neuron. 2002;35:227–42.
2. Niessing J, Ebisch B, Schmidt KE, Niessing M, Singer W, Galuske RA. Hemodynamic signals correlate tightly with synchronized gamma oscillations. Science. 2005;309:948–51.
3. Malmivuo J, Suihko V, Eskola H. Sensitivity distributions of EEG and MEG measurements. IEEE Trans Biomed Eng. 1997;44:196–208.
4. Hamalainen MS. Basic principles of magnetoencephalography. Acta Radiol Suppl. 1991;377:58–62.
5. Vrba J, Robinson SE. SQUID sensor array configurations for magnetoencephalography applications. Supercond Sci Technol. 2002;15:51–89.
6. Okada Y, Lahteenmaki A, Xu C. Comparison of MEG and EEG on the basis of somatic evoked responses elicited by stimulation of the snout in the juvenile swine. Clin Neurophysiol. 1999;110:214–29.
7. Okada Y, Lauritzen M, Nicholson C. MEG source models and physiology. Phys Med Biol. 1987;32: 43–51.
8. Vrba J, Robinson SE. Signal processing in magnetoencephalography. Methods. 2001;25:249–71.
9. Mosher JC, Leahy RM, Lewis PS. EEG and MEG: forward solutions for inverse methods. IEEE Trans Biomed Eng. 1999;46:245–59.
10. Hämäläinen M, Hari R, Ilmoniemi RJ, Knuutila J, Lounasmaa OV. Magnetoencephalography – theory, instrumentation, and applications to noninvasive studies of the working human brain. Rev Mod Phys. 1993;65:413–97.
11. Sekihara K, Nagarajan SS. Adaptive Spatial Filters for Electromagnetic Brain Imaging. Berlin: Springer; 2008.
12. Dalal SS, Guggisberg AG, Edwards E, Sekihara K, Findlay AM, Canolty RT, et al. Five-dimensional neuroimaging: localization of the time-frequency dynamics of cortical activity. Neuroimage. 2008;40:1686–700.
13. Dalal SS, Sekihara K, Nagarajan SS. Modified beamformers for coherent source region suppression. IEEE Trans Biomed Eng. 2006;53:1357–63.
14. Quraan MA, Cheyne D. Reconstruction of correlated brain activity with adaptive spatial filters in MEG. Neuroimage. 2010;49:2387–400.
15. Hinkley LB, Nagarajan SS, Dalal SS, Guggisberg AG, Disbrow EA. Cortical temporal dynamics of visually guided behavior. Cereb Cortex. 2011;21:519–29.
16. Wipf D, Nagarajan S. A unified Bayesian framework for MEG/EEG source imaging. Neuroimage. 2009;44: 947–66.
17. Zumer JM, Attias HT, Sekihara K, Nagarajan SS. A probabilistic algorithm integrating source localization and noise suppression for MEG and EEG data. Neuroimage. 2007;37:102–15.
18. Zumer JM, Attias HT, Sekihara K, Nagarajan SS. Probabilistic algorithms for MEG/EEG source reconstruction using temporal basis functions learned from data. Neuroimage. 2008;41:924–40.
19. Delorme A, Makeig S. EEGLAB: an open source toolbox for analysis of single-trial EEG dynamics including independent component analysis. J Neurosci Methods. 2004;134:9–21.
20. Makeig S, Jung TP, Bell AJ, Ghahremani D, Sejnowski TJ. Blind separation of auditory event-related brain responses into independent components. Proc Natl Acad Sci U S A. 1997;94:10979–84.
21. Wipf DP, Owen JP, Attias HT, Sekihara K, Nagarajan SS. Robust Bayesian estimation of the location, orientation, and time course of multiple correlated neural sources using MEG. Neuroimage. 2010;49:641–55.
22. Hillebrand A, Barnes GR. A quantitative assessment of the sensitivity of whole-head MEG to activity in the adult human cortex. Neuroimage. 2002;16:638–50.
23. Barkley GL, Baumgartner C. MEG and EEG in epilepsy. J Clin Neurophysiol. 2003;20:163–78.
24. Baumgartner C, Pataraia E. Revisiting the role of magnetoencephalography in epilepsy. Curr Opin Neurol. 2006;19:181–6.
25. Knowlton RC, Shih J. Magnetoencephalography in epilepsy. Epilepsia. 2004;45 Suppl 4:61–71.
26. Pataraia E, Simos PG, Castillo EM, Billingsley RL, Sarkari S, Wheless JW, et al. Does magnetoencephalography add to scalp video-EEG as a diagnostic tool in epilepsy surgery? Neurology. 2004;62:943–8.
27. Kaiboriboon K, Nagarajan S, Mantle M, Kirsch HE. Interictal MEG/MSI in intractable mesial temporal lobe epilepsy: spike yield and characterization. Clin Neurophysiol. 2010;121:325–31.
28. Stefan H, Hummel C, Scheler G, Genow A, Druschky K, Tilz C, et al. Magnetic brain source imaging of focal epileptic activity: a synopsis of 455 cases. Brain. 2003;126:2396–405.
29. Wheless JW, Castillo E, Maggio V, Kim HL, Breier JI, Simos PG, et al. Magnetoencephalography (MEG) and magnetic source imaging (MSI). Neurologist. 2004;10:138–53.
30. Wu JY, Sutherling WW, Koh S, Salamon N, Jonas R, Yudovin S, et al. Magnetic source imaging localizes epileptogenic zone in children with tuberous sclerosis complex. Neurology. 2006;66:1270–2.
31. Bast T, Oezkan O, Rona S, Stippich C, Seitz A, Rupp A, et al. EEG and MEG source analysis of single and averaged interictal spikes reveals intrinsic epileptogenicity in focal cortical dysplasia. Epilepsia. 2004;45: 621–31.
32. Fischer MJ, Scheler G, Stefan H. Utilization of magnetoencephalography results to obtain favourable outcomes in epilepsy surgery. Brain. 2005;128:153–7.

33. Genow A, Hummel C, Scheler G, Hopfengartner R, Kaltenhauser M, Buchfelder M, et al. Epilepsy surgery, resection volume and MSI localization in lesional frontal lobe epilepsy. Neuroimage. 2004;21: 444–9.
34. Guggisberg AG, Kirsch HE, Mantle MM, Barbaro NM, Nagarajan SS. Fast oscillations associated with interictal spikes localize the epileptogenic zone in patients with partial epilepsy. Neuroimage. 2008;39: 661–8.
35. Chang EF, Nagarajan SS, Mantle M, Barbaro NM, Kirsch HE. Magnetic source imaging for the surgical evaluation of electroencephalography-confirmed secondary bilateral synchrony in intractable epilepsy. J Neurosurg. 2009;111:1248–56.
36. Stefan H, Scheler G, Hummel C, Walter J, Romstock J, Buchfelder M, et al. Magnetoencephalography (MEG) predicts focal epileptogenicity in cavernomas. J Neurol Neurosurg Psychiatry. 2004;75:1309–13.
37. Jin K, Nakasato N, Shamoto H, Kanno A, Itoyama Y, Tominaga T. Neuromagnetic localization of spike sources in perilesional, contralateral mirror, and ipsilateral remote areas in patients with cavernoma. Epilepsia. 2007;48:2160–6.
38. Iida K, Otsubo H, Mohamed IS, Okuda C, Ochi A, Weiss SK, et al. Characterizing magnetoencephalographic spike sources in children with tuberous sclerosis complex. Epilepsia. 2005;46:1510–7.
39. Gallen CC, Schwartz BJ, Bucholz RD, Malik G, Barkley GL, Smith J, et al. Presurgical localization of functional cortex using magnetic source imaging. J Neurosurg. 1995;82:988–94.
40. Kamada K, Takeuchi F, Kuriki S, Oshiro O, Houkin K, Abe H. Functional neurosurgical simulation with brain surface magnetic resonance images and magnetoencephalography. Neurosurgery. 1993;33:269–72. discussion 272–263.
41. Makela JP, Kirveskari E, Seppa M, Hamalainen M, Forss N, Avikainen S, et al. Three-dimensional integration of brain anatomy and function to facilitate intraoperative navigation around the sensorimotor strip. Hum Brain Mapp. 2001;12:180–92.
42. Gaetz W, Cheyne D, Rutka JT, Drake J, Benifla M, Strantzas S, et al. Presurgical localization of primary motor cortex in pediatric patients with brain lesions by the use of spatially filtered magnetoencephalography. Neurosurgery. 2009;64:177–85. discussion 186.
43. Korvenoja A, Kirveskari E, Aronen HJ, Avikainen S, Brander A, Huttunen J, et al. Sensorimotor cortex localization: comparison of magnetoencephalography, functional MR imaging, and intraoperative cortical mapping. Radiology. 2006;241:213–22.
44. Ossenblok P, Leijten FS, de Munck JC, Huiskamp GJ, Barkhof F, Boon P. Magnetic source imaging contributes to the presurgical identification of sensorimotor cortex in patients with frontal lobe epilepsy. Clin Neurophysiol. 2003;114:221–32.
45. Taniguchi M, Kato A, Ninomiya H, Hirata M, Cheyne D, Robinson SE, et al. Cerebral motor control in patients with gliomas around the central sulcus studied with spatially filtered magnetoencephalography. J Neurol Neurosurg Psychiatry. 2004;75:466–71.
46. Lutkenhoner B, Krumbholz K, Lammertmann C, Seither-Preisler A, Steinstrater O, Patterson RD. Localization of primary auditory cortex in humans by magnetoencephalography. Neuroimage. 2003;18: 58–66.
47. Rowley HA, Roberts TP. Functional localization by magnetoencephalography. Neuroimaging Clin N Am. 1995;5:695–710.
48. Plomp G, Leeuwen C, Ioannides AA. Functional specialization and dynamic resource allocation in visual cortex. Hum Brain Mapp. 2010;31:1–13.
49. Ishibashi H, Morioka T, Nishio S, Shigeto H, Yamamoto T, Fukui M. Magnetoencephalographic investigation of somatosensory homunculus in patients with peri-Rolandic tumors. Neurol Res. 2001;23:29–38.
50. Nagarajan S, Kirsch H, Lin P, Findlay A, Honma S, Berger MS. Preoperative localization of hand motor cortex by adaptive spatial filtering of magnetoencephalography data. J Neurosurg. 2008;109:228–37.
51. Schiffbauer H, Berger MS, Ferrari P, Freudenstein D, Rowley HA, Roberts TP. Preoperative magnetic source imaging for brain tumor surgery: a quantitative comparison with intraoperative sensory and motor mapping. Neurosurg Focus. 2003;15:E7.
52. Kirsch HE, Zhu Z, Honma S, Findlay A, Berger MS, Nagarajan SS. Predicting the location of mouth motor cortex in patients with brain tumors by using somatosensory evoked field measurements. J Neurosurg. 2007;107:481–7.
53. Rezai AR, Hund M, Kronberg E, Zonenshayn M, Cappell J, Ribary U, et al. The interactive use of magnetoencephalography in stereotactic image-guided neurosurgery. Neurosurgery. 1996;39:92–102.
54. Kober H, Nimsky C, Moller M, Hastreiter P, Fahlbusch R, Ganslandt O. Correlation of sensorimotor activation with functional magnetic resonance imaging and magnetoencephalography in presurgical functional imaging: a spatial analysis. Neuroimage. 2001;14: 1214–28.
55. Cheyne D, Bakhtazad L, Gaetz W. Spatiotemporal mapping of cortical activity accompanying voluntary movements using an event-related beamforming approach. Hum Brain Mapp. 2006;27: 213–29.
56. Papanicolaou AC, Simos PG, Castillo EM, Breier JI, Sarkari S, Pataraia E, et al. Magnetocephalography: a noninvasive alternative to the Wada procedure. J Neurosurg. 2004;100:867–76.
57. Doss RC, Zhang W, Risse GL, Dickens DL. Lateralizing language with magnetic source imaging: validation based on the Wada test. Epilepsia. 2009; 50:2242–8.
58. Szymanski MD, Perry DW, Gage NM, Rowley HA, Walker J, Berger MS, et al. Magnetic source imaging of late evoked field responses to vowels: toward an

assessment of hemispheric dominance for language. J Neurosurg. 2001;94:445–53.
59. Hirata M, Kato A, Taniguchi M, Saitoh Y, Ninomiya H, Ihara A, et al. Determination of language dominance with synthetic aperture magnetometry: comparison with the Wada test. Neuroimage. 2004;23: 46–53.
60. Hari R, Aittoniemi K, Jarvinen ML, Katila T, Varpula T. Auditory evoked transient and sustained magnetic fields of the human brain. Localization of neural generators. Exp Brain Res. 1980;40:237–40.
61. Nakasato N, Kumabe T, Kanno A, Ohtomo S, Mizoi K, Yoshimoto T. Neuromagnetic evaluation of cortical auditory function in patients with temporal lobe tumors. J Neurosurg. 1997;86: 610–8.
62. Grummich P, Nimsky C, Pauli E, Buchfelder M, Ganslandt O. Combining fMRI and MEG increases the reliability of presurgical language localization: a clinical study on the difference between and congruence of both modalities. Neuroimage. 2006;32: 1793–803.
63. Kober H, Moller M, Nimsky C, Vieth J, Fahlbusch R, Ganslandt O. New approach to localize speech relevant brain areas and hemispheric dominance using spatially filtered magnetoencephalography. Hum Brain Mapp. 2001;14:236–50.
64. Hirata M, Goto T, Barnes G, Umekawa Y, Yanagisawa T, Kato A, et al. Language dominance and mapping based on neuromagnetic oscillatory changes: comparison with invasive procedures. J Neurosurg. 2010; 112:528–53.
65. Bartolomei F, Bosma I, Klein M, Baayen JC, Reijneveld JC, Postma TJ, et al. Disturbed functional connectivity in brain tumour patients: evaluation by graph analysis of synchronization matrices. Clin Neurophysiol. 2006;117:2039–49.
66. Bartolomei F, Bosma I, Klein M, Baayen JC, Reijneveld JC, Postma TJ, et al. How do brain tumors alter functional connectivity? A magnetoencephalography study. Ann Neurol. 2006;59:128–38.
67. Bosma I, Douw L, Bartolomei F, Heimans JJ, van Dijk BW, Postma TJ, et al. Synchronized brain activity and neurocognitive function in patients with low-grade glioma: a magnetoencephalography study. Neuro Oncol. 2008;10:734–44.
68. Bosma I, Stam CJ, Douw L, Bartolomei F, Heimans JJ, van Dijk BW, et al. The influence of low-grade glioma on resting state oscillatory brain activity: a magnetoencephalography study. J Neurooncol. 2008;88:77–85.
69. Guggisberg AG, Honma SM, Findlay AM, Dalal SS, Kirsch HE, Berger MS, et al. Mapping functional connectivity in patients with brain lesions. Ann Neurol. 2008;63:193–203.
70. Oshino S, Kato A, Wakayama A, Taniguchi M, Hirata M, Yoshimine T. Magnetoencephalographic analysis of cortical oscillatory activity in patients with brain tumors: synthetic aperture magnetometry (SAM) functional imaging of delta band activity. Neuroimage. 2007;34:957–64.

Imaging Metabolic and Molecular Functions in Brain Tumors with Positron Emission Tomography (PET)

8

Beril Gok and Richard L. Wahl

Molecular imaging is the amalgamation of molecular biology and imaging technology in a unique way that enables in vivo observation of molecular biological processes without altering the process or organism being studied. The microscopic classification of brain tumors was described by Bailey and Cushing in 1926, which ultimately led to formalization of the World Health Organization (WHO) classification in 1979 [1]. The data gained from histopathological examination of tumor tissue have been augmented in a 2007 update of the WHO classification, but this has not yet been upgraded to include molecular approaches to a tissue diagnosis.

Positron Emission Tomography (PET) is the most advanced form of molecular imaging suitable for broad application in human [2–4]. PET requires a tracer that is labeled with a positron-emitting radionuclide, which decays by positron emission. The collision of an emitted positron with a nearby electron produces two γ-rays at 511 keV that are separated by 180°. Two scintillation detectors that are separated by 180° transmit a coincident signal. The photon energy that is absorbed by the detectors is reemitted as visible light and then is converted into an electrical current, which is proportional to the incident photon energy. The registered events are reconstructed into a three-dimensional image representing the spatial distribution of the radioactive source in the studied subject [2–4].

Since the brain is substantially immobilized in the cranium it provides an ideal environment for PET imaging, and high resolution of PET can be realized [3, 4]. The tissues surrounding the brain have relatively uniform and predictable X-ray attenuation characteristics at 511 keV, allowing calculated attenuation-correction algorithms to be implemented. Image registration with other imaging modalities such as computed tomography (CT) or magnetic resonance imaging (MRI) is simpler and more accurate for the brain compared to any other parts of the body [2–4].

Regardless of the radiotracer chosen PET is a quantitative imaging method that measures the regional concentration of the tracer with a high level of accuracy at the picomolar level [2, 3]. Changes in tissue radiotracer concentration with time can be measured with dynamic scan or a series of static scans. Standardized uptake values (SUV) provide a quantitative calculation of tumor uptake in brain tumors and this can be used to assess tumors longitudinally [2–4].

PET Radiopharmaceuticals for Imaging Brain Tumors

Since positron-emitting radionuclides of elements such as C, N, O, and F can replace the stable analogues in drugs and biomolecules of

B. Gok, M.D. (✉) • R.L. Wahl, M.D.
Division of Nuclear Medicine, Department of Radiology, Johns Hopkins Hospital, Baltimore, MD, USA
e-mail: bgok1@jhmi.edu

J.J. Pillai (ed.), *Functional Brain Tumor Imaging*, DOI 10.1007/978-1-4419-5858-7_8,

fundamental biochemical principles, it is possible to synthesize PET probes with the same chemical structure as the parent unlabeled molecules without altering their biological activity [2–4, 8, 9]. Fundamental biochemical principles comprise several potential targets including the receptors on the tumor surface, targeting agents based on increased metabolic demands of the cancer, and potentially enzymes or processes which are related to cell growth and survival. Characteristics of the microenvironment of tumors, including tumor perfusion and hypoxia, can also be targeted as well as elements of the tumor stroma.

Due both to intimate relationship between glucose metabolism and malignancy, and the wide availability of this tracer, 2-[^{18}F]-fluoro-2-deoxy-D-glucose (FDG) is the most commonly used radiopharmaceutical for PET and has proven efficacy in whole-body imaging for a variety of malignancies [4–8]. There is a significant increase in the number of functional glucose transporters at the transformed cell's surface, and nearly all mitogens and cellular oncogenes activate glucose transport. FDG enters a cell via glucose transporter proteins where it competes with glucose for hexokinase and is phosphorylated. In contrast to glucose-6-phosphate, FDG-6-phosphate is metabolically trapped within tumor cells in proportion to the glucose metabolic rate [4–8].

In malignant tumor cells, increased amino acid (AA) transport, in addition to increased glucose metabolism, has been shown to be associated with every event in carcinogenesis [9–15]. Many synthetic derivatives have also been shown to enter the cells using AA transport systems, but they are not metabolized. The uptake of AA in normal brain is low and the contrast between tumor and normal brain is generally better with AA scanning as compared to FDG PET [9–15]. The L-type amino acid transporter 1 (LAT1) is a Na^+-independent AA transport system and a major route for the transport of large neutral AAs through the plasma membrane. LAT1 expression has been demonstrated to correlate with the proliferative capacity of glioma cells in vitro and predicts survival in patients with astrocytic brain tumors [10, 13]. Many natural AAs (such as methionine, glycine, tyrosine, phenylalanine, and leucine) and their synthetic analogues have been labeled with radioactive isotopes and have been demonstrated by multiple studies to be a sensitive tool for evaluation of brain neoplasm [8, 9, 16, 17, 23, 24].

Methionine, an essential sulfur AA involved in the pathways of protein synthesis, transsulfuration and transmethylation causes the "methionine dependence" observed in various tumor cell lines in vitro [8–10]. Imaging with L-[methyl-^{11}C]-methionine (MET) has been shown to be of great value for imaging both low-grade and high-grade gliomas. Other tracers labeled with ^{11}C, include leucine and tyrosine for studying amino acid transport and protein synthesis in tumors, however its short half life of 20 min restricts its use to PET centers with an in-house cyclotron facility [8–10]. ^{18}F-labeled (half-life = 110 min) aromatic amino acid analogues have been developed to overcome the short half-life of ^{11}C (20 minutes). Non-metabolizable analogues of AAs, such as O-(2-^{18}Ffluoroethyl)-L-tyrosine (FET), L-3,4-dihydroxy-6-[^{18}F]fluorophenylalanine (FDOPA), and ^{18}F-labeled 1-amino-3-fluro-cyclobutane carboxylic acid (FACBC), have been prepared in high yield by rapid methods that can be easily automated [8, 9, 16, 17, 23, 24].

The ability to measure tumor cell proliferation by noninvasive imaging could improve the diagnosis, grading, and staging of cancer. Tritiated thymidine is the "gold standard" for studying cell proliferation in vitro, and most of the effort to develop PET radiotracers for evaluation of cell proliferation has focused on the thymidine salvage pathway [28–30]. ^{11}C and ^{18}F labeled thymidine appear to have better specificity for tumor proliferation, compared with inflammation, and may therefore have advantages for differentiating recurrent tumors from radiation necrosis [28–30].

Choline has been targeted as a PET imaging molecule, which is integrated into lecithin, a component of cell membrane phospholipids, and indicates increased metabolism and proliferation in tumor cells [31–34]. Cellular uptake of ^{11}C -choline and ^{18}F-fluorocholine (FCH) are thought to be proportional to the rate of tumor duplication, due to increase biosynthesis of cell membranes.

Clinical studies found that choline PET has higher contrast than FDG PET in visualizing various types of cancer, including brain tumors and is useful for the differentiation between malignant and benign tumors [31–34].

Understanding the importance of angiogenesis and hypoxia in tumor biology has led to the investigation of diagnostic imaging methodologies and development of efficacious agents against angiogenesis in primary brain tumors [35, 36]. One of the earliest and most commonly used agents for detection of hypoxia is the PET tracer ^{18}F-fluoromisonidazole (FMISO). It is a derivative of the nitroimidazole group of compounds, which enter cells by passive diffusion and undergo reduction to form a reactive intermediate species. In the presence of oxygen the molecule is reoxidized and the nitroimidazole diffuses back out of the cell. Under hypoxic conditions further reduction occurs, forming covalent bonds with intracellular macromolecules, thus trapping the compound inside the cell. FMISO PET has been linked to pO_2 and FMISO retention is detectable in the range of 2–3 mmHg [35, 36].

Cell surface receptor target imaging is another valuable tool for visualization and characterization of the brain tumors. The somatostatin analogue DOTA-D-Phe(1)-Tyr(3)-octreotide (DOTA-TOC) labeled with ^{68}Ga, DOTATOC-PET/CT is of value for molecular evaluation of patients with SSTR-positive lesions such as neuroendocrine tumors and meningiomas [37].

Clinical Applications of PET in Brain Tumor Imaging

In brain tumors, molecular imaging with PET might allow (1) Differential diagnosis and grading, (2) Determination of prognosis, (3) Determination of the exact localization, extent, and metabolic activity of biologically active brain tumors for establishing the target for therapy, (4) Evaluation of the response to treatment, (5) Differentiation between treatment induced lesions and residual or recurrent tumor tissue, (6) Evaluation of function changes within the surrounding brain tissue which need to be assessed for the determination of the pharmacodynamic and neurotoxicity of therapeutic agents.

The 2007 WHO classification divides central nervous system tumors into those originating from neuroepithelial tissue, lymphomas and hematopoietic neoplasms, tumors originating from meninges, cranial and paraspinal nerves, metastatic tumors, germ cell tumors, and the tumors of the sellar regions [1, 4]. In addition WHO schemes have been notable for their grading of individual tumor classes (I, II, III, and IV) [1]. Specific subtypes of brain tumors will be described below.

Neuroepithelial Tissue Tumors

Neuroepithelial tumors are the most common and lethal primary brain tumors, accounting for approximately 80 % of primary malignant CNS tumors [1, 4, 6]. Molecular information provided by PET has proved helpful in the management of these histologically distinct and challenging to treat brain tumors.

Diagnosis, Grading, and Prognostic Characterization of Brain Tumors

A primary value of FDG PET in evaluating glial and other neuroepithelial tumors is the correlation of FDG metabolism with tumor grade [5–7]. Low-grade astrocytomas appear as hypometabolic areas surrounded by normal high FDG uptake within the cerebral cortex (see Fig. 8.1). Most malignant tumors within the brain have high glucose metabolism and avidly accumulate FDG (see Fig. 8.2). Padma et al. found that 86 % of the patients with low FDG uptake had low-grade gliomas, whereas 94 % with high FDG uptake had high-grade gliomas [5].

Independent of prior therapy for both low- and high-grade astrocytomas, FDG accumulation can yield important information about prognosis. Patronas et al. pioneered the use of FDG PET results as a prognostic factor in gliomas, showing that patients with hypermetabolic tumors had an average survival of 5 months, while patients with eumetabolic or hypometabolic tumors had an average survival of 19 months [6]. In studies of

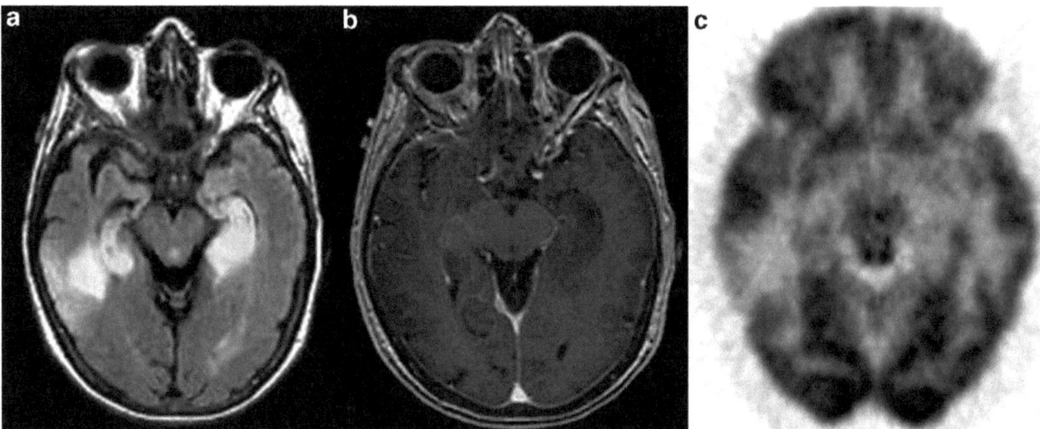

Fig. 8.1 MRI and FDG PET images of a patient with grade 2 astrocytoma, (**a**) The T2–FLAIR image reveals edema. (**b**) There is no enhancement on T1-MRI with Gd, (**c**) A FDG-PET image demonstrates a level of FDG metabolism that is similar to normal white matter, which indicates that it is a low-grade lesion

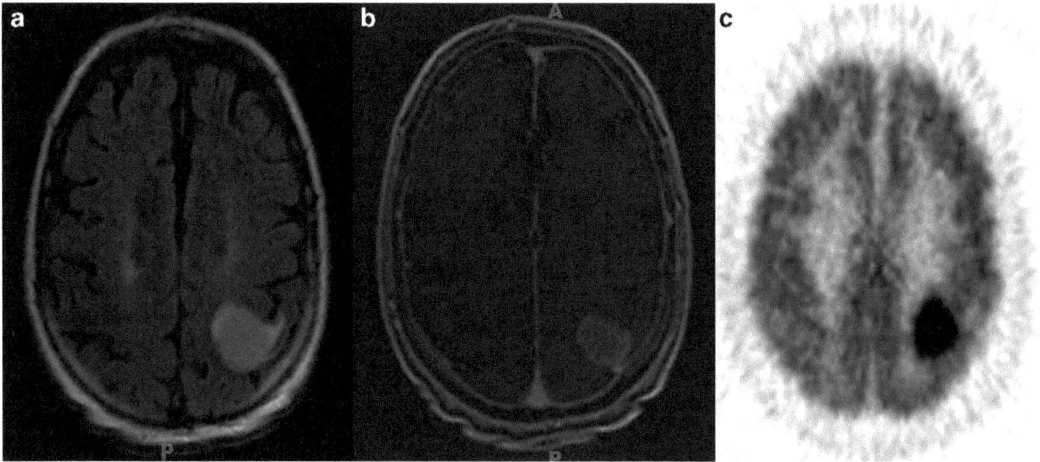

Fig. 8.2 MRI and FDG PET images of a patient with glioblastoma multiforme. (**a**) The T2–FLAIR image reveals edema, (**b**) The T1-MRI with Gd demonstrates a contrast-enhancing tumor, (**c**) A FDG-PET image demonstrates metabolically active tumor

patients with low-grade tumors, the development of focal areas of hypermetabolism has been associated with poorer prognosis [5–7].

The physiological high background FDG accumulation in gray matter structures such as the cerebral cortex and basal ganglia, makes the lesions less conspicuous and limits the ability of FDG PET to detect and characterize small lesions. The uptake of FDG is nonspecific and inflammatory/infectious lesions demonstrate variable FDG uptake [4–7]. Image interpretation can be greatly facilitated by coregistration with MRI and/or databases of FDG uptake in normal brains. A negative FDG PET can also be helpful to exclude a high-grade glioma [4–7].

MET is the most studied PET AA imaging modality for brain tumors, with an overall sensitivity of 76–97 % and specificity of 75–100 % in brain tumor detection and differentiation of benign from malignant lesions [9–15]. Ogawa et al. found 97 % sensitivity for MET-PET in 32 patients with high-grade astrocytomas but only

61 % sensitivity in low-grade astrocytomas [9]. Although the sensitivity is lower compared to the high-grade gliomas, a MET PET scan is particularly useful in detecting low-grade gliomas which are difficult to identify with enhancement characteristics on anatomical images [10, 11]. Ribom et al. reported that 94 % of low-grade gliomas demonstrated increased MET uptake, while only 38 % showed contrast enhancement on CT or MRI [11]. Similar results have been reported for high-grade gliomas. Kracht found that 29 of 53 surgical specimens of grade 3 and 4 astrocytomas presented with no signs of contrast enhancement on MRI but showed increased MET uptake [10]. Furthermore, Chung et al. reported that 89 % of 35 brain tumors with decreased or iso- FDG activity on PET could be detected and differentiated with high sensitivity and good contrast using MET PET [12]. The reported causes of false positives on a MET PET brain scan include demyelination, necrosis, subacute or chronic ischemia, leukoencephalitis, brain abscess, acute infarct, and hematoma. The mechanism of MET accumulation in benign inflammatory lesions is not clear, but thought to be due to the increased methionine uptake in the perivascular mononuclear infiltrate, gliotic reaction, increased blood flow, and blood–brain barrier breakdown [4, 9, 12, 13].

MET uptake correlates with cell proliferation, in vitro Ki-67 expression, proliferating cell nuclear antigen, and microvessel density, making it a potential biomarker for active tumor proliferation [4, 13]. However, unlike FDG PET, MET PET has not revealed a clear predictive value for grading with visual analysis [7, 14, 15]. Although the prognosis depends on the histological tumor grade, MET PET is a significant prognostic factor, even superior to FDG PET, independent of tumor grade and prior treatment. High MET uptake has been shown to be statistically associated with a poor survival time [7, 9–11, 14, 15].

FET is one of the most promising ^{18}F AA radiotracer, which can be produced in large amounts for clinical purposes, and exhibits a similar diagnostic potential to MET [8, 16–18]. Unlike MET and FDG, FET exhibits low uptake in nonneoplastic inflammatory cells [8, 16–18]. The tumor specificity has been the major reason for the specific interest in FET, which was thought to be related to selective uptake of FET via a specific subtype of the LAT system [17, 18]. The sensitivity and specificity of FET were reported to be between 93 and 100 %, and 100 %, respectively, for both low- and high-grade gliomas with higher results for high-grade glioma [8, 16–20]. In a comparative study, MRI had a sensitivity of 96 % for the detection of tumor tissue, but a specificity of only 53 %. In contrast, the combined use of MRI and FET PET increased the specificity to 94 % with a sensitivity of 93 %. The combined use of MRI and FET PET was clearly superior to that of MRI alone for the noninvasive distinction of tumor tissue and peritumoral brain tissue in patients with cerebral gliomas [20]. In a similar study, Floeth et al. demonstrated that sensitivity and specificity for tumor detection were 100 and 81 % for MR spectroscopy (MRS) and 88 and 88 % for FET PET. The accuracy in distinguishing neoplastic from nonneoplastic tissue could be increased from 68 % with the use of MRI imaging alone to 97 % with MRI imaging in conjunction with FET PET and MRS [17].

Assessment of tumor grade with FET PET has been considered of little value because of the individual variability of SUV FET [16, 17, 20–23]. However, the ratio of FET SUV to background has been found to correlate with clinical outcomes in patients with gliomas [22]. Interestingly, nonspecific incidental brain lesions, seen as circumscribed growth patterns on MRI and having normal or low FET uptake, were reported to be strong predictors for a benign course. If there was eventual development of a glioma, a diffuse growth pattern on MRI and increased FET uptake indicated a high risk for the development of a high-grade glioma [23].

FDOPA, is another amino acid analogue that is taken up by normal brain at the blood–brain barrier by the neutral amino acid transporter, trapped in striatum and was thought to be transported into but not trapped in tumors [24–26]. FDOPA has demonstrated a high specificity of 90–100 % for diagnosis of initial and recurrent gliomas in all grades. FDOPA uptake preceded tumor detection on MRI and FDOPA uptake has been reported in gliomas with no enhancement on MRI [26]. FDOPA PET demonstrated higher sensitivity than FDG PET and FDOPA uptake correlated better with Ki-67 values, and was a more powerful predictor of tumor progression and survival compared to FDG PET [25–27]. There are controversial studies related to correlation with neoplastic grade; however, compared to other AA radiotracers, FDOPA uptake kinetics have been demonstrated to correlate better with tumor grade [25–27].

FLT, developed as a PET tracer to evaluate tumor cell proliferation, and the uptake of FLT has been demonstrated to correlate with thymidine kinase-1 (TK1) activity and the proliferation index Ki-67 in gliomas [28, 29]. FLT seems to be superior to MET and FDG in noninvasive tumor grading, assessment of proliferation activity, progression and survival of the patients with gliomas of different grades [24, 30]. However, Jacobs et al. reported 78.3 % sensitivity for FLT PET for the detection of tumors, which was lower than the 91.3 % sensitivity of MET PET, especially for low-grade astrocytomas [30].

Choline has been targeted as a PET imaging molecule, a likely marker of metabolic activity, preferentially taken up by tumor cells, but not by chronic inflammatory cells. In gliomas, FCH uptake has been demonstrated to correlate well with tumor grade [31–34]. Abnormal metabolite profiles of increased levels of choline and decreased levels of *N*-acetyl acetate (NAA) correlate with high-grade intracranial malignancies on MRS. High-grade gliomas are distinguishable from oligodendrogliomas and other low-grade gliomas by higher uptake of choline tracers seen with PET and higher levels of choline metabolites using MRSI. However, with MRS, increased levels of choline metabolites may also be found in demyelinating lesions, which reduces the specificity of MRSI for diagnosing high-grade malignancies [17, 32]. Kwee et al. reported a case in which PET imaging with FCH aided in distinguishing a demyelinating lesion from a suspected high-grade glioma [32].

Hypoxia is the driving force in angiogenesis and it has been shown to be associated with resistance to therapy, poorer survival, and more malignant tumor phenotypes. Cher et al observed FMISO uptake in high-grade gliomas but not in low-grade gliomas. They also found a significant correlation between FMISO uptake and Ki-67 and VEGFR-1 expression [35]. Increased FMISO uptake was also demonstrated to be associated with shorter survival in this patient population [35, 36]. FMISO PET provides a noninvasive assessment of hypoxia in gliomas and is prognostic for treatment outcomes in a majority of patients.

Tumor Delineation for Surgery and Biopsy Planning

FDG PET has limited application in delineation of gliomas. Although distribution FDG has been demonstrated to correlate with tumor borders and histological anaplasia, both AA radiotracers and FLT PET demonstrated better tumor delineation compared to FDG PET [12, 16, 24, 30, 33, 34].

Many studies have demonstrated that the margins of both low- and high-grade brain tumors assessed by MET uptake, are frequently wider than the anatomic boundaries demonstrated by MRI [10, 38–40]. Miwa et al. found that in 100 % of 10 cases, the area of abnormal MET uptake (MET area) was larger than the gadolinium-enhancing area (Gd area). In 90 % of cases, the MET area was located within a 3-cm radius of the Gd area, and the distance was positively correlated with tumor size. In 100 % of the 10 cases, the area of T2 prolongation surrounding the tumor was larger than the MET area, suggesting that peritumoral edema extends beyond the margins of the neoplasm. MET uptake has been reported to correlate with histological tumor spread and to provide a better definition of the true extent of gliomas than CT or MRI [38].

Image guidance with PET scan has been proved to provide independent and complementary information to assess tumor extent and plan tumor resection better than with anatomical imaging guidance alone [10, 29, 31, 38–42]. Pirotte et al. demonstrated that final target contours defined with FDG and MET PET were different from those obtained with MRI alone. Complete resection of the area of increased PET tracer uptake has been demonstrated to prolong the survival of patients with high-grade glioma. Removal of the MRI contrast enhanced area was not correlated with a significantly better survival [39]. Tanaka demonstrated that the addition of MET PET to navigation systems was more effective than the conventional navigation system to decrease the mass of the tumor remnant in the resectable portion of the tumor. They reported that multimodality navigation system-guided surgery benefited patient survival significantly more than the conventional navigation-guided surgery [40].

Although the data is limited, similar results have been published for FET for delineation of the extent of gliomas. Ewelt et al. used FET PET and MRI coregistered data to guide neuronavigated biopsies before resection. FET uptake correlated with biopsy results in 86 % of 17 patients with high-grade gliomas, whereas with Gd enhanced MRI it was only 57 %. In biopsies corresponding to 13 patients with low-grade gliomas, FET was positive in 41 % (7/17), and Gd scans were negative in all but one instance [41]. Stadlbauer et al. demonstrated a correlation between tumor invasion and FET uptake with stereotatic biopsies. They concluded that their findings may help to distinguish between edema versus tumor-associated neurological deficits and could prevent the destruction of important structures during tumor operations by allowing more precise preoperative planning [42].

In addition to poorly defined borders, another characteristic feature of glial tumors is their heterogeneous nature, with frequent geographic variation of tumor grade. Stereotactic biopsies of localizations that are based on PET seem to be more successful to find accurate brain tumor tissue than are biopsy tractories based on CT or MRI [18, 26, 31–33, 38]. Herholz et al. found that cell density, but not nuclear polymorphism, correlated significantly with FDG uptake in both - and high-grade gliomas [43]. MET uptake was shown to directly correlate with tumor viability, endothelial proliferation, and mitotic activity [10–12, 14, 16, 34, 43]. Decreased MET uptake in necrotic parts and high uptake in anaplastic parts of the tumor tissue has been assumed to improve the results of brain tumor biopsies [34]. Similar results have been published for DOPA and FET PET, which have been demonstrated to be superior to FDG-PET for biopsy guidance and treatment planning in both low- and high-grade gliomas [8, 20, 21, 24, 25, 27]. Although FLT PET is unable to identify the margins of gliomas, an increase in FLT uptake was found to correlate with contrast enhancement seen on MRI, and the maximum uptake of FLT correlated with the highest MIB-1 labeling index within the tumor [24, 27–30]. Planning of biopsy trajectories has been improved with the use of FLT, particularly in low-grade astrocytomas [24, 27–30].

Tumor Delineation for Radiotherapy and Radiosurgery Planning

Radiation therapy (RT) improves survival in high-grade gliomas but most patients relapse, usually within the radiation fields. This is thought to be due to uncertainties in target delineation and difficulties in identifying radioresistant regions for dose escalation. Coregistration of PET has been demonstrated to enable the visualization of the metabolically active components of brain tumors during planning for RT and radiosurgery (RS) [44–48]. Koga et al. reported that coregistration of FDG PET, MRI and diffusion-tensor tractography decreased the treated volume and the maximal dose to the white matter tracts [44].

PET based on AA tracers is currently the best choice, and the most data are available for the use of MET in radiation treatment planning [45, 46]. Grosu et al. reported that of the 39 patients undergoing RT planning for malignant gliomas after surgical resection, 74 % had a MET defined tumor volume larger than the contrast-enhanced T1-weighted MRI-defined volume. The region of increased MET uptake extended up to 45 mm beyond the Gd enhanced area. They reported that patients with high-grade gliomas who were reirradiated using MET-PET in the treatment planning had statistically significant longer survival times in comparison to patients whose treatments were based on MRI/CT alone [45].

Similar results were reported for FET, the size and geometrical location of tumor volume defined with FET PET was different than the tumor volume described with MRI in 100 % of 19 patients [47]. Weber et al. reported that using biological and morphological target volumes during the RT

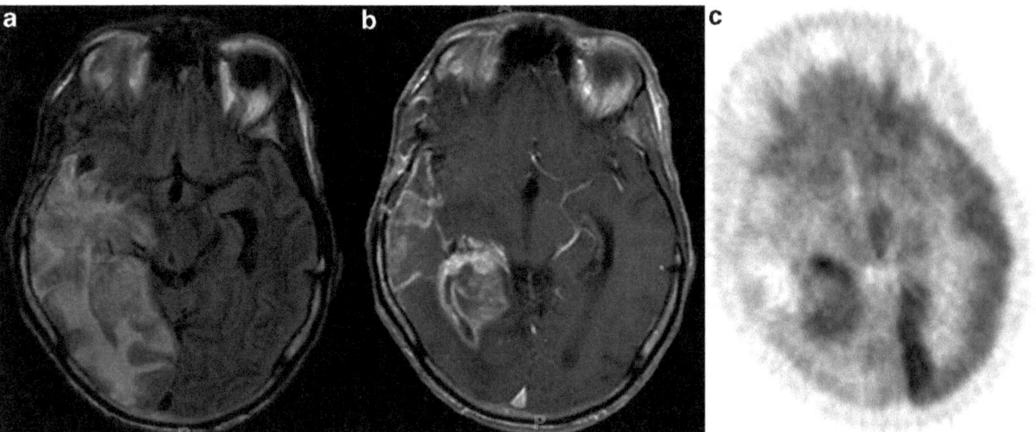

Fig. 8.3 A glioblastoma multiforme was removed surgically and followed with radiation therapy. (**a**) The signal hyperintensities on the T2–FLAIR MRI overestimate the real tumor size by also delineating perifocal but nontumoral changes, (**b**) The T1-MRI with Gd shows the contrast-enhancing area and seems to underestimate the tumor size, (**c**) A FDG-PET image demonstrates the metabolically active part of the tumor, which is essential for biopsy or for following the response to treatment. The entire cortex and the adjacent gray matter structures appear hypometabolic, which suggests edema in the adjacent cortex

planning process a 66 % reduction in non-central tumor failure could be achieved [48].

Hypoxia is one of the resistance mechanisms to the cytotoxic therapies such as chemotherapy and radiation. Preliminary clinical data suggest that FMISO PET images provide a spatial description of hypoxia in brain tumors that is independent of blood–brain barrier disruption and tumor perfusion. Since hypoxic tissue is relatively resistant to radiation therapy, perfusion–hypoxia patterns may lead to a better prediction of treatment response in patients with gliomas [35, 36].

Monitoring Treatment Response and Diagnosis of Recurrence

After intensive irradiation or chemotherapy for brain tumors, the basic assumption for imaging is to visualize the biological activity of the tumor. Early detection of recurrent or residual tumor is of particular interest since the treatment course will be changed if residual or recurrent tumor is present.

Conventional imaging strategies can be nonspecific and not a direct measurement of tumor activity [49–54]. Since PET activity reflects tumor metabolic activity, using PET to guide treatment and assess residual recurrent tumor has been demonstrated to be helpful to differentiate between tumor and nonspecific postoperative changes [49–54]. Increased FDG uptake after treatment is compatible with residual high-grade tumor (see Fig. 8.3). In a study of 47 patients with primary and metastatic brain tumors who underwent stereotactic radiosurgery, Chao et al. found FDG PET to have a sensitivity of 75 % and specificity of 81 % for differentiating recurrent tumor from radiation necrosis [49].

The feasibility and usefulness of MET PET for of assessment of response to therapy have been demonstrated in several studies. A stable or decreased MET uptake is seen in patients with no evidence of disease or stable disease; an increased uptake is seen in patients with progressive disease (see Fig. 8.4). Compared to MRS, MET PET has been demonstrated to be a powerful tool for diagnosis of recurrent tumor [50]. MET PET was able to differentiate tumor recurrence from necrosis in 4 of 9 patients with elevated Choline on MRS [50]. Van Laere et al. demonstrated pathologically increased MET uptake in 28 of 30 patients and FDG uptake in 17 of 30 of the same patients with recurrence or progression of primary brain tumors after previous therapy, and they considered MET the agent of choice because of its high sensitivity and clearer delineation of the suspected recurrence [51].

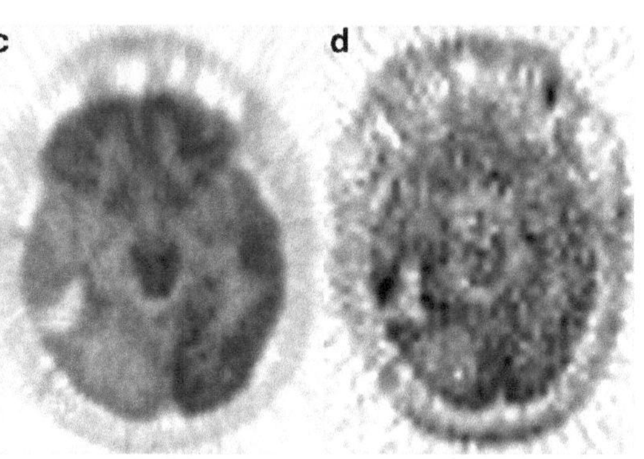

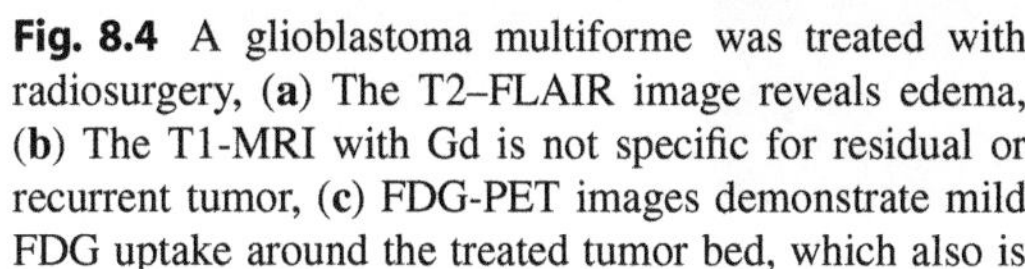

Fig. 8.4 A glioblastoma multiforme was treated with radiosurgery, (**a**) The T2–FLAIR image reveals edema, (**b**) The T1-MRI with Gd is not specific for residual or recurrent tumor, (**c**) FDG-PET images demonstrate mild FDG uptake around the treated tumor bed, which also is not specific for residual or recurrent tumor, (**d**) [^{11}C] Methionine (MET) PET images demonstrate increase MET uptake around the tumor bed, which indicates a metabolically active tumor

Similarly, FET PET has been demonstrated to be a sensitive tool to predict treatment response after radiation and chemotherapy. Piroth et al. that a decrease in FET uptake significantly correlated with a longer median disease-free survival and overall survival in patients with glioblastoma after radiochemotherapy [52]. FET uptake has been reported to represent an early indicator of response to chemotherapy in low-grade gliomas. The authors concluded that the assessment of response based on only MR should be reconsidered [53].

The most promising use for PET imaging with thymidine and its analogues is in monitoring the response to treatment. Chen et al. demonstrated that a reduction of more than 25 % in the tumor FLT SUV was predictive of a metabolic response after bevacizumab and irinotecan treatments. Metabolic responders lived three times as long as nonresponders, and a FLT PET response was a more significant predictors of overall survival compared to a MRI response [54].

Central Nervous System Lymphomas and Hematopoietic Neoplasms

Primary central nervous system lymphoma (PCNSL) accounts for approximately 3 % of all primary brain tumors and 1 % of all non-Hodgkin lymphomas, and mainly observed in immunocompromised patients [55–57]. FDG-PET scanning has been reported to be useful in the differential diagnosis of intracranial mass lesions in immunocompromised patients (see Fig. 8.5). Lymphoma in the central nervous system is typically very metabolically active, whereas nonmalignant etiologies such as toxoplasmosis do not demonstrate high metabolic activity [4, 8, 55–57]. Kawase et al. reported 100 % sensitivity of MET PET and FDG PET for the detection of primary lesions in patients with PCNSL [55].

FDG uptake may have prognostic value in newly diagnosed PCNSL. The overall survival time of patients with PCNSL with low to moderate FDG uptake was significantly longer than that of patients with high FDG uptake. The progression free survival was also significantly longer in patients with low to moderate FDG uptake compared to the patients with high FDG uptake [56].

Detection of systemic spread of PCNSL, although rare (4 %), is very important since therapy is usually modified. Karantanis et al. suggested that whole body FDG PET/CT may be a useful examination in the detection and monitoring of systemic spread in patients with PCNSL [57].

Meningioma

Meningiomas are the most common nonglial primary brain tumors, accounting for approximately

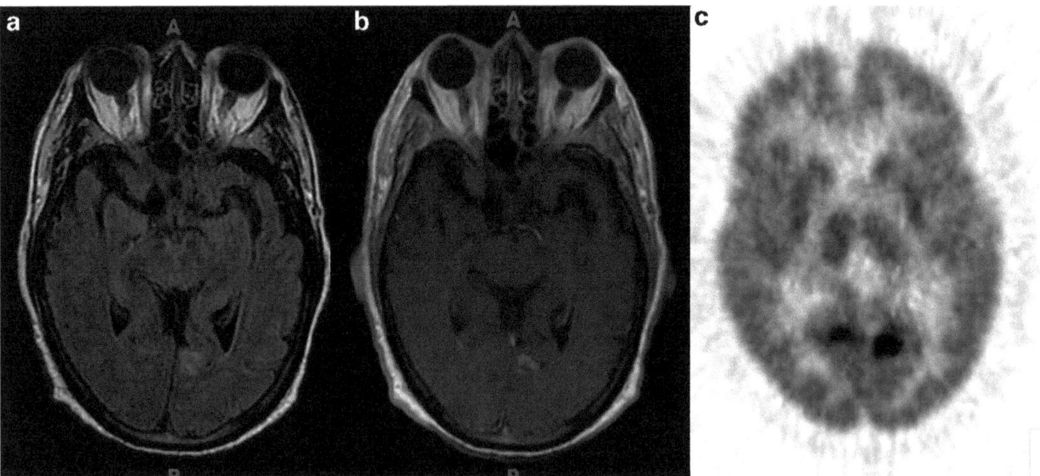

Fig. 8.5 MRI and FDG PET images of a patient with primary central nervous system lymphoma. (**a**) A T2-weighted FLAIR image reveals cytotoxic edema, (**b**) The T1-weighted MRI with Gd demonstrates an enhancement pattern suggestive of a vascular lesion, (**c**) A FDG-PET image demonstrates intense FDG activity, revealing metabolically active tumor

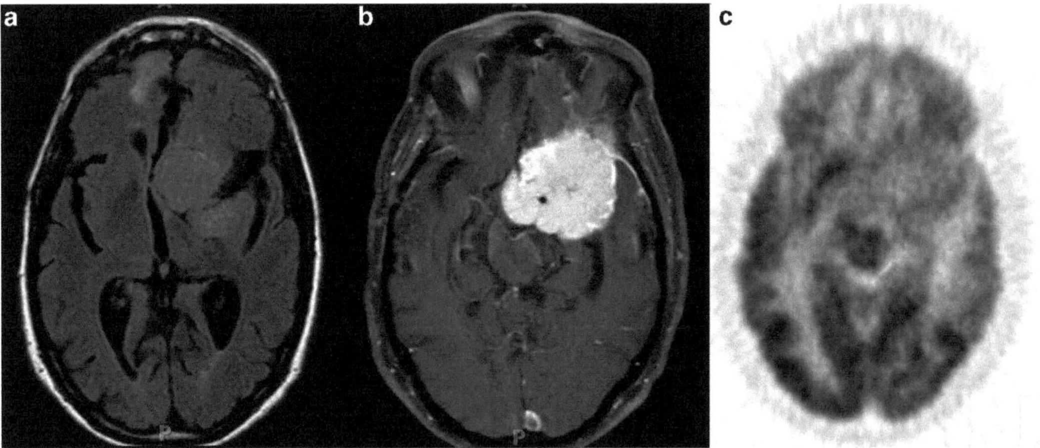

Fig. 8.6 MRI and FDG PET images of a patient with a low-grade meningioma, (**a**) The T2- FLAIR image reveals an iso-intense extra-axial mass lesion, (**b**) This tumor demonstrates intense enhancement on T1-MRI with Gd, (**c**) A FDG-PET image demonstrates a level of FDG metabolism that is similar to normal white matter and indicates that this is likely a low-grade lesion

14–20 % of all brain tumors in adults. More than 90 % of meningiomas are benign and curable; however, they can occasionally recur and demonstrate aggressive behaviors. FDG PET has been demonstrated to predict tumor grade and tumor recurrence (see Fig. 8.6) [4, 8, 58]. Even differentiation of grade I from grade II to III meningiomas has been reported to be possible using FDG-PET [4, 8, 58].

MET uptake has also been demonstrated to be significantly correlated with the Ki-67 index and histological indexes of the proliferative activity of meningiomas [58, 59]. The initial results indicate that MET PET may contribute to the evaluation, treatment planning, and follow-up of patients with skull base meningiomas and neuromas [4, 59].

Meningiomas demonstrate expression of a variety of receptors, including somatostatin receptor subtype 2 (SSTR2), which offers the possibility of receptor-targeted imaging. DOTATOC PET/CT provides high meningioma to background ratios, and has been demonstrated to be helpful in the differentiation between meningioma, neurinoma/neurofibromas, and metastases. DOTATOC PET/CT information may strongly complement patho-anatomical data from MRI and CT in patients with complex meningiomas and is helpful for improved delineation of target volume, especially for skull base manifestations and recurrent disease after surgery. DOTATOC-PET has also been shown to be helpful in detection of additional lesions in patients with multiple meningiomas [37].

Cranial and Paraspinal Nerves

Benign plexiform neurofibromas (PNfib), especially those occurring in patients with neurofibromatosis type 1, are at a significant risk of progressing to a malignant peripheral nerve sheath tumor (MPNST). MPNSTs are difficult to diagnose, metastasize widely and frequently herald a poor prognosis. An SUV obtained with FDG has been reported to have high sensitivity and specificity for the diagnosis of malignant transformation and PNfib related MPNSTs [60, 61].

Metastatic Brain Tumors

Intracranial metastatic tumors are far more common than primary brain tumors. Soft tissue metastases in the brain and elsewhere in the body generally have high glucose metabolism and demonstrate the same image characteristics as high-grade gliomas. Brain FDG PET/CT has been reported to have a sensitivity of 50 % and specificity of 93 % for detection of brain metastases, whole-body FDG PET could be helpful in detecting the primary lesion, with a sensitivity of 79.2 % and specificity of 94.0 % [62, 63].

MET PET and FET MET have been demonstrated to be useful in differentiating recurrent metastatic tumor from post radiotherapy changes, with a sensitivity of 91 % and specificity of 100 %, as well as delineation of gliomas [64].

Positron Emission Tomography in Pediatric Brain Tumors

Pediatric tumors differ from adult brain tumors in many ways, and studies of PET imaging of brain tumors in children are limited. Some studies, however, have demonstrated that FDG uptake is correlated with tumor grade, prognosis, and response to chemotherapy [65]. More data is available related to the efficacy of PET imaging for treatment planning in pediatric patients with brain tumors. Pirotte et al. have reported that in 85 pediatric patients with brain tumors where MRI images were unable to assist in the treatment strategy, FDG and/or MET PET influenced surgical decisions or procedures in all cases. It has been reported that the use of PET is helpful to better differentiate indolent from active components in complex lesions, improve target selection and the diagnostic yield of stereotactic biopsies, reduce the amount of tissue needed for biopsy sampling in brainstem lesions, provide better delineation of tumor and lead to a significantly increased the amount of tumor tissue removed in cases in which total resection influenced survival, and avoid unnecessary reoperation [66, 67].

Future Directions in PET Imaging of Brain Tumors

New developments in molecular imaging with PET/CT aim toward (1) earlier detection of tumor genesis at "pre-disease states" with the detection of brain tumor stem cells and imaging of tumor-specific signal transduction pathways (2) highly specific tumor visualization with the design of tumor-specific antigens, (3) glioma angiogenesis and neovascularization, (4) detailed evaluation of tumor pathophysiology including the characterization of apoptotic pathways, and (5) radiolabeling of drugs to measure specific pharmacodynamic endpoints and identify specific targets, and (6) therapeutic genes to allow direct assessment of therapeutic gene expression. Along with the advances in molecular biology, the effectiveness of PET with noninvasive biomarkers will become increasingly important.

References

1. Rousseau A, Mokhtari K, Duyckaerts C. The 2007 WHO classification of tumors of the central nervous system—what has changed? Curr Opin Neurol. 2008;21:720–7.
2. Li Z, Conti PS. Radiopharmaceutical chemistry for positron emission tomography. Adv Drug Deliv Rev. 2010;62:1031–51.
3. Oriuchi N, Higuchi T, Ishikita T, Miyakubo M, Hanaoka H, Iida Y, Endo K. Present role and future prospects of positron emission tomography in clinical oncology. Cancer Sci. 2006;97:1291–7.
4. Fischman AJ. PET Imaging of Brain Tumors. In: Blake MA, Kalra MK, editors. Imaging in oncology. Boston, MA: Springer; 2008. p. 67–92.
5. Padma MV, Said S, Jacobs M, et al. Prediction of pathology and survival by FDG PET in gliomas. J Neurooncol. 2003;64(3):227–37.
6. Patronas NJ, Di Chiro G, Kufta C, et al. Prediction of survival in glioma patients by means of positron emission tomography. J Neurosurg. 1985;62:816–22.
7. Francavilla TL, Miletich RS, Di Chiro G, et al. Positron emission tomography in the detection of malignant degeneration of low-grade gliomas. Neurosurgery. 1989;24:1–5.
8. Lau EW, Drummond KJ, Ware RE, et al. Comparative PET study using F-18 FET and F-18 FDG for the evaluation of patients with suspected brain tumour. J Clin Neurosci. 2010;17(1):43–9. Epub 2009 Dec 9.
9. Ogawa T, Kanno I, Shishido F, et al. Clinical value of PET with 18F-fluorodeoxyglucose and L-methyl-11C-methionine for diagnosis of recurrent brain tumor and radiation injury. Acta Radiol. 1991;32: 197–202.
10. Kracht LW, Miletic H, Busch S, Jacobs AH, et al. Delineation of brain tumor extent with [11C] L-methionine positron emission tomography: local comparison with stereotactic histopathology. Clin Cancer Res. 2004;10:7163–70.
11. Ribom D, Schoenmaekers M, Engler H, et al. Evaluation of 11C-methionine PET as a surrogate endpoint after treatment of grade 2 gliomas. J Neurooncol. 2005;71:325–32.
12. Chung JK, Kim YK, Kim S, et al. Usefulness of 11C-methionine PET in the evaluation of brain lesions that are hypo- or isometabolic on 18F-FDG PET. Eur J Nucl Med Mol Imaging. 2002;129:176–82.
13. Okubo S, Zhen HN, Kawai N, et al. Correlation of L-methyl-11C-methionine (MET) uptake with L-type amino acid transporter 1 in human gliomas. J Neurooncol. 2010;99:217–25.
14. Kameyama M, Shirane R, Itoh J, et al. The accumulation of 11C-methionine in cerebral glioma patients studied with PET. Acta Neurochir (Wien). 1990;104:8–12.
15. Kim S, Chung JK, Im SH, Jeong JM, Lee DS, Kim DG, Jung HW. Lee MC 11C-methionine PET as a prognostic marker in patients with glioma: comparison with 18F-FDG PET. Eur J Nucl Med Mol Imaging. 2005;32:52–9.
16. Weber WA, Wester HJ, Grosu AL, et al. O-(2-[18F] fluoroethyl)-L-tyrosine and L-[methyl-11C]methionine uptake in brain tumours: initial results of a comparative study. Eur J Nucl Med. 2000;27:542–9.
17. Floeth FW, Pauleit D, Wittsack HJ, et al. Multimodal metabolic imaging of cerebral gliomas: positron emission tomography with [18F]fluoroethyl-L-tyrosine and magnetic resonance spectroscopy. J Neurosurg. 2005;102(2):318–27.
18. Heiss P, Mayer S, Herz M, et al. Investigation of transport mechanism and uptake kinetics of O-(2-[18F] fluoroethyl)-L-tyrosine in vitro and in vivo. J Nucl Med. 1999;40:1367–73.
19. Benouaich-Amiel A, Lubrano V, Tafani M, et al. Evaluation of O-(2-[18F]-Fluoroethyl)-L-Tyrosine in the Diagnosis of Glioblastoma. Arch Neurol. 2010;67(3):370–2.
20. Pauleit D, Floeth F, Hamacher K, et al. O-(2-[18F] fluoroethyl)-L-tyrosine PET combined with MRI improves the diagnostic assessment of cerebral gliomas. Brain. 2005;128:678–87.
21. Pöpperl G, Kreth FW, Mehrkens JH, et al. FET PET for the evaluation of untreated gliomas: correlation of FET uptake and uptake kinetics with tumour grading. Eur J Nucl Med Mol Imaging. 2007;34:1933–42.
22. Thiele F, Ehmer J, Piroth MD, et al. The quantification of dynamic FET PET imaging and correlation with the clinical outcome in patients with glioblastoma. Phys Med Biol. 2009;54:5525–39.
23. Floeth FW, Sabel M, Stoffels G, et al. Prognostic value of 18F-fluoroethyl-L-tyrosine PET and MRI in small nonspecific incidental brain lesions. J Nucl Med. 2008;49:730–7.
24. Tripathi M, Sharma R, D'Souza M, et al. Comparative evaluation of F-18 FDOPA, F-18 FDG, and F-18 FLT-PET/CT for metabolic imaging of low grade gliomas. Clin Nucl Med. 2009;34:878–83.
25. Schiepers C, Chen W, Cloughesy T, et al. 18F-FDOPA kinetics in brain tumors. J Nucl Med. 2007;48: 1651–61.
26. Ledezma CJ, Chen W, Sai V, et al. 18F-FDOPA PET/MRI fusion in patients with primary/recurrent gliomas: initial experience. Eur J Radiol. 2009;71:242–8.
27. Fueger BJ, Czernin J, Cloughesy T, et al. Correlation of 6-18F-fluoro-L-dopa PET uptake with proliferation and tumor grade in newly diagnosed and recurrent gliomas. J Nucl Med. 2010;51:1532–8.
28. Backes H, Ullrich R, Neumaier B, Kracht L, et al. Noninvasive quantification of 18F-FLT human brain PET for the assessment of tumour proliferation in patients with high-grade glioma. Eur J Nucl Med Mol Imaging. 2009;36:1960–7.
29. Price SJ, Fryer TD, Cleij MC, et al. Imaging regional variation of cellular proliferation in gliomas using 3′-deoxy-3′-[18F]fluorothymidine positron-emission tomography: an image-guided biopsy study. Clin Radiol. 2009;64:52–63.
30. Jacobs AH, Thomas A, Kracht LW, et al. 18F-fluoro-L-thymidine and 11C-methylmethionine as markers of increased transport and proliferation in brain tumors. J Nucl Med. 2005;46:1948–58.

31. Hara T, Kondo T, Hara T, Kosaka N. Use of 18F-choline and 11C-choline as contrast agents in positron emission tomography imaging-guided stereotactic biopsy sampling of gliomas. J Neurosurg. 2003;99:474–9.
32. Kwee SA, Coel MN, Lim J, Ko JP. Combined use of F-18 fluorocholine positron emission tomography and magnetic resonance spectroscopy for brain tumor evaluation. J Neuroimaging. 2004;14:285–9.
33. Tian M, Zhang H, Oriuchi N, et al. Comparison of 11C-choline PET and FDG PET for the differential diagnosis of malignant tumors. Eur J Nucl Med Mol Imaging. 2004;31:1064–72.
34. Kato T, Shinoda J, Nakayama N, et al. Metabolic assessment of gliomas using 11C-methionine, [18F] fluorodeoxyglucose, and 11C-choline positron-emission tomography. AJNR Am J Neuroradiol. 2008;29:1176–82.
35. Cher LM, Murone C, Lawrentschuk N, et al. Correlation of hypoxic cell fraction and angiogenesis with glucose metabolic rate in gliomas using 18F-fluoromisonidazole, 18F-FDG PET, and immunohistochemical studies. J Nucl Med. 2006;47: 410–8.
36. Szeto MD, Chakraborty G, Hadley J, et al. Quantitative metrics of net proliferation and invasion link biological aggressiveness assessed by MRI with hypoxia assessed by FMISO-PET in newly diagnosed glioblastomas. Cancer Res. 2009;69:4502–9.
37. Nyuyki F, Plotkin M, Graf R, et al. Potential impact of (68)Ga-DOTATOC PET/CT on stereotactic radiotherapy planning of meningiomas. Eur J Nucl Med Mol Imaging. 2010;37:310–8.
38. Miwa K, Shinoda J, Yano H, et al. Discrepancy between lesion distributions on methionine PET and MR images in patients with glioblastoma multiforme: insight from a PET and MR fusion image study. J Neurol Neurosurg Psychiatry. 2004;75:1457–62.
39. Pirotte B, Goldman S, Massager N, et al. Comparison of 18F-FDG and 11C-methionine for PET-guided stereotactic brain biopsy of gliomas. J Nucl Med. 2004;45:1293–8.
40. Tanaka Y, Nariai T, Momose T, et al. Glioma surgery using a multimodal navigation system with integrated metabolic images. J Neurosurg. 2009;110:163–72.
41. Ewelt C, Floeth FW, Felsberg J, et al. Finding the anaplastic focus in diffuse gliomas: The value of Gd-DTPA enhanced MRI, FET-PET, and intraoperative, ALA-derived tissue fluorescence. Clin Neurol Neurosurg. 2011;113(7):541–7.
42. Stadlbauer A, Pölking E, Prante O, et al. Detection of tumour invasion into the pyramidal tract in glioma patients with sensorimotor deficits by correlation of (18)F-fluoroethyl-L: -tyrosine PET and magnetic resonance diffusion tensor imaging. Acta Neurochir (Wien). 2009;151:1061–9.
43. Herholz K, Pietrzyk U, Voges J, et al. Correlation of glucose consumption and tumor cell density in astrocytomas. A stereotactic PET study J Neurosurg. 1993;79:853–8.
44. Koga T, Maruyama K, Igaki H, et al. The value of image coregistration during stereotactic radiosurgery. Acta Neurochir (Wien). 2009;151:465–71. discussion 471.
45. Grosu AL, Weber WA, Franz M, et al. Reirradiation of recurrent high-grade gliomas using amino acid PET (SPECT)/CT/MRI image fusion to determine gross tumor volume for stereotactic fractionated radiotherapy. Int J Radiat Oncol Biol Phys. 2005;63:511–9.
46. Nuutinen J, Sonninen P, Lehikoinen P, et al. Radiotherapy treatment planning and long-term follow-up with [(11)C]methionine PET in patients with low-grade astrocytoma. Int J Radiat Oncol Biol Phys. 2000;48:43–52.
47. Weber DC, Zilli T, Buchegger F, et al. [(18)F] Fluoroethyltyrosine- positron emission tomography-guided radiotherapy for high-grade glioma. Radiat Oncol. 2008;3:44.
48. Weber DC, Casanova N, Zilli T, et al. Recurrence pattern after [(18)F]fluoroethyltyrosine-positron emission tomography-guided radiotherapy for high-grade glioma: a prospective study. Radiother Oncol. 2009;93:586–92.
49. Chao ST, Suh JH, Raja S, et al. The sensitivity and specificity of FDG PET in distinguishing recurrent brain tumor from radionecrosis in patients treated with stereotactic radiosurgery. Int J Cancer. 2001;96:191–7.
50. Nakajima T, Kumabe T, Kanamori M, et al. Differential diagnosis between radiation necrosis and glioma progression using sequential proton magnetic resonance spectroscopy and methionine positron emission tomography. Neurol Med Chir (Tokyo). 2009;49:394–401.
51. Van Laere K, Ceyssens S, Van Calenbergh F. at al. Direct comparison of 18F-FDG and 11C-methionine PET in suspected recurrence of glioma: sensitivity, inter-observer variability and prognostic value. Eur J Nucl Med Mol Imaging. 2005;32:39–51.
52. Piroth MD, Pinkawa M, Holy R, et al. Prognostic value of early (18)f]fluoroethyltyrosine positron emission tomography after radiochemotherapy in glioblastoma multiforme. Int J Radiat Oncol Biol Phys. 2011;80:176–84.
53. Wyss M, Hofer S, Bruehlmeier M, et al. Early metabolic responses in temozolomide treated low-grade glioma patients. J Neurooncol. 2009;95:87–93.
54. Chen W, Delaloye S, Silverman DH, et al. Predicting treatment response of malignant gliomas to bevacizumab and irinotecan by imaging proliferation with [18F] fluorothymidine positron emission tomography: a pilot study. J Clin Oncol. 2007;25:4714–21.
55. Kawase Y, Yamamoto Y, Kameyama R, et al. Comparison of (11)C-Methionine PET and (18) F-FDG PET in Patients with Primary Central Nervous System Lymphoma. Mol Imaging Biol. 2011;13(6): 1284–9.
56. Kawai N, Zhen HN, Miyake K, et al. Prognostic value of pretreatment 18F-FDG PET in patients with primary central nervous system lymphoma: SUV-based assessment. J Neurooncol. 2010;100:225–32.

57. Karantanis D, O'Neill BP, Subramaniam RM, et al. Contribution of F-18 FDG PET-CT in the detection of systemic spread of primary central nervous system lymphoma. Clin Nucl Med. 2007;32:271–4.
58. Lippitz B, Cremerius U, Mayfrank L, et al. PET-study of intracranial meningiomas: correlation with histopathology, cellularity and proliferation rate. Acta Neurchir Suppl. 1996;65:108–11.
59. Nyberg G, Bergström M, Enblad P, et al. PET-methionine of skull base neuromas and meningiomas. Acta Otolaryngol. 1997;117:482–9.
60. Warbey VS, Ferner RE, Dunn JT, et al. [18F]FDG PET/CT in the diagnosis of malignant peripheral nerve sheath tumours in neurofibromatosis type-1. Eur J Nucl Med Mol Imaging. 2009;36: 751–7.
61. Benz MR, Czernin J, Dry SM, et al. Quantitative F18-fluorodeoxyglucose positron emission tomography accurately characterizes peripheral nerve sheath tumors as malignant or benign. Cancer. 2010;11: 451–8.
62. Kitajima K, Nakamoto Y, Okizuka H, et al. Accuracy of whole-body FDG-PET/CT for detecting brain metastases from non-central nervous system tumors. Ann Nucl Med. 2008;22(7):595–602.
63. Jeong HJ, Chung JK, Kim YK, et al. Usefulness of whole-body (18)F-FDG PET in patients with suspected metastatic brain tumors. J Nucl Med. 2002;43(11):1432–7.
64. Grosu AL, Astner ST, Riedel E, et al. An Interindividual Comparison of O-(2- [(18)F] Fluoroethyl)-L-Tyrosine (FET)- and L-[Methyl-(11) C]Methionine (MET)-PET in Patients With Brain Gliomas and Metastases. Int J Radiat Oncol Biol Phys. 2011;81(4):1049–58.
65. Holthoff VA, Herholz K, Berthold F, et al. In vivo metabolism of childhood posterior fossa tumors and primitive neuroectodermal tumors before and after treatment. Cancer. 1993;72:1394–403.
66. Pirotte BJ, Lubansu A, Massager N, et al. Clinical impact of integrating positron emission tomography during surgery in 85 children with brain tumors. J Neurosurg Pediatr. 2010;5:486–99.
67. Pirotte B, Acerbi F, Lubansu A, et al. PET imaging in the surgical management of pediatric brain tumors. Childs Nerv Syst. 2007;23:739–51.

Proton Magnetic Resonance Spectroscopy and Spectroscopic Imaging of Primary Brain Tumors

9

Lester Kwock

Introduction

Brain tumors comprise 2–5 % of all neoplastic lesions in adults and remain a significant cause of cancer morbidity and mortality in the USA. The estimated incidence of brain tumors is 14 per 100,000 people/year with 40–60 % of these individuals being diagnosed with having gliomas [1, 2]. Unfortunately, because of the aggressive infiltrative nature of these tumors, most gliomas continue to result in significant disability and death despite the use of the best therapies currently available [3]. Clinical oncologists face a significant challenge in attempting to implement a treatment protocol that not only will effectively treat the patient's central nervous system tumor to improve survivability but also must maintain the patient's neurological functions and avoid any major treatment-associated morbidity. The advent of magnetic resonance imaging (MRI) techniques for the diagnosis and follow-up of brain tumors has greatly aided the oncologist in the clinical management of these lesions. The capability of MRI to obtain anatomical images in any orientation and to vary between T1- and T2-weighted contrast has greatly aided in identifying regions containing tumor, and in the planning and monitoring of surgical and radiotherapeutic treatment. Furthermore, the use of intravenous gadolinium-containing (Gd) magnetic resonance contrast agents along with perfusion and water diffusion MRI techniques have allowed more accurate differentiation of tumor from edematous regions.

However, confirming the presence and the extent of malignant disease is still problematical. This is especially true of highly diffuse primary brain tumors. For instance, not all visible Gd-contrast enhancement may correspond to the presence of active tumor. Other biological processes besides the presence of a tumor can cause breakdown of the blood–brain barrier (BBB) which leads to contrast enhancement. Tumefactive processes and radiation-induced necrosis are known to cause breakdown in the BBB, leading to a radiologic MR appearance suggestive of an active tumor process [4]. In addition, an absence of Gd-contrast enhancement does not always indicate that a tumor is not present. WHO Grade 2 gliomas commonly do not exhibit Gd-contrast enhancement [5], and furthermore the heterogeneity of high grade gliomas suggests that some regions of the tumor may enhance while other regions of the same tumor may not [6, 7]. Therefore, treatments that rely on Gd-contrast enhanced T1-weighted MRI to delineate the extent of the tumor may not be targeting the full extent of the tumor and/or the most active regions of the tumor [8]. Similar ambiguities with T2-weighted and FLAIR MR tumor imaging have also been found [8, 9].

L. Kwock, Ph.D. (✉)
Department of Radiology, University of North Carolina, School of Medicine, CB# 7510, Chapel Hill, NC 27544-7510, USA
e-mail: kwock@med.unc.edu

J.J. Pillai (ed.), *Functional Brain Tumor Imaging*, DOI 10.1007/978-1-4419-5858-7_9,

Accurate diagnosis and delineation of tumor extent is critical to the clinical management of patients with intracranial tumors. Both the surgical and radiotherapy (RT) tumor treatment plans are based on the MR imaging techniques described above and have been shown to be inadequate by themselves to accurately diagnosis and delineate tumor extent. Depending on the tumor type, these MRI techniques can only diagnosis intracranial lesions with a 30–90 % success rate [10, 11]. A biopsy is still considered the "gold standard" for determining the cancer type and degree of malignancy. Once the lesion is diagnosed as a malignant brain tumor, planning of the surgical and radiotherapy treatments is based solely on the anatomical abnormalities observed on the conventional imaging studies. These conventional MR imaging studies, as indicated earlier, do not always provide an accurate picture of the extent or location of the tumor [8, 9, 12, 13]. This is especially true in determining the zone(s) of tumor infiltration with low to moderate rates of proliferation, regions of non-migrating, actively proliferating tumor, and regions of quiescent pseudopalisading migrating tumor cells adjacent to necrotic regions [3, 14]. Usually, large uniform surgical and radiotherapy margins between 1 and 4 cm are treated to account for these regions [9, 12, 13]. These margins may underestimate the extent of tumor infiltration, treat areas devoid of tumor which increases the risk for normal tissue toxicity events, and/or undertreat tumor cells which are not actively proliferating in the planned treatment volumes.

To obtain the most benefit from the newer neurosurgical and radiotherapy treatment approaches, such as computer guided stereotactic neurosurgical techniques and the use of intensity modulated and conformal radiotherapy treatment techniques, it is critical that regions identified for special attention be defined accurately. Areas of active tumor proliferation need to be identified from areas suspicious for tumor extension which are less proliferative but more infiltrative from areas which contain quiescent pseudopalisading migratory tumor cells around regions of necrosis. Noninvasive techniques need to be utilized which can provide information to improve our ability to characterize the genetic and molecular differences in the tumor populations present in a lesion and delineate the spatial extent of each population. This information, especially in high grade glioma patients, could improve our ability to treat these lesions more accurately with the techniques now available and aid in the development of more "targeted" therapies to obtain better patient outcomes.

One such noninvasive technique is three-dimensional (3D) multivoxel magnetic resonance spectroscopy imaging (MRSI). This technique provides information about tumor activity based upon the biochemical profile of the lesion [15, 16]. The earliest magnetic resonance spectroscopy (MRS) studies showed clear differences between the proton (1H) spectra of brain tumors and normal brain tissue based upon the cellular metabolite levels of choline (Cho), creatine (Cr), *N*-acetylaspartate (NAA), and lactate/lipid (Lac/Lip). This chapter focuses on the application of 1H-MRSI in gliomas and how it is applied to: (1) characterizing the malignant character of the glioma (i.e., grade of lesion), (2) defining and delineating the extent of tumor cell populations within the observed glioma lesion, and (3) monitoring the response of the glioma to treatment.

Biochemical Features of Tumors: Use in Tumor Grading

As indicated in the Introduction, gliomas are the most common primary tumors of the central nervous system. Histological grading of gliomas is important since the grade of the lesion will determine how the lesion is clinically managed and in the assessment of prognosis [17, 18]. Patients diagnosed with Grade 2 gliomas have a median survival of 2–8 years, and patients with Grade 3 or 4 have approximately 12–18 months with one of the worst 5 year survival rates among human cancers [19]. The prognosis of these patients is directly related to the initial histologic grading of their tumors. Direct tissue sampling and histological evaluation continues to be the "gold standard" used in the treatment staging of these patients. Unfortunately, the gross resection needed to obtain large portions of the tumor or multiple biopsies in different areas of the tumor are often not feasible. This is due to the appearance of gliomas which tend to be heterogeneous in nature and may contain different histological grade tumor cells within the lesion; thus, a single biopsy sample may not reflect the true grade of the lesion. The observance of mitotic activity in just one biopsy sample obtained from the patient is sufficient to upgrade a tumor from Grade 2 to Grade 3. This upgrade will lead to a dramatic difference in the post-surgical management of this tumor. Grade 3 and 4 lesions are normally treated aggressively with a combined regimen of radiotherapy and chemotherapy approaches, whereas Grade 2 lesions may be treated with chemotherapy alone or receive no further treatment beyond surgical biopsy or resection until there is a suspicion of recurrence or progression. Because of the sampling problems encountered with surgical biopsies, use of a noninvasive imaging based tumor grading technique to guide the clinician to biopsy sites which characterize the whole lesion would clearly improve our ability to select an appropriate target site(s) to biopsy and allow greater confidence that the presumed tumor process is properly categorized by the resulting tissue samples obtained.

Proton MR spectroscopy, especially multivoxel proton magnetic resonance spectroscopic imaging (1H MRSI), can be used to noninvasively assess the overall grade of the tumor and to identify areas in the tumor which have clusters of low grade and high grade components [20–25]. The typical 1H MR spectroscopy features of gliomas obtained using a TE = 135 ms compared to the normal brain proton spectrum, shown in Fig. 9.1, is a reduction in the levels of *N*-acetylaspartate (NAA), creatine (Cr), and an elevation of choline (Cho). These changes in metabolite levels are not specific for gliomas but are observed in other tumors [26] and active metabolic processes such as inflammation and astrogliosis [27].

In an early application of MRS, Tsien et al. [28] in a single voxel study using a TE = 270 ms, showed that Grade 4 lesions had lower NAA and Cr levels and higher Cho levels when compared to lower grade lesions. In a similar study using a TE = 135 ms, Kwock et al. [29]. found the same correlation; but in addition, they found that as long as the lesion had not been treated, the level of myoinositol (MI) observed at 3.5–3.6 ppm (using a short TE of 20 or 30 ms) could also aid in differentiating low from high grade gliomas (Fig. 9.2 and Table 9.1). These investigators found that there was a trend towards lower MI levels as the glioma became more malignant, namely, Grade 4 had barely detectable levels of MI, Grade 3 had levels equal to or less than found in surrounding brain tissue, and Grade 2 had elevated levels of MI compared to normal surrounding tissue. This observation was confirmed in high resolution magic angle spinning (HRMAS) "ex vivo" nuclear magnetic resonance spectroscopy studies of glioma tissue [23, 30]. The decrease in myoinositol to creatine (MI/Cr) ratio was shown to be due to a decrease in the level of myoinositol (MI) as the histological grade of the lesion increased (Fig. 9.3) [23].

In a similar study, using a single voxel MRS technique, Moller-Hartmann and colleagues [31] assessed 164 patients with suspected brain tumors. Comparing Cho/Cr peak intensity ratios obtained from the MRS studies with the anatomical MRI data of the lesions, they found that addition of proton MRS data to the MRI evaluation lead to a 15 % increase in the number of correct diagnoses with respect to the grade and type of lesion, 6.2 % fewer incorrect diagnoses, and 16 % fewer equivocal diagnoses. In addition, they found that the Cho/Cr peak intensity ratios (Table 9.2) increased with the grade of the glioma similar to what was reported by Kwock et al. [29] and Magalhases et al. [32].

The reduction of NAA indicates a loss of neurons as they are destroyed or substituted by tumor. Reduction of Cr is related to an altered energy metabolism; with decreased Cr levels indicating more active metabolism whereas increased levels indicate hypometabolism [33]. The marked increase in Cho intensity in these malignant tumors has been attributed to increased activity of plasma membrane components involved in cellular proliferative [34] and migratory processes [35] within these tumors.

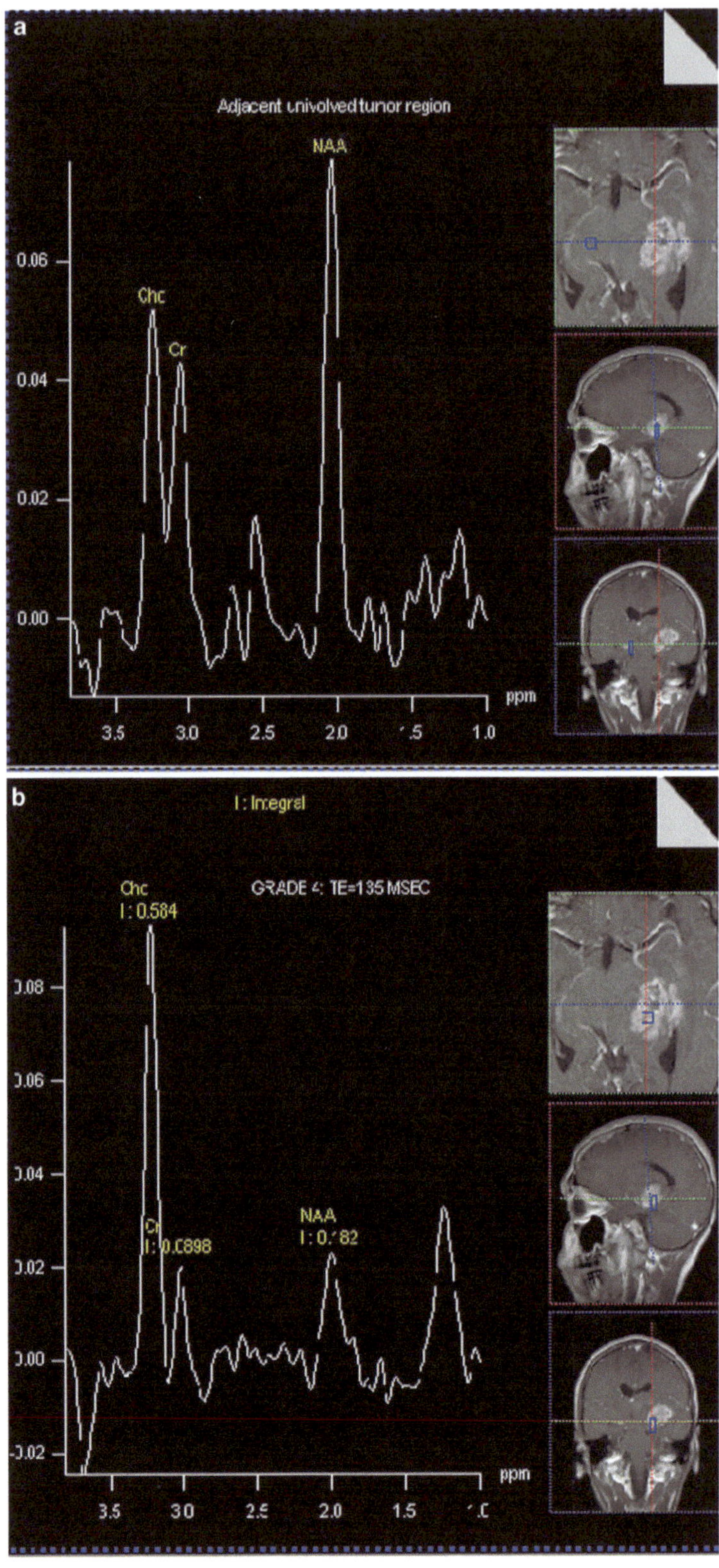

Fig. 9.1 Proton MR spectra of Normal (**a**) and Grade 4 glioma (**b**): TE = 135 ms

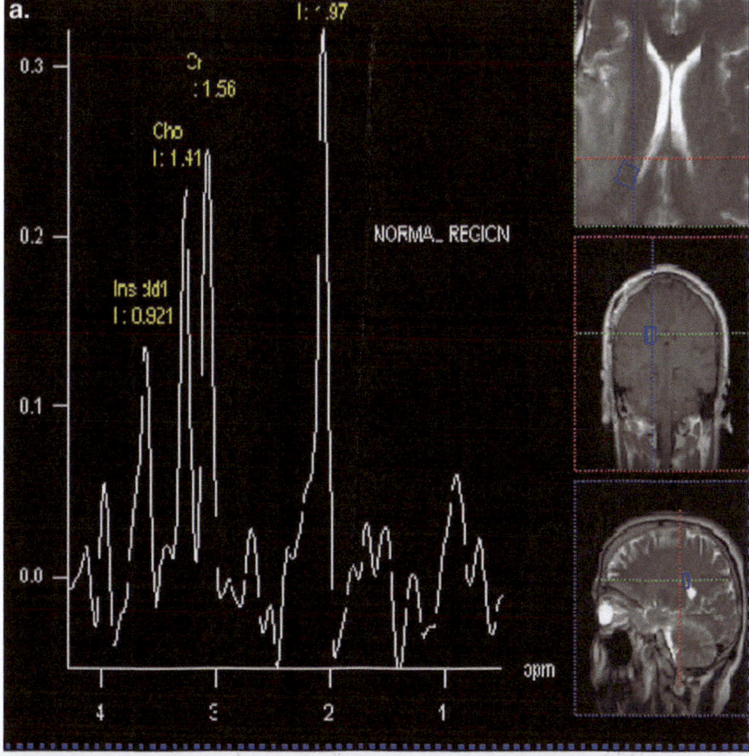

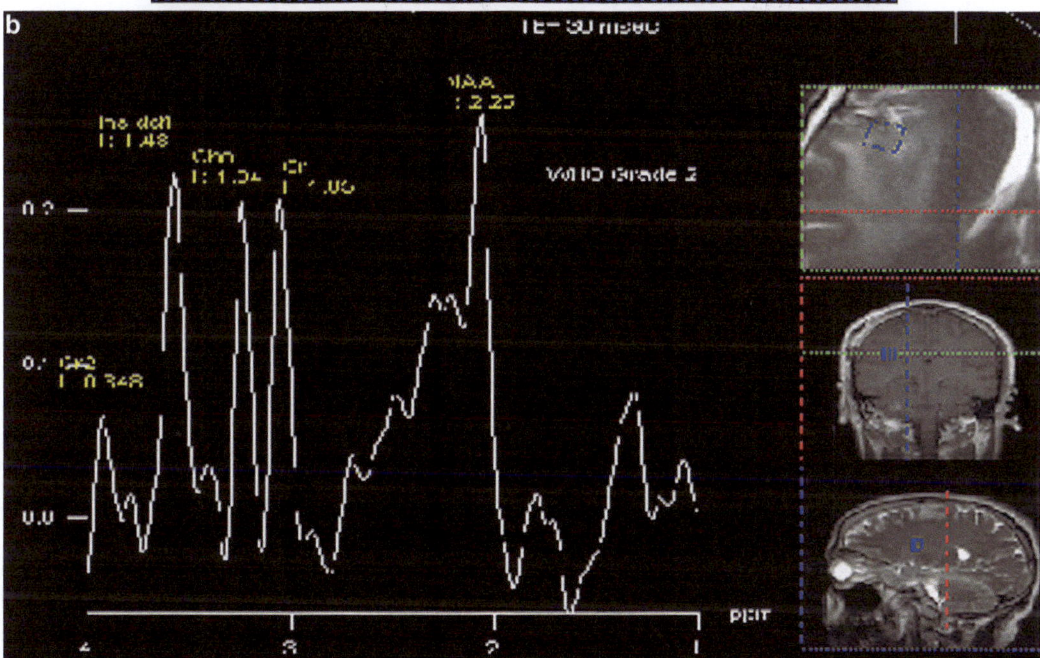

Fig. 9.2 Proton MR spectra of (**a**) normal brain, (**b**) Grade 2 glioma, and (**c**) grade 4 glioma: TE = 30 ms

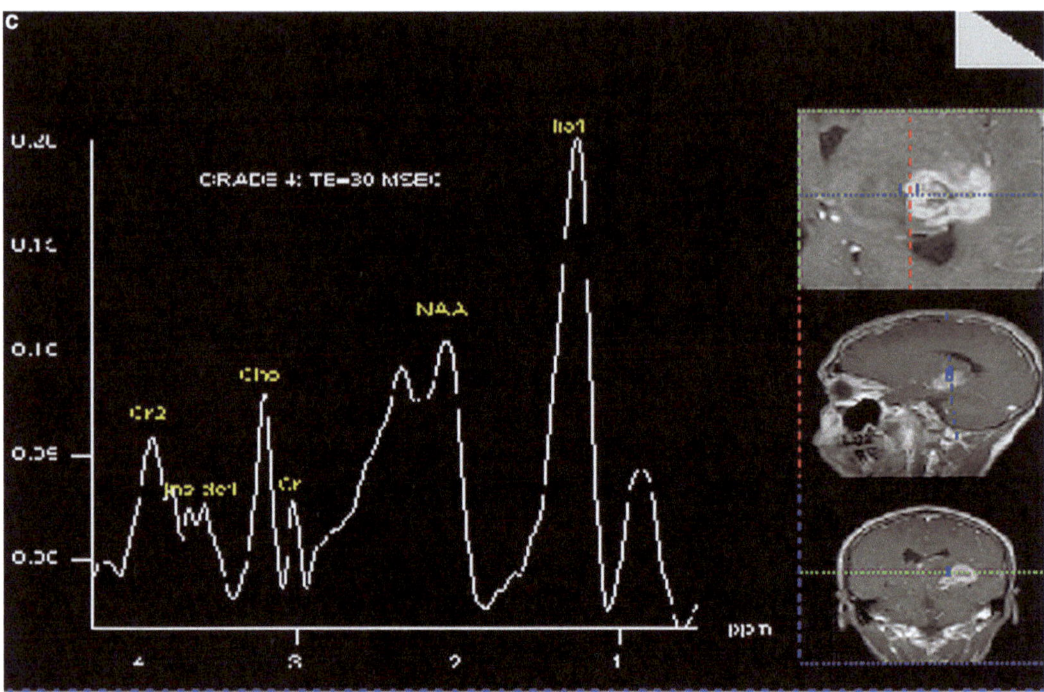

Fig. 9.2 (continued)

Table 9.1 Choline/Creatine (Cho/Cr) and Myoinositol/Creatine (Myo/Cr) Proton Metabolite Peak Area Ratios in Normal brain and Gliomas

	TE = 135 ms	TE = 30 ms	
	Cho/Cr	Cho/Cr	Myo/Cr
1. Normal Brain (n = 20)	1.08 ± 0.19	0.91 ± 0.15	0.42 ± 0.16
2. WHO Grade 2 (n = 5)	1.66 ± 0.28	1.28 ± 0.63	1.02 ± 0.13
3. WHO Grade 3 (n = 5)	2.72 ± 0.49	2.06 ± 0.36	0.49 ± 0.21
4. WHO Grade 4 (n = 10)	3.23 ± 1.06	2.15 ± 0.66	0.33 ± 0.17

In clinicopathological studies, proton MRS spectral patterns obtained in MRSI studies of gliomas have shown to be able to differentiate high-grade from low grade lesions throughout the tumor [20–25]. Pruel and colleagues [25] applied linear discriminate analysis to the "in vivo" MRS metabolite to creatine (metabolite/Cr) signal-intensity ratio spectral profiles obtained from brain lesions and found that the MRS spectral profiles could be used to not only distinguish the grade of the glioma but also could distinguish the type of brain lesion (i.e., benign vs. malignant and primary brain tumor vs. metastatic lesion). The spectral profiles were correlated with biopsies obtained from these lesions with greater than 90 % accuracy. In 104 of 105 MR samples analyzed, the grade and type of malignant disease were classified correctly using the MRS spectral profiles, whereas conventional preoperative clinical diagnosis misclassified 20 of 91 lesions.

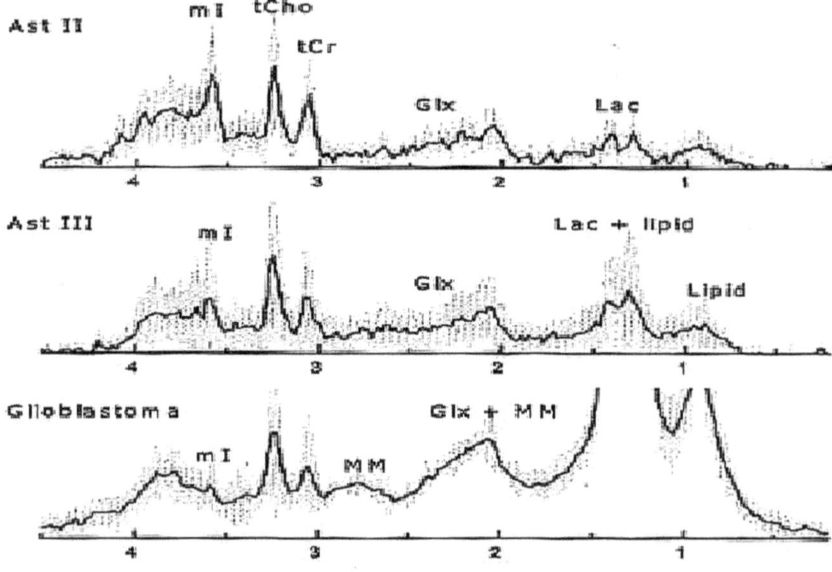

Fig. 9.3 In Vitro High Resolution Proton Magnetic Resonance Spectroscopy of Primary Brain Tumors (Reprinted with permission [31])

Table 9.2 Choline to Creatine proton peak intensity ratios(Cho/Cr) of gliomas: TE = 135 ms

WHO Classificartion:	Grade 2	Grade 3	Grade 4
1. Moller-Hartmann et al. [31]	1.33 ± 0.08	2.13 ± 0.12	3.93 ± 0.64
2. Magalhaes et al. [32]	1.50 ± 0.32	1.62 ± 0.38	3.34 ± 1.15
3. Kwock et al. [29]	1.66 ± 0.28	2.72 ± 0.49	3.23 ± 1.06

Along with Cho/Cr ratios, Choline to *N*-acetylaspartate ratios (Cho/NAA) have also been used to "histologically" grade primary brain tumors. In initial studies conducted by Dowling et al. [36] when Cho levels were found to be elevated by more than 2 SD above the norm and the NAA levels decreased by at least 2 SDs from the norm, regions biopsied for histological evaluation always contained tumor. Using this as a criterion, McKnight et al. [37] and Stadlbauer et al. [38] showed that a combination of increased concentrations of Cho and decreased concentrations of NAA (Cho/NAA metabolic ratios) were associated with the presence of metabolically active tumor cells which correlated positively with the grade of the lesion (Grade 2: Cho/NAA = 0.40 ± 0.16 and Grade 3: Cho/NAA = 0.81 ± 0.46 [38]). However of major importance was that these studies also showed that Cho/NAA maps could be co-registered with MR images and used to determine the location and spatial distribution of the most metabolically active tumor population within the lesion (Fig. 9.4) [38]. This metabolite map could then be used, not only for guiding tumor biopsy procedures to obtain tissue for histological analysis, but also for neurosurgical and radiotherapy treatment planning.

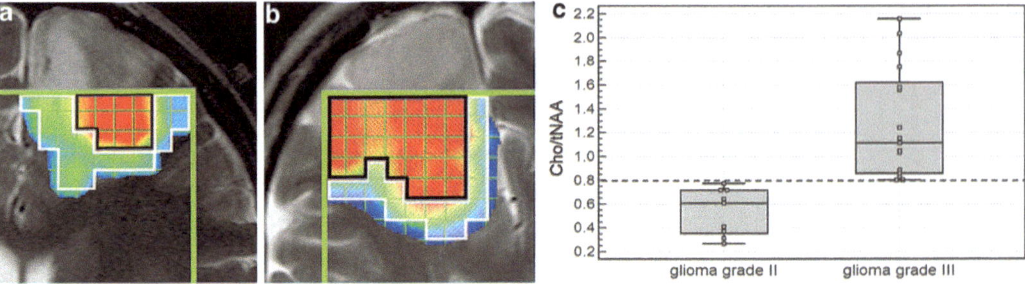

Fig. 9.4 (**a**, **b**) Transverse T2-weighted (6,490/98) MR images in (**a**) patient 6 (astrocytoma grade II) and (**b**) patient 7 (oligodendroglioma grade III) superimposed with color-coded segmented Cho/NAA ratio image. Voxels in predominantly red areas (enclosed by *black line*) were determined as voxels in the tumor center; all other voxel positions were determined as voxels in the tumor border (enclosed by *white line*). *Green lines* show volume of interest of the MR spectroscopic examination. Violet and blue minimum value, *red* maximum value. (**c**) Box plot shows a significant and definite difference (*P* 0.001) for quantified Cho/tNAA ratio averaged over the tumor center between patients with glioma grades II (*n*9) and III (*n*17). The *central box* represents values from lower to upper quartile (25–75 percentile), the middle line represents the median, and vertical bars extend from minimum to maximum value. Small *black squares* show individual data points. (Reprinted with permission [38])

Defining and Delineating Metabolically Different Tumor Regions with Proton MRS

Surgical and radiation therapy (XRT) treatment planning based solely upon conventional anatomical MR imaging is one of the reasons for the dismal prognosis of high grade gliomas (Grade 3 and 4; HGG). The extent of neurosurgical resection is a significant prognostic factor in HGG, and with the aid of computer assisted neuronavigation systems have improved the neurosurgical procedures for the resection of HGGs [39–41]. Patients receiving gross total resection live longer and have improved functional abilities than do patients who undergo subtotal tumor resection [40]. However, HGGs are morphologically and phenotypically heterogeneous and extensively infiltrate brain parenchyma. The MR techniques currently used to plan the surgical resection of the lesion or selecting specific surgical biopsy targets, as previously indicated have been shown [8, 9, 12, 13] to be inadequate of accurately delineating both the extent of tumor infiltration and/or defining and locating the different intratumoral populations within the lesion [namely, (1) the active proliferating tumor population, (2) the migratory tumor population, and (3) the quiescent psuedopalisading hypoxic tumor population]. Establishing the extent of tumor process is one of the major problem areas in HGG neurosurgical planning. Surgical resection is currently targeted to areas based on gadolinium (Gd) enhancement observed on T1-weighted MR images following intravenous injection of gadolinium-DPTA (Gd-DPTA). Enhancement is attributed to BBB breakdown associated with increased tumor angiogenesis in regions of active tumor growth [4, 6]. However, Gd- enhancement, as previously indicated, is not always a reliable indicator of viable tumor due to the presence of non-enhancing tumor regions and contrast-enhancing necrosis [4, 5, 12]. In addition because of the infiltrative nature of HGG, it has been demonstrated that it can extend, nonuniformly, several centimeters beyond regions of contrast enhancement [5]. Thus, reliance on Gd-enhanced MR images for neurosurgical planning can underestimate tumor volume and lead to subtotal resections of the lesion.

Surgical resection is then followed by concomitant adjuvant XRT and chemotherapy. Prior to the availability of computerized X-ray tomography (CT), whole brain or large field external beam XRT techniques were used to treat HGG since conventional imaging techniques were unable to accurately assess the extent of tumor [13].

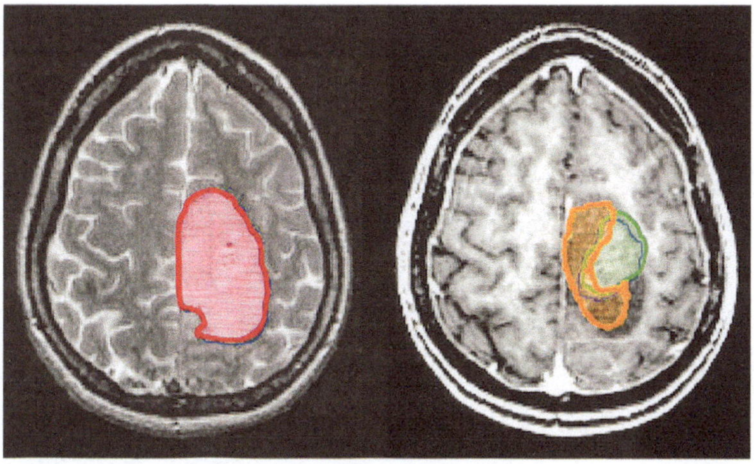

Fig. 9.5 Comparison of lesion extent measured using T2 weighted MRI (*red*), T1 weighted MRI following injection of contrast agent (*green*), and MRS to measure high Cho/NAA (*orange*) for a patient with a grade 4 glioma (with permission [45])

Consequently XRT toxicity to normal brain tissue within the treatment field was common and dose-limiting. With the advancements in 3D conformal XRT techniques, the therapeutic index of XRT in tumor versus normal brain has been substantially increased [42, 43]. However, conformal XRT treatment of HGG especially intensity modulated radiation therapy (IMRT) and radio-surgical XRT techniques require a more accurate definition of the extent and location of the target volumes if these techniques are to be used effectively. Incorrect definition of target volumes can lead to recurrences either at the edge of the target volumes or within the lesion if incorrectly defined.

Currently, the Radiation Therapy Oncology Group (RTOG) recommends using CT and/or MRI to identify tumor volumes for radiotherapy treatment planning [44]. For MRI, fluid attenuated inversion recovery (FLAIR) and T2-weighted MR images are the recommended imaging sequences to use for planning the radiation treatment paradigm. Essentially the same MR imaging methods utilized to delineate the tumor volumes prior to the advent of the more precise RT targeting techniques. Generally, the standard conformal radiotherapy plan targets the abnormal MR imaging area plus a uniform margin of between 1 and 4 cm in all directions to account for tumor infiltration [12, 13]. Using either T2-weighted or contrast enhanced T1-weighted MR images to define target volumes, Price et al. [8] found that in 20 patients, "both T2- and gadolinium-enhanced T1 weighted images missed 1 region of gross tumor. In the infiltrating tumor region, enhanced T1-weighted imaging could identify only 11 of 20 regions and T2-weighted could identify 12 of 20." Similarly, in a study comparing T2 and FLAIR imaging for target delineation in HGG, Stall et al. [9] found that the FLAIR clinical target volumes (CTV) and the planning target volumes (PTV) were significantly larger than the T2 CTVs and PTVs. In addition, they found that the different sequences showed a discordant location for the target volumes (Fig. 9.5; [45]).

The primary therapeutic goal in neuro-oncology is the complete eradication of tumor; therefore, for patients diagnosed with HGG, to obtain the maximum benefit from these new radiotherapeutic and neuro-navigational surgical techniques, it is essential to know as accurately as possible the extent of the tumor borders. However, by utilizing just the conventional MR and CT imaging techniques to plan the radiotherapeutic and/or neurosurgical approaches, as recommended by the RTOG guidelines, we have not improved our ability to define tumor boundaries nor our ability to more accurately assess the degree of tumor infiltration to treat the tumor or normal brain more effectively.

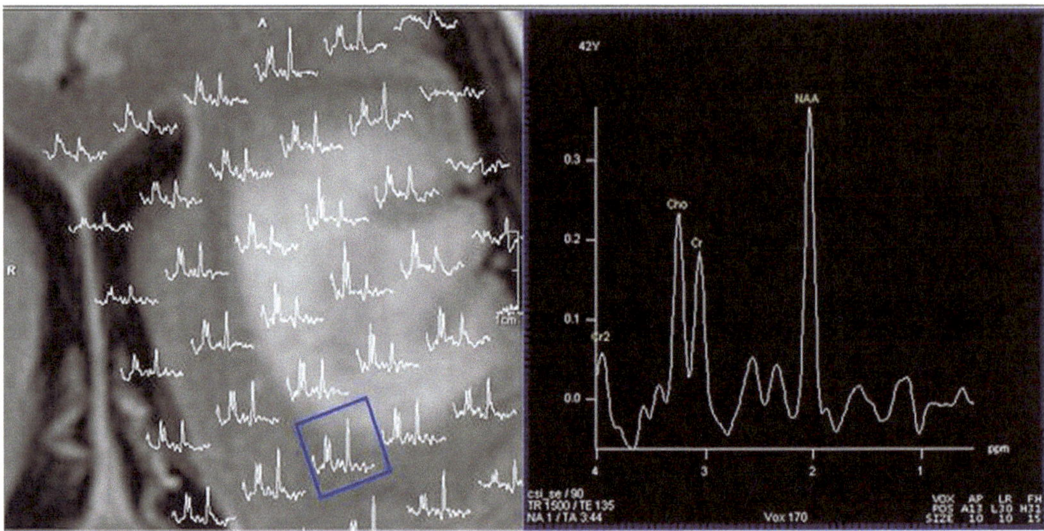

Fig. 9.6 Proton MRSI of uninvolved brain region adjacent to low grade lesion. (Note level of NAA in abnormal FLAIR tumor region vs. uninvolved tumor region shown in *square*)

To achieve the goal of "complete eradication of the tumor" or at least better local tumor control, better noninvasive imaging techniques must be employed to (1) not only delineate the extent of the tumor better for neurosurgical and radiotherapy treatment planning but also to (2) determine the extent and characterize the differences in the major intratumoral populations within the lesion. The latter is needed to identify the tumor populations that are responsible for the recurrence and/or resistant to the HGG treatment paradigm used, so that once identified, treatment strategies can be developed to target this tumor population within the lesion.

In 2001, Dowling et al. [36] took an important step in establishing MRS as a potential technique to map tumor extension. Utilizing a 3-dimensional (3D) MRS technique, they evaluated the 3D MR spectra obtained from 28 brain tumor patients and correlated the histological findings from specific sites to the corresponding MR spectral voxels. Their results showed the following:

1. If the level of NAA is normal, the tissue within that voxel is normal. Conversely, abnormal levels of NAA correlate with abnormal tissue regardless of the underlying histological findings (Figs. 9.6 and 9.7).
2. When a lesion contains a Cho peak area intensity greater than the peak area intensity of NAA and larger than the normal peak area intensity of Cho, tumor was always present (Figs. 9.6 and 9.7).
3. The peak area intensity of Cho correlated with percentage of tumor in the sampled voxel.
4. Non-detectable to near-normal levels of NAA and Cho are seen in areas of gliosis and necrosis).
5. Image areas with similar appearance and enhancement may show different spectral patterns and histological characteristics (Fig. 9.8).

On the basis of these data, 3D MRSI may be an important method that can be used to map tumor margins, identify areas with the highest proliferative fractions for targeted therapy and biopsy, and identify post therapy sites of tumor recurrence.

In a patient study of 34 HGG, Pirzkall et al. [12] determined whether the metabolic information provided by MRSI defined volumes could improve the accuracy of target volumes for RT treatment planning compared to target volumes defined by MRI. Using elevated Cho and decreased NAA as criteria, Pirzkall et al. [12], compared the MRSI defined volumes to that

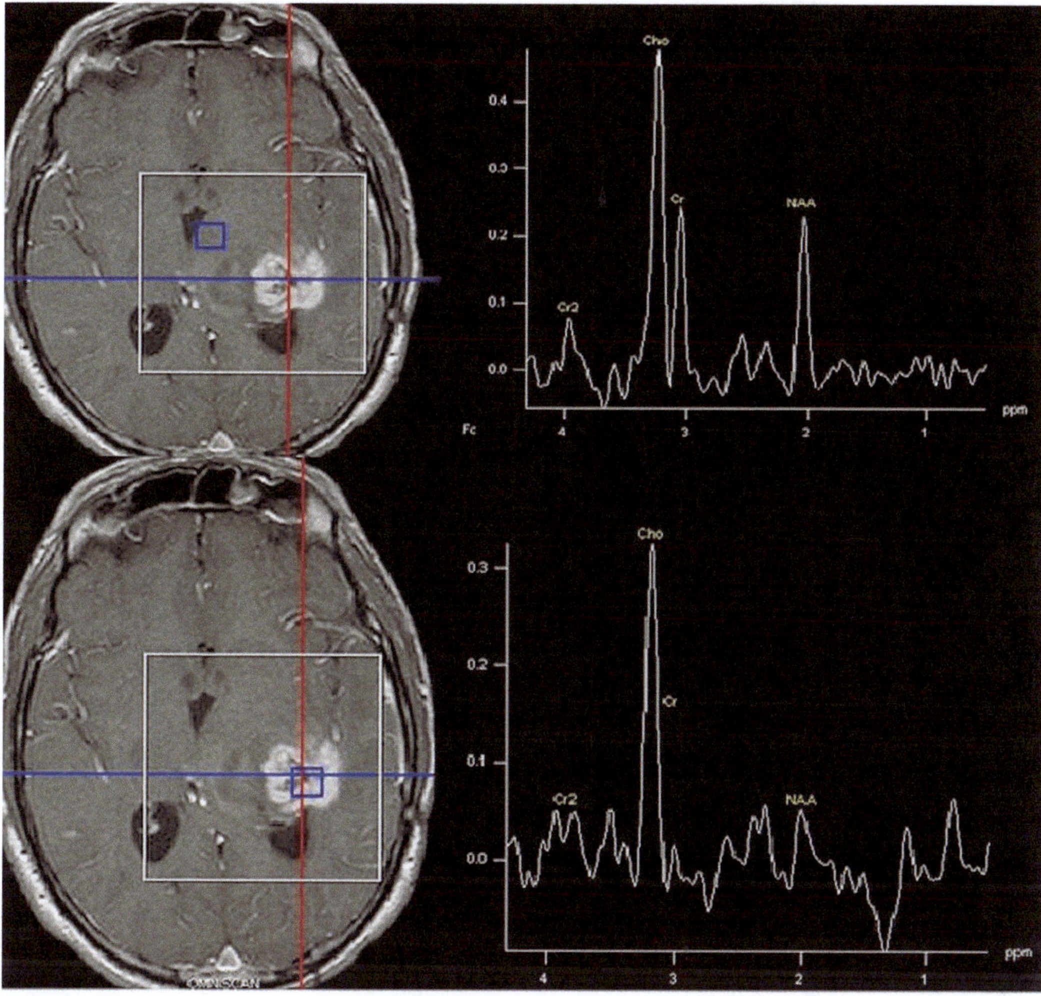

Fig. 9.7 Infiltrative Grade 4 Glioma: Note level of Cho relative to Cr and NAA in enhancing and non-enhancing brain regions. Both spectra indicative of tumor being present

defined by the Gd-enhanced T1 and T2-weighted MRI studies. They found that the T2 studies estimated, as judged by the volume of the hyperintense T2 region, the region at risk of containing microscopic disease as being as much as 50 % greater than by MRSI. On the other hand, the Gd-enhanced T1 studies suggested a lesser tumor volume and different location of active disease compared to MRSI studies (see Fig. 9.4). They concluded that "the use of MRSI to define target volumes for RT treatment planning would increase, and change the location of the volume receiving a boost dose as well as reduce the volume receiving a standard dose." This study suggests that the inclusion of MRSI data into the treatment planning process could potentially improve tumor control while reducing normal tissue radiation complications. This was clearly shown to have occurred in a XRT study of 26 patients with grade 4 gliomas by a study conducted by Chan et al. [46]. Patients with MRSI abnormalities (i.e., elevated Cho/NAA levels) outside of the MRI defined target volume had decreased median survival times relative to those with MRSI abnormalities inside the MRI defined target volumes (10.4 vs. 15.7 months).

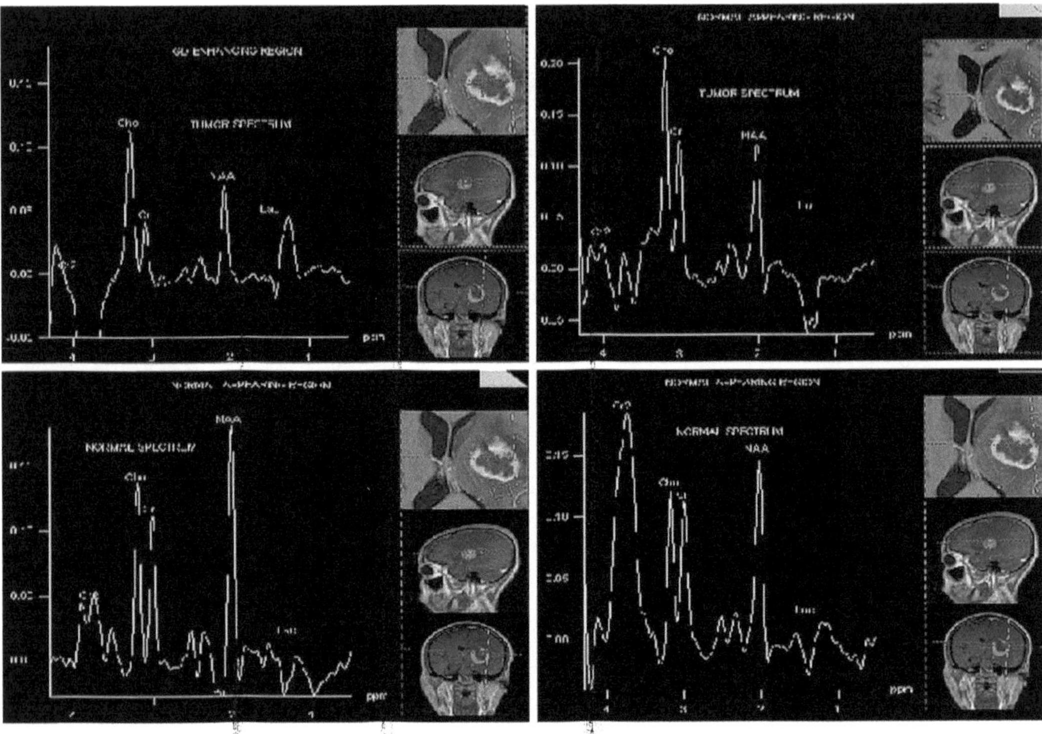

Fig. 9.8 MR Images with similar appearance but show either same spectral patterns or different spectral patterns suggesting different histological characteristics

MRS Spectral Profile of (a) Proliferative, (b) Hypoxic/Psuedopalisading, and (c) Infiltrating Glioma Populations

Another factor that contributes to the poor therapy outcome in HGG patients is the subjective grouping of all HGGs by only its histological characteristics without considering the differences in molecular and genetic character of the different tumor populations within the observed HGG lesion, namely, the main proliferating and stationary tumor body, the infiltrative population of HGG which has a lower proliferation rate, and the quiescent psuedopalisading migratory tumor population adjacent to necrotic regions of the lesion. The molecular and/or genetic character of these population can affect different proliferative and/or infiltrative signaling pathways that are not normally considered when designing the patient's treatment plan. For example, with RT treatment of HGG, concomitant temozolomide chemotherapy is delivered with the XRT treatment. The reason for this is due to the mechanism of action of this drug. Temozolomide is a DNA alkylating agent which induces nicks in DNA, and if not repaired in daughter cells can inhibit replication in the daughter cells leading to increased apoptosis and increased radiation sensitivity. The inhibition of cellular replication occurs in the G2-M phase of the cell cycle [47], i.e., the most radiosensitive phase of the reproductive cell cycle. Thus, the major effect of temozolomide is on tumor cells in the most radio-responsive position of the cell cycle. However, the level of response to temozolomide has been shown to be dependent on the genetic character of the HGG [48]. Deletion on chromosome 10 (PTEN) of the phosphatase and tensin homolog leads to increased sensitivity to temozolomide. PTEN is a lipid phosphatase which plays a basic role in attenuating the phosphatidylinositol 3-kinase (P13K)/Akt-1 signaling pathway; hence, loss of PTEN can affect major oncogenic events during gliomagenesis [48]. Loss of PTEN occurs in about 36 % of patients diagnosed with Grade 4 gliomas; thus, only about a third of the patients diagnosed with HGG will benefit from temozolomide treatment.

However, what about the two other tumor populations present in the HGG lesion in patients who respond to temozolomide, namely, the psuedopalisading migratory cells adjacent to necrotic regions and diffusively infiltrating tumor cells? Both of these tumor types should be refractory to temozolomide since neither type rapidly proliferate [3].

Around areas of necrosis in HGG, the tumor cells show psuedopalisading [3]. Data suggests that the pseudopalisading zone is the result of tumor cells migrating away from the necrotic region, and that necrosis selects for tumor cells that are more aggressive and more resistant to apoptosis-inducing therapeutic regimens [49]. Similarly, data indicates that glioma cells that migrate out of the main tumor body have a decreased proliferative capacity and decreased susceptibility to apoptosis [50]. These two populations may be the tumor cells that are responsible for regrowth and recurrence of the HGG. Thus, more information that can be obtained which characterizes molecular signaling pathways that are activated in these populations will allow for more effective therapies to be developed. For instance, in the case of the migratory HGG cell population, evidence indicates that treatment of glioma cells with inhibitors of migration, does not affect apoptosis of migration restricted/stationary glioma cells, but can sensitize migrating glioma cells to cytotoxic agents [50].

Proliferative Glioma Population: Cho/NAA Ratio Profiles

At the present time, the major role of MRSI in the surgical treatment planning of HGG is in guiding the neurosurgeon to regions which show high metabolic activity to biopsy, namely, regions with elevated Cho levels and low NAA levels relative to normal brain tissue [36, 37].

McKnight et al. [21] has shown that the Cho/NAA but not the Cho/Cr ratios correlates significantly with the proliferation index as determined by MIB-1 immunostaining ($p<0.001$) and the cell density measurements ($p<0.001$) of the biopsy obtained voxel sample. This finding suggests that voxels containing elevated Cho/NAA ratios have the highest probability of being a region that has "high cell density, high proliferative fraction, and/or high ratio of cell proliferation to cell death" [21].

Hypoxic/Psuedopalisading Tumor Population: MRS Metabolic Profile

However as previously indicated, the active proliferating glioma population is not the only tumor population that needs to be examined or treated in the HGG lesion. Two other populations that can lead to the possible recurrence and/or resistance of the tumor to the therapy used also needs to be evaluated, namely, the quiescent psuedopalisading migratory tumor population adjacent to necrotic regions and the active infiltrating tumor populations migrating from the main tumor body [3, 14].

Regions with low Cho and NAA levels relative to normal brain normally indicate necrosis, astrogliosis, macrophage infiltration, or mixed tissue [36]. However, these regions which appear to be necrotic may also contain quiescent, psuedopalisading migratory tumor cells adjacent to necrotic centers [3, 14] especially if they show spectra (obtained at TE = 30 ms) which have elevated choline levels relative to NAA and Cr, lipid/lactate resonances, and possible lower overall levels of metabolites relative to normal tissue (Figs. 9.9 and 9.16). This spectral profile, in fact, may represent the most aggressive tumor population within the HGG lesion and the major population responsible for the resistance and recurrence of the tumor [14, 49].

In a study conducted by Martin et al. [51] to determine the efficacy of MRSI in guiding biopsy, they found that in 17 out of 21 patients who had histological confirmed biopsy tumor samples, the Cho levels were elevated relative to normal levels. However in four patients with low Cho levels similar to those observed in necrotic

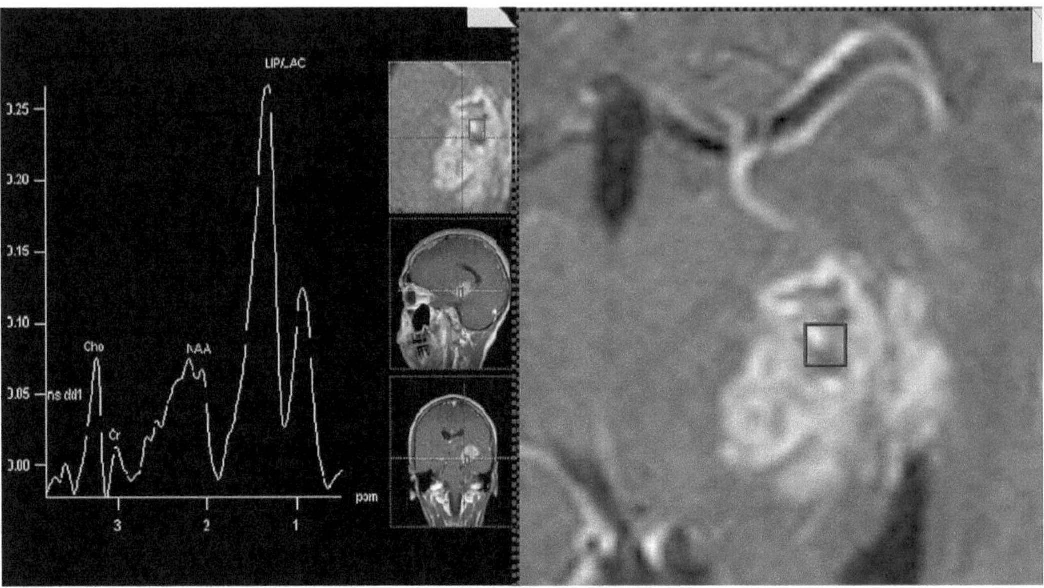

Fig. 9.9 MRSI volume showing necrosis (Lip/Lac) and tumor spectrum (Note elevated Cho/Cr levels)

regions, the histological evaluation of the biopsy sampled showed tumor. The representative MRSI spectra of one of these patients (Fig. 9.10) shows relatively elevated Cho/Cr and Cho/NAA ratios and an elevated lipid/lactate resonance. In addition, the spectra show overall lower levels of all metabolites (compare with Fig. 9.17 of a recurrent anaplastic astrocytoma). Both spectra at our institution would have been considered as suspicious for the possible presence of tumor and monitored serially for changes in choline levels to indicate recurrence of tumor.

Infiltrative Glioma Population: Cho/Cr and Cho/NAA Ratio Profiles

The infiltrating tumor population which originates from the primary stationary actively dividing tumor population and invades the normal brain parenchyma also needs to be characterized and delineated. If this population is not treated appropriately, it can also lead to the recurrence of the tumor. To determine the usefulness of MRSI in assessing the degree of tumor infiltration, Ganslandt et al. [53] performed MRSI studies on seven patients with untreated grade 2 and 3 gliomas. The MRSI data sets were fused with the 3D MRI data sets and integrated into a frameless stereotactic system for image guided interactive neuro-navigation surgery. Tissue samples were obtained from three regions based on the Cho/NAA ratios found in the MRSI study, namely, (1) normal appearing brain region, (2) zone between spectroscopically pathological and suspicious for infiltrating tumor volumes, and (3) maximum spectroscopically pathological volumes. The implementation of the MRSI data set into the frameless stereotactic system was successful in all cases, and stereotactic biopsies were obtained from the MRSI defined regions. In this study, a relationship between the tumor cell density and Cho/NAA metabolic changes were found (60–100 % in the maximum pathological areas to 5–15 % in the border zones suspicious for infiltrating tumor). Another important finding of this study was that the tumor areas defined by the metabolic maps, which were confirmed histopathologically, exceeded the T2-weighted signal change in all cases by 6–32 %. However, in four patients, biopsies obtained with normal Cho/NAA ratio showed the presence of tumor infiltration. It was suggested that the false negative finding in these patients was due to the low resolution of MRSI with respect to the glioma borders. However another explanation could be that the Cho/NAA ratio reflects primarily the proliferative capacity of the tumor cells and not necessarily

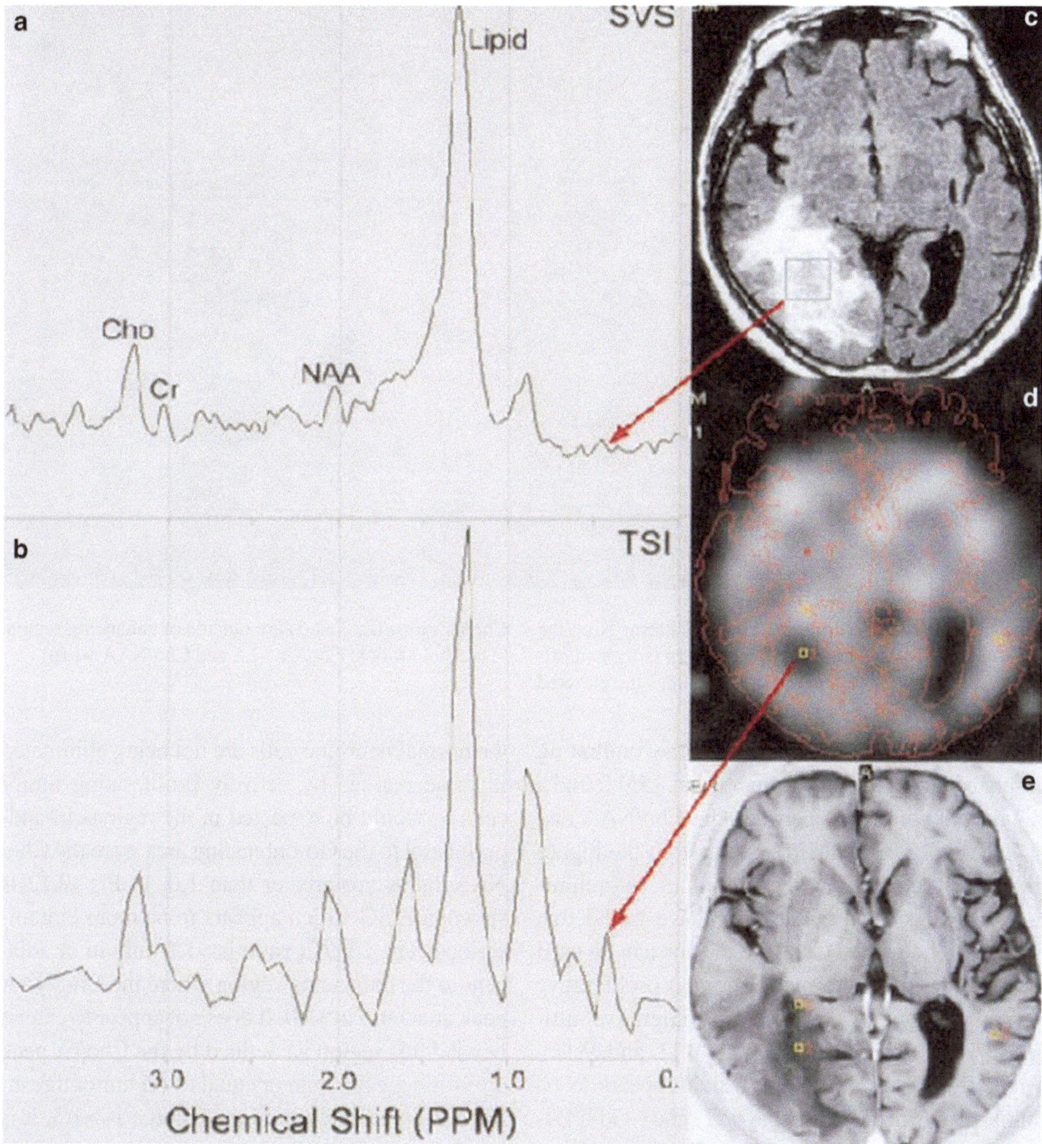

Fig. 9.10 The patient had prominent lipid resonance and otherwise reduced metabolic levels on both SVS and MRSI. While a modest degree of Cho elevation is evident on both spectra, it is difficult to definitively infer the presence of tumor. However, on biopsy this area was confirmed to be recurrent glioblastoma. (Reprinted with permission [51])

the migratory capacity. Thus, in infiltrative tumor zones, Cho/NAA levels maybe normal or only slightly elevated because tumor cells are not dividing and/or displacing or destroying normal neural cells. Highly infiltrative cells normally only proliferate at vascular branch points [3] therefore in infiltrative white matter tumor regions the Cho/NAA ratios may not be elevated. However, the Cho/Cr ratios may be elevated.

The infiltrating tumor pattern of gliomas is closely associated with the expression of matrix metalloproteinase-2 (MMP-2) [54]. Invasion of glioma cells involves the attachment of invading cells to the extracellular matrix (ECM), disruption of the ECM components, and subsequent penetration of the invading cell into adjacent brain structures. This is accomplished in part by the secretion of MMPs by the invading glioma cell to break-

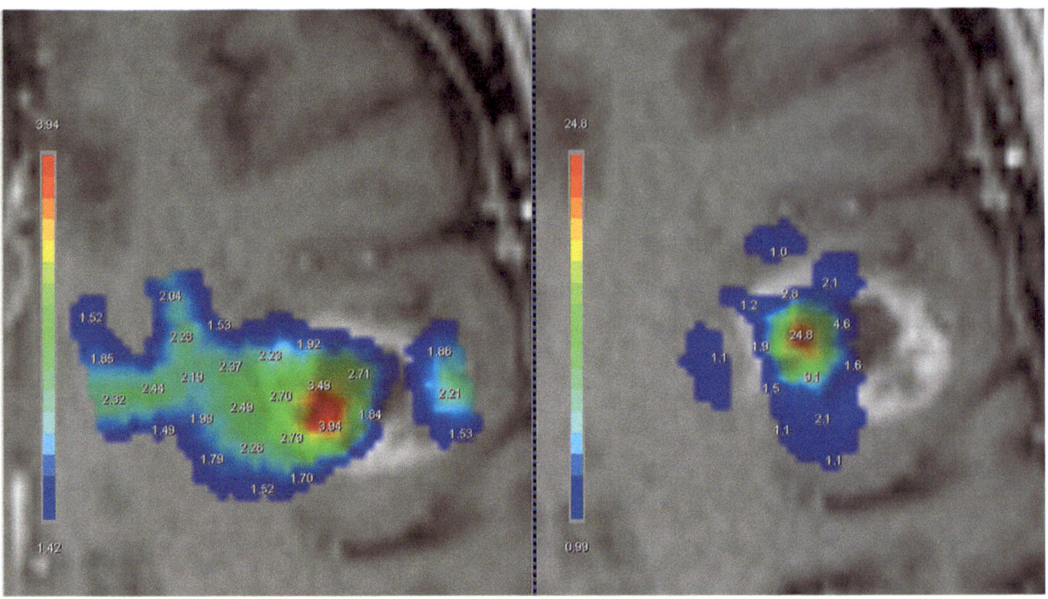

Fig. 9.11 MRSI of Migratory Tumor Pattern: Note the elevated Cho/NAA ratio (i.e., >1.0) pattern is located primarily in enhancing region of tumor whereas the elevated Cho/Cr ratios (i.e., >1.5) are outside of enhancing region. [Threshold ratios: Cho/Cr >1.5 and Cho/NAA >1.0)]

down the ECM barrier impeding the infiltrating tumor cell [54]. Recently, Zhang et al. [55] found a significant correlation between the Cho/NAA and Cho/Cr ratios and MMP-2 expression; the higher the ratios the more invasive the tumor. In preliminary MRSI glioma studies, we have found that both the Cho/Cr and Cho/NAA ratios can be used to delineate the more metabolic and proliferative tumor population from the less proliferative infiltrating tumor population (Figs. 9.11 and 9.12). Figure 9.11 shows a tumor which appears to be infiltrating into areas beyond the Gd-T1w-enhancing regions of tumor. The Cho/Cr peak area ratios in these areas are greater or equal to 1.5. This region outside of the enhancing area also shows Cho/NAA peak area ratios less than or equal to 1.0. This data suggests that in areas outside of the Gd-enhancing or T2w hyperintense areas, in which Cho/Cr ratios >1.5 and Cho/NAA levels of <1.0 (Fig. 9.11) may be regions containing infiltrating tumor cells with lower rates of proliferation; whereas in the area of enhancement or extending just beyond this area, were the MRSI Cho/Cr ratios are >1.5 and the Cho/NAA ratios are >1.0, are areas of active tumor proliferation (Fig. 9.11).

Cho/NAA ratios, we postulate, should be low in areas of tumor infiltration (namely, <1.0) since the normal neuronal cells are not being eliminated in these regions by actively proliferating tumor cells as would be expected in the regions in-and-peripheral to the Gd-enhancing area were the Cho/NAA ratios are greater than 1.0. In Fig. 9.12 is shown a HGG which appears to be more circumscribed. The Cho/Cr ratio is >1.5 only in or adjacent to the enhancing region where the Cho/NAA peak area ratio is >1.0. It does not appear to extend beyond this region as defined by the Cho/Cr peak area ratio greater than or equal to 1.5 tumor threshold ratio (namely, where the Cho/Cr is >1.5, it is highly probable that tumor is present in this voxel). This observed Cho/Cr and Cho/NAA ratio pattern may suggest that the tumor is expanding via a more proliferative rather than an infiltrative pathway due to the more cortical location of this lesion in Fig. 9.12 compared to the tumor shown in Fig. 9.11 [3, 21]. These preliminary studies agree with the study of Stadlbauer et al. [56] who found that ratios of Cho/Cr showed a moderate and statistically significant positive linear correlation to tumor infiltration and tumor cell number.

The data presented in this section suggest that 1H MRSI may be useful in combination with the frameless stereotactic neuro-navigation system compared to conventional anatomic MRI alone to

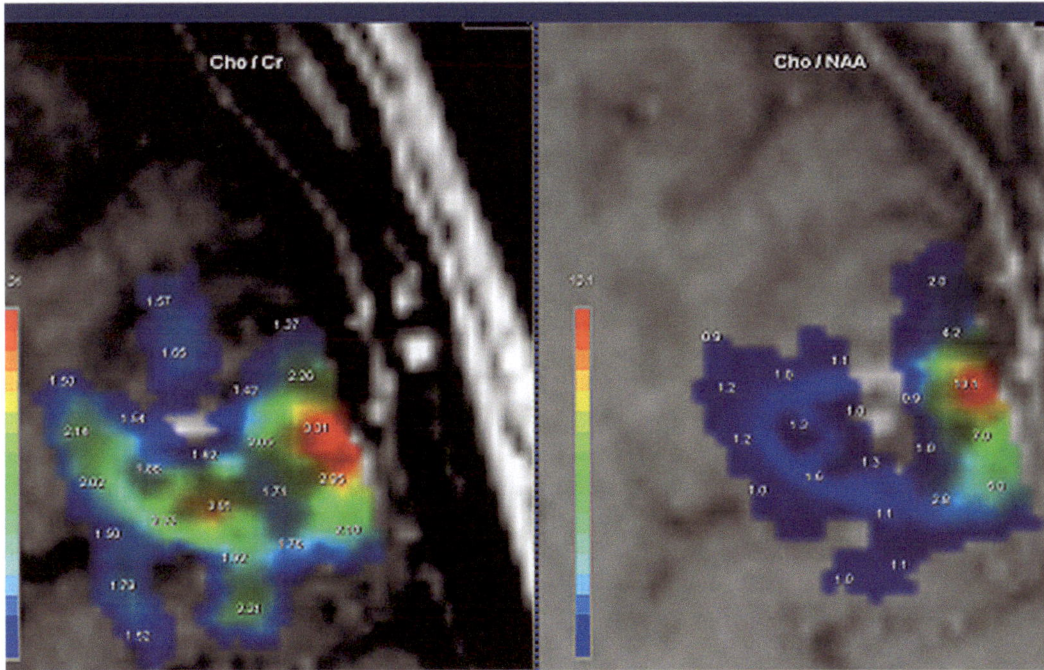

Fig. 9.12 MRSI of Proliferative Glioma Pattern: Note both Cho/Cr and Cho/NAA patterns are similar. (Threshold ratios: Cho/Cr >1.5 and Cho/NAA >1.0)

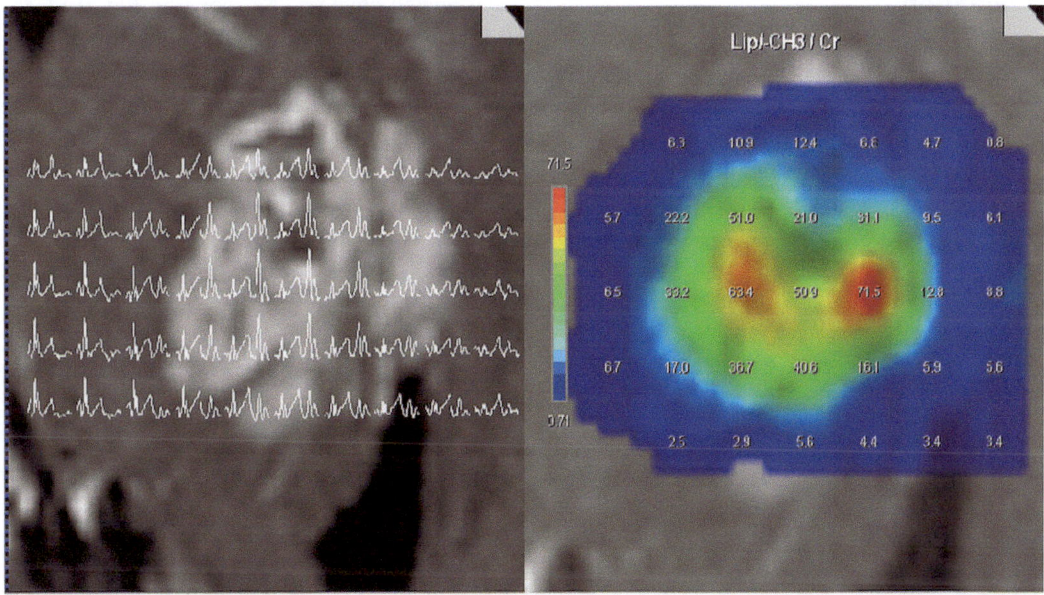

Fig. 9.13 MR spectral pattern and spectroscopic image of Lipid/Cr peak area intensity ratios: Note lipid resonances fall off at edge of enhancing lesion

define more exactly the tumor infiltration and more metabolically active tumor zone [51]. In addition, 1H MRSI may aid in defining the quiescent psuedopalisading migratory tumor zone within the observed lesion for surgical resection as defined by the Lip/Lac resonance (0.8–1.5 ppm), Cho/Cr, and Cho/NAA levels (Figs. 9.9a, and 9.13; [14, 49]). Neurosurgical intervention will undoubtedly continue to be important in the role of treating cerebral gliomas; however, the only possibility of significantly improving patient survival in patients diagnosed with HGG will come with a better understanding of HGG tumor biology and the development of therapies which will take advantage of this better biological understanding of the genetic and metabolic makeup of HGGs. We suggest that the most important use of MRSI maybe in its use to define intratumoral biopsy target sites within the lesion to obtain tissue for not just histological characterization but also for genomic, proteomic, and metabolomic analysis of the aberrant signaling pathways involved in the different tumor populations in patients diagnosed with HGG. The information from these analyses can then be used for the development of "targeted" treatment paradigms of these different tumor populations in the malignant lesion.

Role of MRSI in the Monitoring of Therapy and Post-Therapy Evaluation

Most brain tumors, especially gliomas, are treated with primary or adjuvant radiotherapy. Delivery of radiation normally involves a high dose boost to the central core of the tumor and a lower second radiation dose to all signal intensity abnormalities observed by MR imaging. Radiation induced injury is histopathologically characterized by damage to the vascular endothelium resulting in vessel occlusion, ischemia, and necrosis [57]. Radiation necrosis can occur as early as 3 months or as late as 10 years post-therapy. The typical MR imaging appearance of the treated region is a hyperintense T2-weighted MRI and increased Gd-enhancement T1-weighted MR image suggestive of recurrent/residual tumor. This is illustrated in Fig. 9.14 which shows a patient diagnosed with a grade 3 anaplastic astrocytoma that extended into the medulla of the brain stem. The region had been treated with radiation therapy up to a dose of 5,400 cGy, and was undergoing temozolomide chemotherapy. The patient's clinical status continued to worsen during treatment and a single volume spectroscopy study was performed over the Gd-enhancing lesion to determine if the patients worsening symptoms were due to non-response of the tumor to the treatments or due to radiation/chemotherapy related changes. As shown in Fig. 9.14, the MRS study only showed a single broad peak between 0.5 and 2 ppm suggestive of radiation necrosis [58–60]. No other metabolites were observed within this enhancing region. The patient was taken off of chemotherapy and over

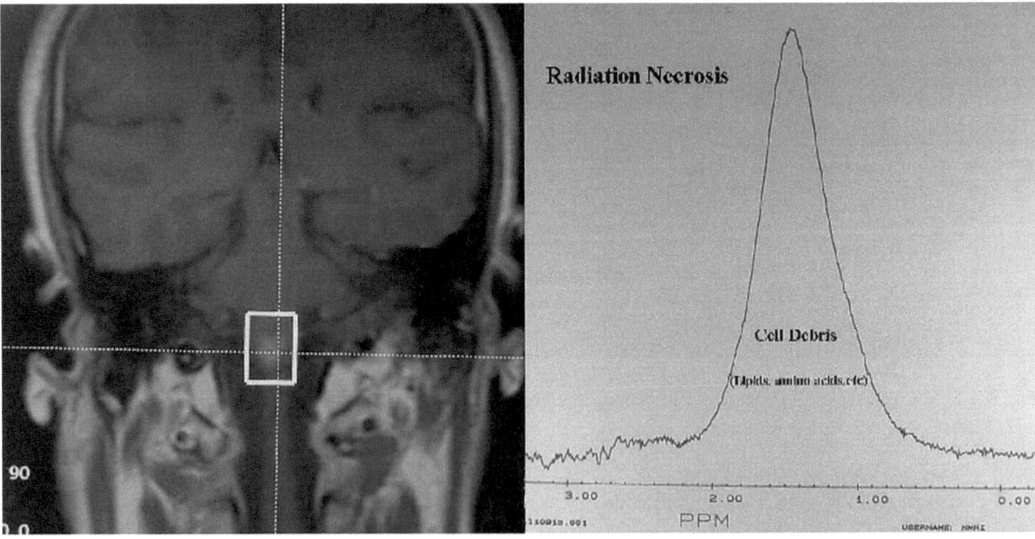

Fig. 9.14 Radiation response of patient diagnosed with Grade 3 glioma

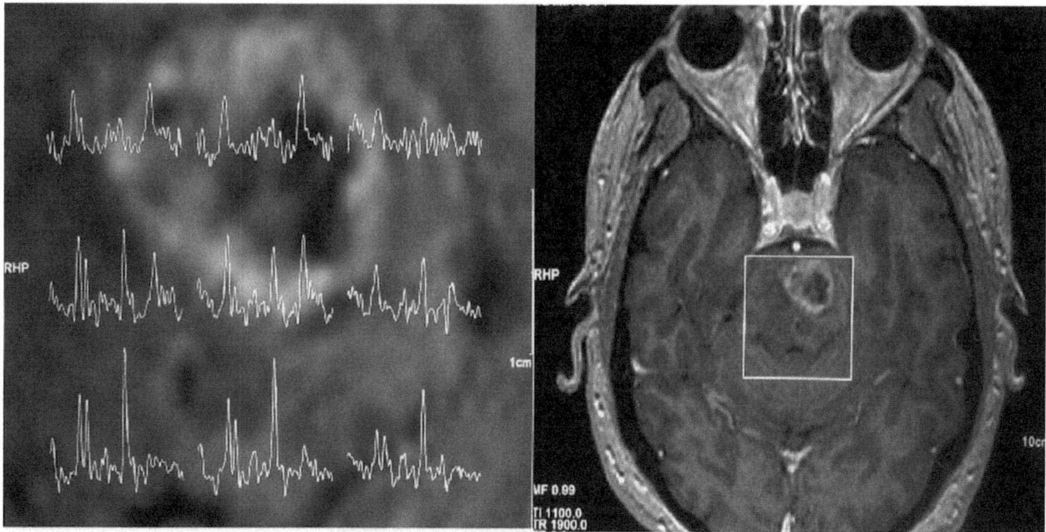

Fig. 9.15 Metastatic Lesion Pre-radiosurgery

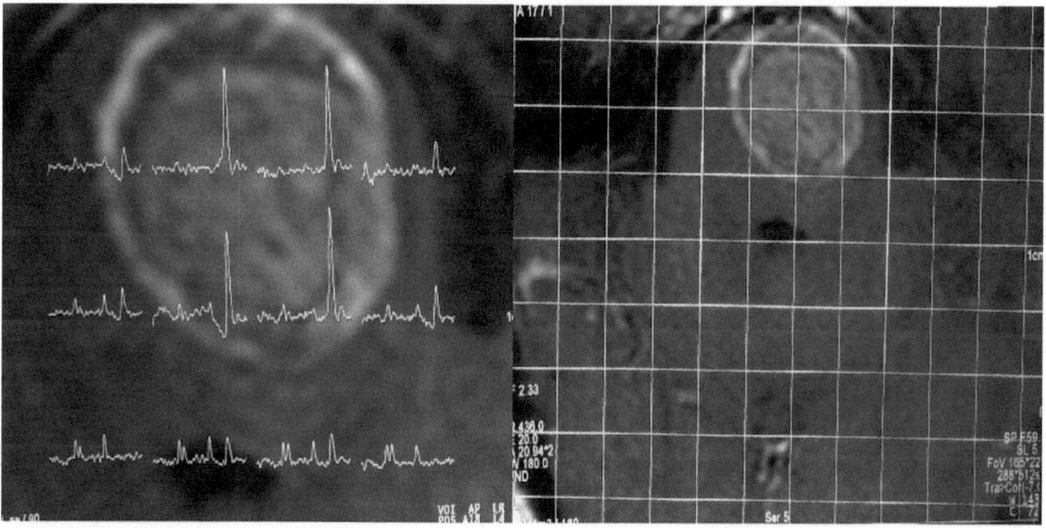

Fig. 9.16 Metstatic Lesion 6 months Post-radiosurgery

the next few weeks the patients clinical symptoms dramatically improved and the Gd-enhancement decreased and became more focal.

Typically what is observed in a tumor that responds to radiation and/or chemotherapy is a decrease in the choline resonance at 3.2 ppm and increases in resonance intensity associated with lipids and lactate at 0.9–1.5 ppm [61–64]. This is illustrated in Figs. 9.15 and 9.16 from a patient with a metastatic lesion located in the brainstem and treated with radiosurgery. Note the large decrease in choline resonance and large increase in lipids similar to that observed in the patient with the brainstem glioma shown in Fig. 9.14. This type of pattern is suggestive of apoptosis induced cell death [58–60] On subsequent follow-up the only metabolite observed was the lipid/lactate resonance peak at 0.9–1.5 ppm (data not shown). Now compare this study with what is shown in Fig. 9.17. This is a patient with a brainstem glioma

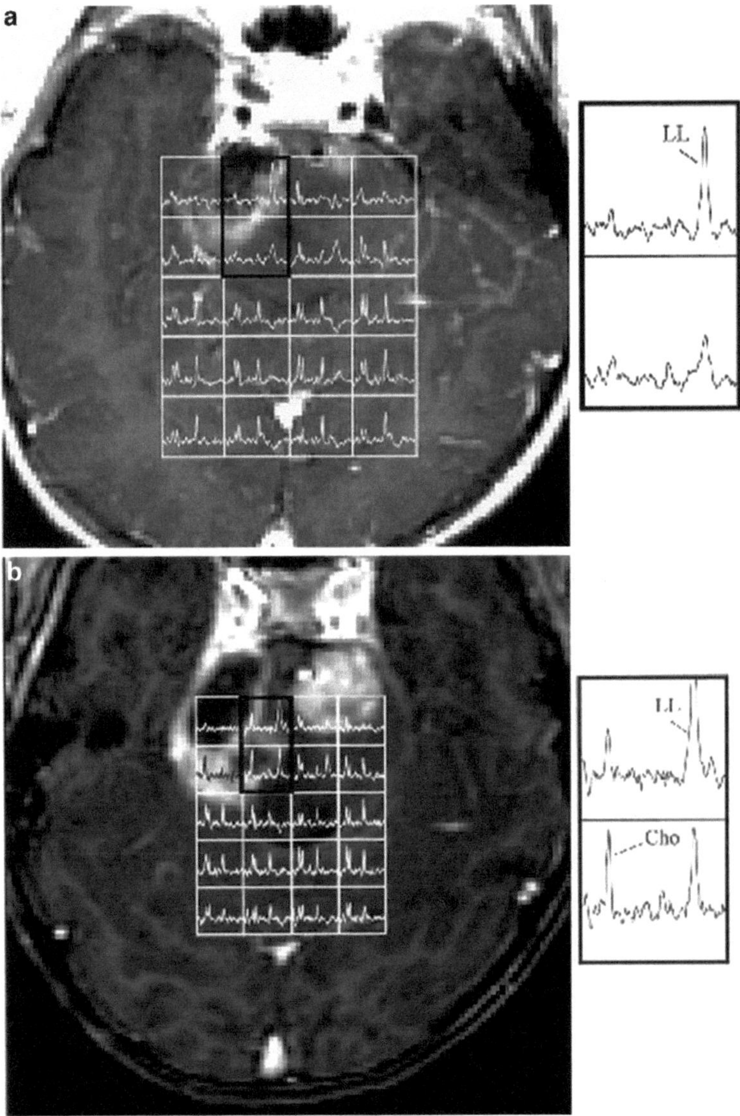

Fig. 9.17 Conventional gadolinium-enhanced T1 weighted images and proton MRSI at 1 month post-RT and at 2 months post RT of a girl age 4 years diagnosed with a diffuse brain stem glioma. (**a**) At one month follow-up, Cho is low, as well as NAA and Cr, but an Lip-Lac(LL) peak appears inside the rim enhancement. (**b**) At (lower image), 2 months follow-up, LL peak persist, and high Cho peaks appear, along with clinical progression and progression of MRI abnormalities (including increased contrast enhancement and increased size of T2-weighted images. (Reprinted with permission [52])

treated with XRT [52]. One month after XRT the MRSI study of this patient showed, predominantly, a large Lip/Lac peak (LL; Fig. 9.17a) suggestive of necrosis. Overall, the metabolite levels relative to surrounding normal voxels appear decreased; however, the Cho/Cr and Cho/NAA ratios were found to be elevated. At this time, the patient's clinical status was stable on examination. However, 1 month later the clinical symptoms of the patient worsened. Both MRI and MRSI studies showed that the tumor had recurred (Fig. 9.17b). Note the large increase in Cho levels and increased Gd-enhancement in the brainstem region. Compare this spectrum with the spectrum in

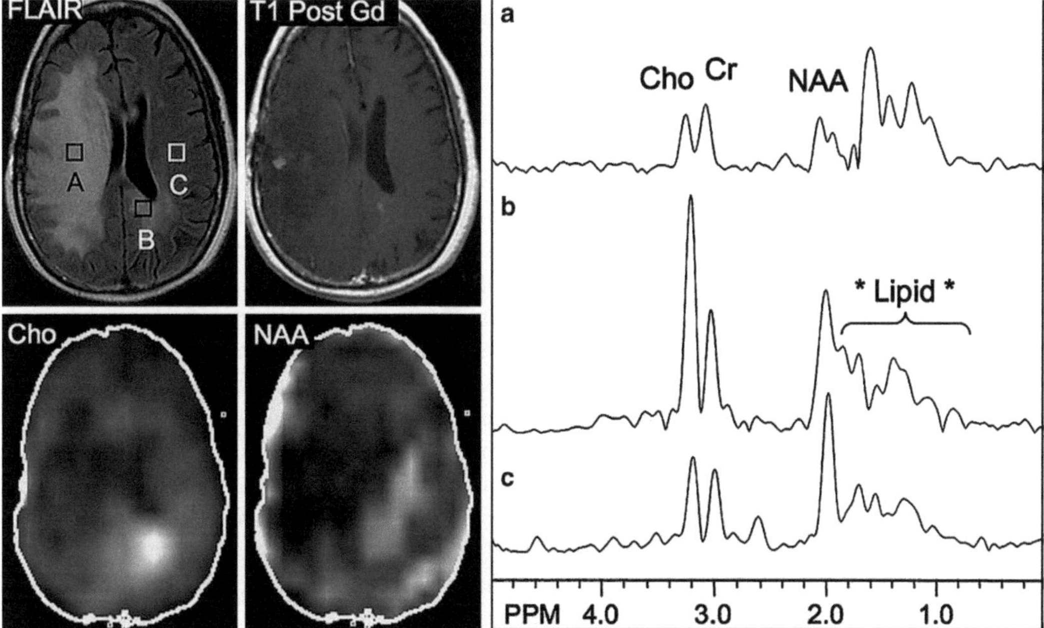

Fig. 9.18 MR imaging (FLAIR, T1, post-Gd) and MRSI (Cho, NAA) in a 53-year-old female with a right frontal anaplastic astrocytoma previously treated with surgery and radiation. The T2 hyperintense large right hemisphere lesion is characterized by reduced levels of all metabolites (**a**), consistent with radiation necrosis, while high Cho is observed in the splenium of the corpus callosum crossing into the left hemisphere, consistent with tumor growth (**b**). A spectrum from a normal-appearing region in the left hemisphere is shown in (**c**) for comparison. Note that the lipids seen in (**a**–**c**) most likely artifacts resulting from head motion during the scan, and also affect the reconstructed NAA image. Small nodules of contrast enhancement are seen in the right hemisphere and the left side of the corpus callosum. The MRSI results were in good accordance with 19F-fluorodeoxyglucose (FDG)-positron emission tomography scan performed contemporaneously (Reprinted with permission [65])

Fig. 9.18a in a patient with a large right hemisphere HGG that has undergone a full course of radiotherapy treatment [65]. Figure 9.18a shows a spectrum more consistent with radio-necrosis; note the level of Cho is not elevated relative to Cr in this spectrum compared to the spectrum shown in Fig. 9.17a. For the most part, the MRSI study showed spectra containing low metabolite signals, consistent with a tumor response to the radiotherapy treatment. Unfortunately, in this patient, tumor spectra were observed throughout the area of the splenium of the corpus callosum and have apparently crossed midline into the contralateral hemisphere (Fig. 9.18).

As demonstrated in the above examples, significantly reduced levels of Cho and Cr and elevation of lipids/lactate levels are suggestive of treatment induced cell death (necrosis or apoptosis) [58–60]. However, if Cho is still present and elevated (evaluated either as elevated Cho signal in tumor to Cho signal in normal tissue, Cho/Cr or Cho/NAA ratios) may suggest that tumor is still present, and that the patient should be monitored carefully for signs of tumor recurrence. It is possible that what one is observing when we see the pattern shown in Fig. 9.17a are the quiescent psuedopalisading tumor cells that are resistant to the radiation dose delivered and will cause recurrence of the tumor (Fig. 9.17b). However, if on follow-up, only the lipid/lactate is visible then this is an indication that this region only contains necrotic products.

Tzika et al. [66] in studies on pediatric brain tumors found that changes in the peak areas of Cho and Cr could be used to discriminate between a responding and non-responding tumor. In eight brain tumors that showed response to either radiation or chemotherapy, all exhibited lower levels of Cho and higher levels of Cr and lower lipid/lactate levels compared to 16 tumors that were treated with only surgery or did not respond to treatment. Similarly, in a pediatric brain study conducted by Taylor et al. [62], only the peak areas of Cho and Cr proved useful in differentiating delayed radiation necrosis from recurrent/residual brain tumor. Although, these studies differ with respect to the use of the lipid/lactate peak as a marker for tumor treatment response, they are all in agreement that increases in choline peak resonance signal indicates recurrent/residual tumor and that decreases in the choline peak resonance signal indicates tumor response. Only if the choline peak levels remain low relative to the other resonances can one say that a complete response has been achieved.

Conclusions

The use of magnetic resonance spectroscopy in the diagnosis and monitoring of treatment response to brain tumors has been documented extensively and shown to be of clinical benefit in a large number of cases. However, it has not been widely accepted as a routine clinical tool outside of major academic medical centers. From the studies presented in this chapter, MRS techniques have improved dramatically because of better magnetic field shimming algorithms, MRS acquisition sequences, and better hardware (i.e., coils, higher field clinical systems, etc.). However what has lagged behind has been the development of robust and automated MRS procedures which can be performed by a radiological MR technologist to collect, analyze and display the results of the MRS study in a timely and routine fashion to the radiologist. This is normally performed by trained and experienced individuals at major academic centers performing routine MRS studies. Additionally for MRS to be accepted as a useful clinical tool, radiologists must be trained to interpret the MRS patterns found for disease processes similar to their training in interpreting the anatomical patterns found on MRI studies of disease processes. Finally, MRS should not be used by itself for the diagnosis but should be integrated and correlated with both conventional and functional MRI studies performed on the patient to maximize the diagnostic benefit of these techniques [22, 26, 67, 68].

In the case of brain tumors, we believe that proton MRSI should not be used just to diagnose the lesion but be used to: (1) delineate the location and the extent of heterogeneous tumor populations within the lesion, (2) define target biopsy sites from which to obtain tissue for histological, genomic [69–71], proteomics [72], and metabolomics [73, 74] for characterization of the tumor, and (3) establishing baseline MRS metabolic characteristics of the MRSI tumor voxels which can be used to monitor, along with conventional and functional MRI techniques, the effectiveness of the therapy paradigm developed to treat all tumor subpopulations comprising the whole lesion.

References

1. CBTRUS Statistical Report. Primary Brain Tumors in the United States, 1995–1999, Hinsdale, IL: Central Brain Tumor Registry of the United States, 2002.
2. Davisa FG, Kupelian V, Freels S, et al. Prevalence estimates for primary brain tumors in the United States by behavior and major histology groups. Neuro Oncol. 2001;3:152–8.
3. Claes A, Idema AJ, Wesseling P. Diffuse glioma growth: a guerilla war. Acta Neuropathol. 2007;114: 443–58.
4. Felix R, Schorner W, Laniado M, et al. MR imaging and gadolinium-DPTA. Radiology. 1985;156:681–8.
5. DeAngelis LM. Brain tumors. N Engl J Med. 2001;344:114–23.
6. Pronin IN, Holodny AI, Petraikin AV. MRI of high grade glial tumors: correlation between the degree of contrast enhancement and the volume of surrounding edema. Neuroradiology. 1997;39:348–50.
7. Li X, Lu Y, Pirzkall A, et al. Analysis of the spatial characteristics of metabolic abnormalities in newly diagnosed glioma patients. J Magn Reson Imaging. 2002;16:229–37.
8. Price SJ, Jena R, Burnet NG, et al. Improved delineation of glioma margins and regions of infiltration with the use of diffusion tensor imaging: An image-guided biopsy study. AJNR Am J Neuroradiol. 2006;27: 1969–74.
9. Stall B, Zach L, Ning H, et al. Comparison of T2 and FLAIR imaging for target delineation in high grade gliomas. Radiat Oncol. 2010;5:5. http//www.ro-journal.com/content/5/1/5.

10. Yu X, Liu Z, Tian Z, et al. Stereotactic biopsy for space-occupying lesions: clinical analysis of 550 cases. Stereotact Funct Neurosurg. 2000;75:103–8.
11. Alesch F, Pappaterra J, Trattig S, Koos WT. The role of stereotactic biopsy in radiosurgery. Acta Neurochir Suppl (Wien). 1995;63:20–4.
12. Pirzkall A, McKnight TR, Graves EE, et al. MR-spectroscopy guided target delineation for high grade gliomas. Int J Radiat Oncol Biol Phys. 2001;50(4):915–28.
13. Lee SW, Benedick BA, Marsch LH, et al. Patterns of failure following high dose 3-D conformal radiotherapy for high grade astrocytomas: a quantitative dosimetric study. Int J Radiat Oncol Biol Phys. 1999;43(1):79–88.
14. Brat DJ, Castellano-Sanchez AA, Hunter SB. Psuedopallisades in glioma are hypoxic, express extracellular matrix proteases, and are formed by an actively migrating cell population. Cancer Res. 2004;64:920–7.
15. Ross B, Michaelis T. Clinical applications of magnetic resonance spectroscopy. Magn Reson Q. 1994;10:191–247.
16. Howe FA. Magnetic resonance spectroscopy *in vivo*. In: Markisz JA, Whalen JP, editors. Principles and practice of MRI: selected topics. Stamford, Conn: Appleton and Lange; 1998. p. 17–107.
17. Chang SM, Prados MD. Chemotherapy for gliomas. Curr Opin Oncol. 1995;7:207–13.
18. Krauseneck P, Muller B. Chemotherapy of malignant gliomas: recent results. Cancer Res. 1994;135:135–47.
19. Krex D, Klink B, Hartman von Deimling A, et al. Long-term survival with glioblastoma multiforme. Brain. 2007;130:2596–606.
20. Toyooka M, Kimura H, Uematsu H, et al. Tissue characterization of glioma by proton magnetic resonance spectroscopy and perfusion-weighted magnetic resonance imaging: glioma grading and histological correlation. Clin Imaging. 2008;32:251–8.
21. McKnight TR, Lamborn KR, Love TD, et al. Correlation of magnetic resonance spectroscopic and growth characteristics within Grade II and III gliomas. J Neurosurg. 2007;106:660–6.
22. Law M, Yang S, Hao Y, et al. Glioma grading: Sensitivity, specificity, and predictive values of perfusion MR imaging and proton MR spectroscopic imaging compared with conventional MR imaging. AJNR Am J Neuroradiol. 2003;24:1989–98.
23. Howe FA, Barton SJ, Cudlip SA, et al. Metabolic profiles of human brain tumors using quantitative in vivo 1H magnetic resonance spectroscopy. Magn Reson Med. 2003;49:223–32.
24. Croteau D, Scarpace L, Hearshen D, et al. Correlation between magnetic resonance spectroscopy imaging and image-guided biopsies: Semiquantitative and qualitative histopathological analyses of patients with untreated glioma. Neurosurgery. 2001;49(4):823–9.
25. Pruel MC, Caramanos Z, Collins DL, et al. Accurate, noninvasive diagnosis of human brain tumors by using proton magnetic resonance spectroscopy. Nat Med. 1996;2(3):323–5.
26. Huang BY, Kwock L, Castillo M, Smith JK. Association of choline levels and tumor perfusion in brain metastases assessed with proton MR spectroscopy and dynamic susceptibility contrast-enhanced perfusion weighted MRI. Technol Cancer Res Treat. 2010;9(4):327–38.
27. Howe FA, Opstad KS. 1H MR spectroscopy of brain tumours and masses. NMR Biomed. 2003;16: 123–31.
28. Tsien RD, Lai PH, Smith JS, Lazeyras F. Single voxel proton brain spectroscopy exam (PROBE/SV) in patients with primary brain tumors. Am J Roentgenol. 1996;167:201–9.
29. Kwock L, Smith JK, Castillo M, et al. Clinical role of proton magnetic resonance spectroscopy in oncology: brain, breast, and prostate cancer. Lancet Oncol. 2006;7:859–68.
30. Cheng LL, Chang IW, Louis DN. Gonzalez RG, correlation of high-resolution magic angle spinning proton magnetic resonance spectroscopy with histopathology of intact human brain tumor specimens. Cancer Res. 1998;58:1825–32.
31. Moller-Hartmann W, Herminghaus S, Krings T. Clinical application of proton magnetic resonance spectroscopy in the diagnosis of intracranial mass lesions. Neuroradiology. 2002;44:371–81.
32. Magalhaes A, Godfrey W, Shen Y, et al. Proton magnetic resonance spectroscopy of brain tumors correlated with pathology. Acta Radiol. 2005;12:51–7.
33. Alger JR, Frank JA, Bizzi A, et al. Metabolism of human gliomas: assessment with H-1 MR spectroscopy and F-18 fluorodeoxyglucose PET. Radiology. 1990;177:633–41.
34. Ramirez de Molina A, Gallego-Ortega D, Sarmentero-Estrada J, et al. Choline kinase as a link connecting phospholipid metabolism and cell cycle regulation: Implications in cancer therapy. Int J Biochem Cell Biol. 2008;40:1753–63.
35. Umezu-Goto M, Kishi Y, Taira A, et al. Autotaxin has lysopholipase D activity leading to tumor cell growth and motility by lysophosphatidic acid production. J Cell Biol. 2002;158(2):227–33.
36. Dowling C, Bollen AW, Noworolski SM, et al. Preoperative proton MR spectroscopic imaging of brain tumors: correlation with histopathologic analysis of resection specimens. AJNR Am J Neuroradiol. 2001;22:604–12.
37. McKnight TR, von dem Bussche MH, Vigneron DB, et al. Histopathological validation of a three-dimensional magnetic resonance spectroscopy index as a predictor of tumor presence. J Neurosurg. 2002;97: 794–802.
38. Stadlbauer A, Gruber S, Nimsky C, et al. Preoperative grading of gliomas by using metabolite quantification with high-spatial resolution proton MR imaging. Radiology. 2006;238(3):958–69.
39. Laws ER, Parney IF, Huang W, et al. Survival following surgery and prognostic factors for recently diagnosed malignant glioma: data from the Glioma Outcomes Project. J Neurosurg. 2003;99:467–73.

40. Lacroix M, Abi-Said D, Fourney DR, et al. A multivariate analysis of 416 patients wih glioblastoma multiforme: Prognosis, extent of resection, and survival. J Neurosurg. 2001;95:190–8.
41. Devaux BC, O'Fallon JR, Kelly PJ. Resection, biopsy, and survival in malignant glial neoplasms. A retrospective study of clinical parameters, therapy, and outcome. J Neurosurg. 1993;78:767–75.
42. Sandler HM. 3-D conformal radiotherapy for brain tumors: the university of Michigan experience. Front Radiat Ther Oncol. 1996;29:250–4.
43. Thorton AF, Hegarty TJ, Ten-Haken RK, et al. Three dimensional treatment planning of astrocytomas: a dosimetric study of cerebral irradiation. Int J Radiat Oncol Biol Phys. 1991;20:1309–15.
44. Radiation Therapy Oncology Group. Active Brain Protocols. 2012. http://rtog.org/ClinicalTrials/ProtocolTable.aspx. Accessed 16 April 2012.
45. Nelson SJ, Graves E, Pirzkall A, et al. In vivo molecular imaging for planning radiation therapy of gliomas: an application of 1H MRSI. J Magn Reson Imaging. 2002;16:464–76.
46. Chan A, Lau A, Pirzkall A, et al. Proton magnetic resonance spectroscopy imaging in the evaluation of patients undergoing gamma knife surgery for Grade IV glioma. J Neurosurg. 2004;101:46–475.
47. Phillips HS, Kharbanda S, Chen R, et al. Molecular subclasses of high grade glioma predict prognosis, delineate a pattern of disease progression, and resemble stages in neurogenesis. Cancer Cell. 2006;9(3):157–73.
48. McEllin B, Camacho CV, Mukherjee B, et al. PTEN loss compromises homologous recombination repair in astrocytes: implications for glioblastoma therapy with temozolomide or poly(ADP-ribose) polymerase inhibitors. Cancer Res. 2010;70(13):5457–64.
49. Raza SM, Lang FF, Aggarwal BB. Necrosis and glioblastoma: a friend or a foe? A and hypothesis. Neurosurgery. 2002;51(1):2–13. review.
50. Joy AM, Beaudry CE, Tran NL, et al. Migrating glioma cells activate the P13K pathway and display decreased susceptibility to apoptosis. J Cell Sci. 2003;116(21):4409–17.
51. Martin AJ, Liu H, Hall WA, Truwit CL. Preliminary assessment of turbo spectroscopic imaging for targeting in brain biopsy. AJNR Am J Neuroradiol. 2001;22:959–68.
52. Laprie A, Pirzkall A, Haas-Kogan DA, et al. Longitudinal multivoxel MR spectroscopy study of pediatric diffuse brainstem gliomas treated with radiotherapy. Int J Radiat Oncol Biol Phys. 2005; 62:20–31.
53. Ganslandt O, Stadlbauer A, Fahlbusch R, et al. Proton magnetic resonance spectroscopic imgaging integrated into image-guided surgery: Correlation to standard magnetic resonance imaging and tumor cell density. Neurosurgery. 2005;56(Supplement 2):291–8.
54. Chintala SK, Tonn JC, Rao JS. Matrix metalloproteases and their biological function in human gliomas. Int J Dev Neurosci. 1999;17:495–502.
55. Zhang K, Li C, Liu Y. Evaluation of invasiveness of astrocytoma using ^{1}H-magnetic resonance spectroscopy: correlation with expression of matrix metalloproteinase-2. Neuroradiology. 2007;49:913–9.
56. Stadlbauer A, Nimsky C, Buslei R, et al. Proton magnetic resonance spectroscopic imaging in the border zone of gliomas: correlation of metabolic and histological changes at low tumor infiltration-initial results. Invest Radiol. 2007;42:218–23.
57. Rubin DB, Greim ML. The histopathology of irradiated endothelium. In: Rubin DB, editor. The radiation biology of the vascular endothelium. Boca Raton, FL: CRC Press; 1998. p. 13–38.
58. Bezabeth T, Mowat MRA, Greenberg AH, Smith ICP. Detection of drug-induced apoptosis and necrosis in human cervical cells using 1H NMR spectroscopy. Cell Death Differ. 2001;8:219–24.
59. Shih C-M, Ko W-C, Yang L-Y, et al. Detection of apoptosis and necrosis in normal human lung cells using 1H NMR specteroscopy. Ann N Y Acad Sci. 2005;1042:488–96.
60. Lyng H, Sitter B, Bathen TF, et al. Metabolic mapping by use of high resolution magic angle spinning 1H MR spectroscopy for assessment of apoptosis in cervical carcinomas. BMC Cancer. 2007;7:1–12. http://www.biomedcentral.com/1471-2407/7/11, Accessed Nov 4, 2012.
61. Pruel MC, LeBlanc R, Caramanos Z, et al. Magnetic resonance spectroscopy guided brain tumor resection: differentiation between recurrent glioma and radiation change in two diagnostically difficult cases. Can J Neurol Sci. 1998;25(1):13–22.
62. Taylor JS, Langston JW, Reddick WE, et al. Clinical value of proton magnetic resonance spectroscopy for differentiating recurrent or residual brain tumor from delayed cerebral necrosis. Int J Radiat Oncol Biol Phys. 1996;36(5):1251–61.
63. Wald LL, Nelson SJ, Day MR, et al. Serial proton magnetic resonance imaging of glioblastoma multiforme after brachytherapy. J Neurosurg. 1997;87(4):525–34.
64. Chernov MF, Hayashi M, Izawa M, et al. Multivoxel proton RS for differentiation of radiation-induced necrosis and tumor recurrence after gamma knife radiosurgery for brain metastases. Brain Tumor Pathol. 2006;23(1):19–27.
65. Horska A, Barker PB. Imaging of brain tumors: MR spectroscopy and metabolic imaging. Neuroimaging Clin N Am. 2010;20(3):294–310.
66. Tzika AA, Strakas LG, Zarifi MK, et al. Spectroscopic and perfusion magnetic resonance imaging predictors of progression in pediatric brain tumors. Cancer. 2004;100:1246–56.
67. Catalaa I, Henry R, Cillon WP, et al. Perfusion, diffusion, and spectroscopy values in newly diagnosed cerebral gliomas. NMR Biomed. 2006;19:463–75.
68. Goebell E, Fiehler J, Ding X-O, et al. Disarrangement of fiber tracts and decline of neuronal density correlate in glioma patients. A combined diffusion tensor imaging and 1H-MR spectroscopy study. AJNR Am J Neuroradiol. 2006;27:1426–31.

69. Pope WB, Chen JH, Dong J, et al. Relationship between gene expression and enhancement in glioblastoma multiforme: Exploratory DNA microarray analysis. Radiology. 2008;249(1):268–77.
70. Kanu OO, Hughes B, Di C, et al. Glioblastoma multiforme oncogenomics and signaling pathways. Oncology. 2009;3:39–52.
71. Verhaak RG, Hoadley KA, Purdom E, et al. Integrated genomic analysis identifies clinically relevant subtypes of glioblastoma characterized by abnormalities in PDGFRA, IDH1, EFGR, and NF1. Cancer Cell. 2010;17:98–110.
72. Brennan C, Momota H, Hambardzumyan D, et al. Glioblastoma subclasses can be defined by activity among signal transduction pathways and associated genomic pathways. PLoS One. 2009;4(11):1–10. e7752.
73. Cheng LL, Anthony DC, Comite AR, et al. Quantification of microheterogeneity in glioblastoma multiforme with ex vivo high resolution magic angle spinning (HRMAS) proton magnetic resonance spectroscopy. Neuro Oncol. 2000;2:87–95.
74. Tzika AA, Astrakas L, Cao H, et al. Combination of high-resolution magic angle spinning proton magnetic resonance spectroscopy and microscale genomics to type brain tumor biopsies. Int J Mol Med. 2007;30:199–208.

Part III

Future Directions in Physiologic Brain Tumor Imaging

Role of Amide Proton Transfer (APT)-MRI of Endogenous Proteins and Peptides in Brain Tumor Imaging

10

Silun Wang, Samson Jarso, Peter C.M. van Zijl, and Jinyuan Zhou

Introduction

A variety of tissue contrast mechanisms are currently utilized in MR imaging of brain tumors, each having its own inherent strengths and weaknesses in clinical applications. The primary exogenous contrast agent used in clinical MR imaging is gadolinium (Gd)-DTPA. It can improve the sensitivity and specificity of MRI in detecting, localizing, and grading brain tumors. However, Gd enhancement essentially reflects the disruption of the blood–brain barrier (BBB), but not necessarily the presence of the aggressive tumor cells [1]. Indeed, approximately 20 % of high-grade gliomas do not enhance [2, 3], while low-grade gliomas occasionally enhance [4], which sometimes makes it difficult to distinguish between high- from low-grade gliomas. Recently, Gd-induced renal toxicity has received much attention. Specifically, life-threatening nephrogenic systemic fibrosis is strongly associated with Gd-DTPA, especially in the patients with end-stage kidney disease, acute kidney injury, or chronic kidney disease [5, 6]. If a suitable endogenous tissue MRI contrast mechanism were available to assess tumor properties, such possible complications could be avoided.

Amide proton transfer (APT) imaging [7, 8] is a new MRI technique that indirectly detects endogenous, low-concentration mobile proteins and peptides, such as those in the cytoplasm, through changes in the water signal used in MRI. In this imaging technique, amide protons in the peptide bonds of such proteins and peptides are selectively saturated. Chemical exchange of the amide protons transfers this saturation to the bulk water signal, the intensity reduction of which will depend on the concentration and exchange rate of the amide protons. APT imaging is currently under investigation to determine its clinical significance in cancer [8–12] and stroke imaging [13, 14]. Preliminary preclinical and clinical investigations have shown that APT imaging provides molecular information that has potential to be used as a new biomarker for brain tumors. The primary goals of brain tumor imaging can be classified into three categories: first, to detect, diagnose, and grade tumors; second, to guide biopsy, tumor resection, and radiation; third, to monitor treatment response and complications. This chapter introduces the basic principle of APT imaging and provides a brief overview of its current applications for brain tumor assessment. We focus on discussing how this unique molecular diagnostic information could help to elucidate the biological features in brain tumors.

S. Wang, Ph.D.
Department of Radiology, Johns Hopkins University School of Medicine, 720 Rutland Avenue, Trailer 217, Baltimore, MD 21287, USA

S. Jarso, Ph.D. • P.C.M. van Zijl, Ph.D. (✉)
J. Zhou, Ph.D. (✉)
Department of Radiology, Johns Hopkins University School of Medicine, 720 Rutland Avenue, Trailer 217, Baltimore, MD 21287, USA

F.M. Kirby Research Center for Functional Brain Imaging, Kennedy Krieger Institute, Baltimore, MD, USA
e-mail: pvanzijl@jhu.edu; jzhou@mri.jhu.edu

J.J. Pillai (ed.), *Functional Brain Tumor Imaging*, DOI 10.1007/978-1-4419-5858-7_10,

Amide Proton Transfer MR Imaging Principle

APT imaging is based on the so-called chemical exchange saturation transfer (CEST) sensitivity enhancement mechanism. Saturation transfer experiments were first performed in 1963 by Forsen & Hoffman, who used the method to measure proton transfer rates between salicylaldehyde and water [15]. In 2000, Ward and coworkers demonstrated that the process of saturation transfer between many diamagnetic molecules and water protons can be used to detect low-concentration solutes with great sensitivity enhancement based on the properties of exchangeable protons [16]. A simple two-pool model is commonly used to explain the CEST-MRI principle. In this model, Pool W represents the high-concentration (around 110 M) water protons, and Pool S the low-concentration (μM to mM range) solute exchangeable protons, such as hydroxyl, amine, or amide protons. To generate CEST effects, a low-power irradiation RF pulse will be applied at the resonance frequency of protons in Pool S. Because protons in Pool W are in exchange with the saturated protons in Pool S, there will be transfer of saturation from Pool S to Pool W, leading to a minute decrease (μM to mM range) in the signal intensity of the protons in Pool W. It should be noticed that such a single transfer of saturation would not be sufficient to produce significant water signal saturation in Pool W due to the much larger concentration of water protons in Pool W compared to Pool S (dynamic range problem for detection). However, because the water pool is much larger than the saturated solute proton pool, each exchanging saturated solute proton is replaced by a non-saturated water proton, which is then again saturated. If the solute protons in Pool S have a sufficiently fast exchange rate (tens of Hz or more) and if the T_1 of water is sufficiently long (sec range), prolonged irradiation leads to accumulation of this saturation effect on Pool W, inducing detectable water signal reduction. CEST-MRI opens the door for the discovery of endogenous and exogenous molecular contrast agents. To better understand the basic mechanism of CEST-MRI, we refer the readers to some recent reviews [17–20].

APT imaging is a special application of CEST using selective irradiation at 3.5 ppm downfield of the water resonance to saturate amide protons in tissue. Similar to CEST-MRI, the APT imaging signal intensities can be quantified using the saturation percentage of the water signal, which can be used to elucidate the concentration of endogenous mobile proteins and peptides. Unfortunately, when performing RF saturation, there typically are multiple saturation effects induced in tissue, including well-known direct water saturation and conventional magnetization transfer, and the APT signal must be separated out. The sum of all saturation effects is generally called the magnetization transfer ratio, $\mathrm{MTR} = 1 - S_{sat}/S_0$, where S_{sat} and S_0 are the signal intensities with and without selective irradiation. The APT image is quantified by the MTR asymmetry at ±3.5 ppm by the following equation [7, 8]:

$$\begin{aligned}\mathrm{MTR}_{asym}(3.5\ \mathrm{ppm}) &= S_{sat}(-3.5\ \mathrm{ppm})/S_0 - S_{sat}(+3.5\ \mathrm{ppm})/S_0 \\ &\approx \mathrm{MTR}'_{asym}(3.5\ \mathrm{ppm}) + \mathrm{APTR}\end{aligned}, \tag{10.1}$$

where APTR is the APT ratio, calculated by the following equation:

$$\mathrm{APTR} = \frac{k[\text{amide proton}]}{[\text{water proton}]R_{1w}}\left(1 - e^{-R_{1w}t_{sat}}\right), \tag{10.2}$$

in which k is the normalized proton exchange rate between the amide proton and water proton pools, [amide proton] and [water proton] indicate the concentrations, R_{1w} is the spin-lattice relaxation rate of water, and t_{sat} is the length of the saturation time. It should be noted that values of APT signal in the normal brain tissue may appear to be negative due to the occurrence of an asymmetry in the conventional MT effect (MTR'_{asym}(3.5 ppm)) with respect to the water resonance [21]. This may confuse the results, and it is therefore important to have a baseline signal established based on a certain RF irradiation power and length. What is currently done is to optimize the experiment to give approximately zero total MTR_{asym} in normal tissue so that increases and decreases can be detected [14]. According to (10.1) and (10.2), the higher concentration of mobile amide protons in tissue will lead to higher MTR_{asym} effects [8]. It is well known that brain tumors, especially high aggressive tumors, usually over-express higher concentrations of many proteins and peptides compared to normal tissue [22, 23]. Therefore, the APT imaging signal becomes an excellent candidate biomarker to explore the brain tumor tissue at the molecular level in vivo.

APT Imaging of Gliomas in Preclinical Models

APT imaging was first applied to an intracranial glioma rat model in 2003 by Zhou et al. [8, 24]. Figure 10.1 shows the imaging features of conventional MRI and APT imaging in 9L gliosarcomas (Fig. 10.1a) and human glioblastoma xenografts (Fig. 10.1b) implanted in the rat brain. In both tumor models, due to higher water content, the tumor masses are hyperintense on T_2, T_1, and apparent diffusion coefficient (ADC) images and hypointense on MTR images compared to contralateral normal brain. On the APT images, the tumor mass can be clearly identified as hyperintensity with a distinct separation from the peritumoral edema and adjacent white matter. The quantitative results indicate that APT contrast between the tumor core and contralateral brain tissue is about 3.9 % of water intensity (1.5 % ± 0.7 % vs. −2.4 % ± 0.2 %) for 9L gliosarcomas (Fig. 10.1a). This contrast reduces to 1.6 % (−1.2 % ± 0.6 % vs. −2.8 % ± 0.4 %) for the human glioblastoma xenografts (Fig. 10.1b). It should be noted that hyperintense (T_2, T_1, ADC) or hypointense (MTR) regions on conventional MR images are generally larger than those on the APT image. These regions may be associated with peritumoral edema, which is a common finding in brain tumors. Although the tumor mass is visible in all of the MR images, the tumor contour is much clearer in the APT images compared to conventional MR images. The hyperintense regions on the APT images have good correspondence with hematoxylin and eosin (H&E)-stained tumor sections. 9L gliosarcomas reveal a homogeneous mass from the tumor core to the boundary. High-density spindle-shaped tumor cells can be observed in the tumor core without necrosis or cystic changes. Human glioblastoma xenografts contain necrotic zones surrounded by a pseudopalisading rim, which is a hallmark of highly aggressive human glioblastomas. These regions of necrosis are distinctly absent from the 9L gliosarcomas. These results indicate that the APT imaging is able to identify the most active components in glioma animal models and to differentiate the tumor core from the adjacent peritumoral edema and normal-appearing white matter.

APT Imaging of Gliomas in Patients

The primary goal of the treatment of malignant gliomas is maximizing tumor removal while minimizing damage to surrounding brain tissue to preserve neuronal function. Optimal neurosurgery and radiotherapy rely on accurate information of the local extent of a tumor and its infiltration into the brain parenchyma. These factors determine the treatment strategy. For example, radiotherapy is delivered to the gross tumor volume with a 2–3-cm margin for the clinical target volume [25]. Therefore, one of the major goals of brain tumor imaging is tumor localization and infiltration characterization [26]. Microstructural tissue characteristics in malignant gliomas vary significantly. Pseudopalisading necrosis is a neuropathological hallmark of glioblastoma multiforme. Typically the necrotic lesion is surrounded by radially arranged anaplastic cells along with

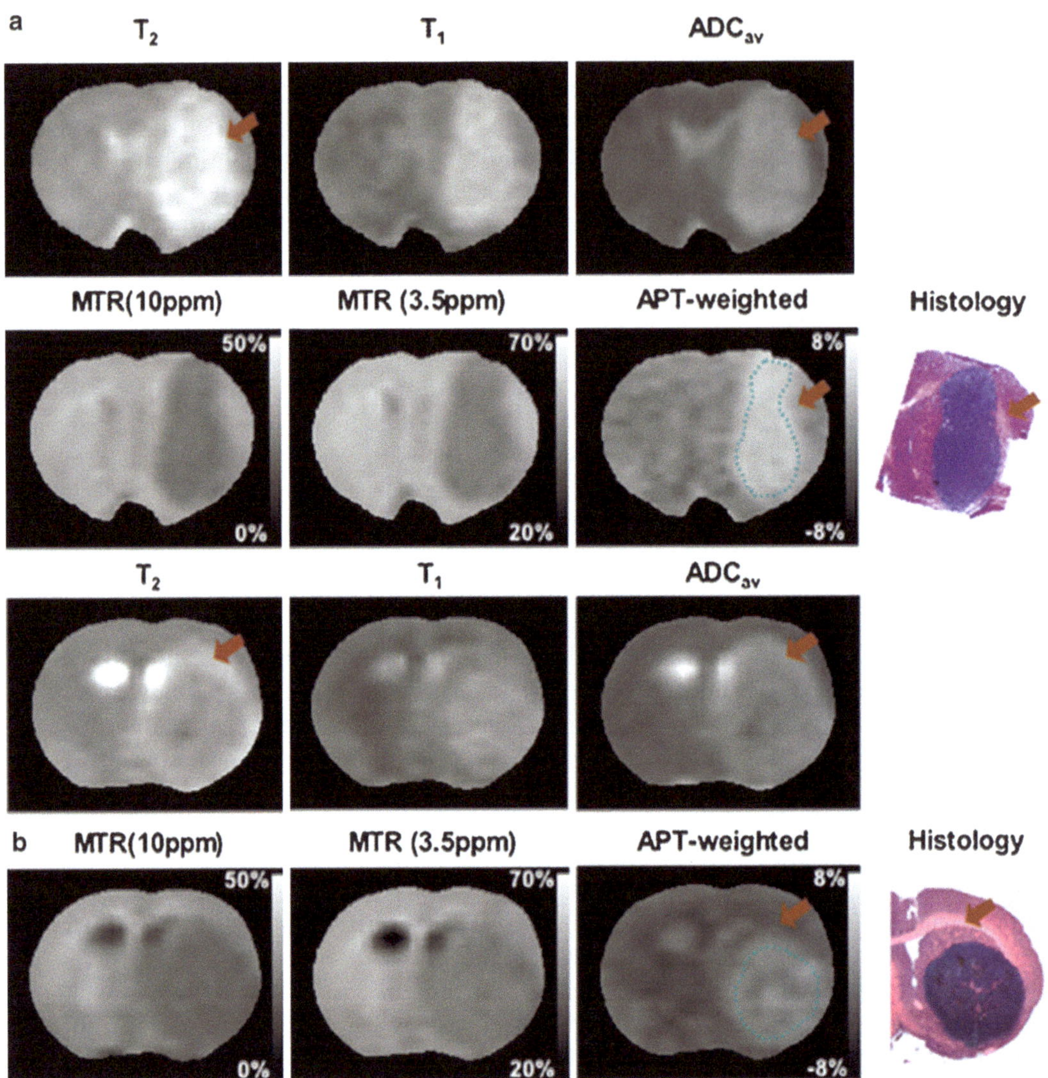

Fig. 10.1 Examples of MR images and histology for 9L gliosarcoma (**a**) and human glioblastoma xenograft (**b**) models. On the APT images, both tumors show hyperintense lesions compared to contralateral normal brain. The APT images appear to more accurately identify the tumor contour compared to conventional MRI. Some T_2-hyperintense regions (*orange arrow*) are white matter edema, not a tumor mass. Histology confirms higher cellularity of tumor cells in the 9L gliosarcoma and necrosis in the human glioblastoma xenografts (reproduced, with permission, from Salhotra A, et al. NMR Biomed. 2008;21:489–497)

tumor cell infiltration, vascular or cytotoxic edema, and reactive gliosis in the peritumoral edema [27]. These components in malignant brain tumors modify the sensitivity to ionizing radiation, affecting the prognosis. It has been indicated that the overall survival time after radiotherapy for brain tumors is decreased by 27 % in patients with necrosis compared with the patients without necrosis [28]. Therefore, determination of cellular components is another major aim of brain tumor imaging.

Preliminary clinical investigations have shown the potential advantages of APT imaging to identify the histological components of gliomas and determine the relationships between the tumor core and adjacent structures, such as peritumoral edema and normal-appearing white matter [10–12]. Figure 10.2a shows MR images for a 35-year-old

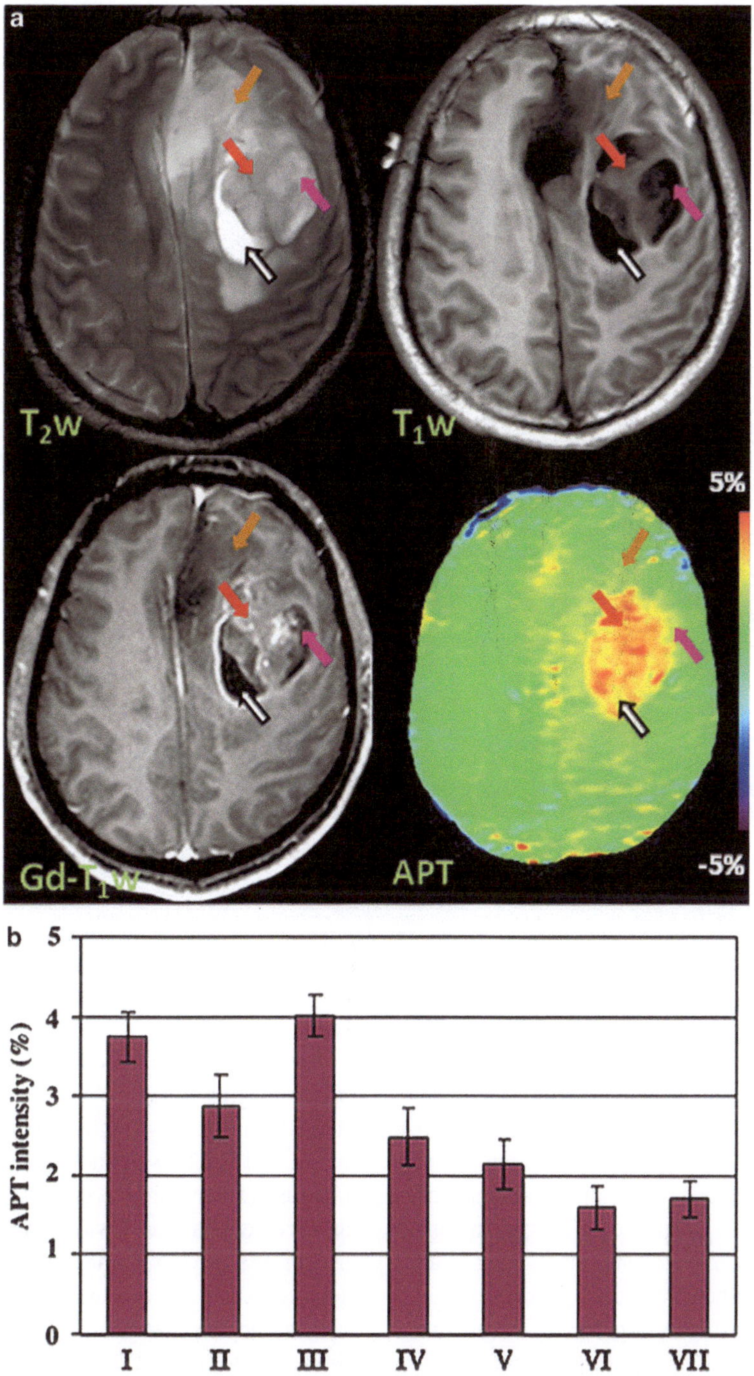

Fig. 10.2 (**a**) Example of clinical APT imaging of glioblastoma. Tumor core (*red arrow*) and cystic cavity (*black arrow*) show APT hyperintensity, compared to the contralateral brain tissue. Necrosis (*pink arrow*) also shows APT hyperintensity, while peritumoral edema (*orange arrow*) has very limited APT signal enhancement compared to normal white matter. (**b**) Quantitative analysis of the APT signal intensities ($n = 12$). (I) tumor core; (II) necrosis; (III) cystic component; (IV) immediate edema; (V) peritumoral edema; (VI) ipsilateral normal-appearing white matter; (VII) contralateral normal-appearing white matter. The APT intensity is the percentage of the bulk water signal (reproduced, with permission, from Wen Z, et al. NeuroImage 2010;51:616–622)

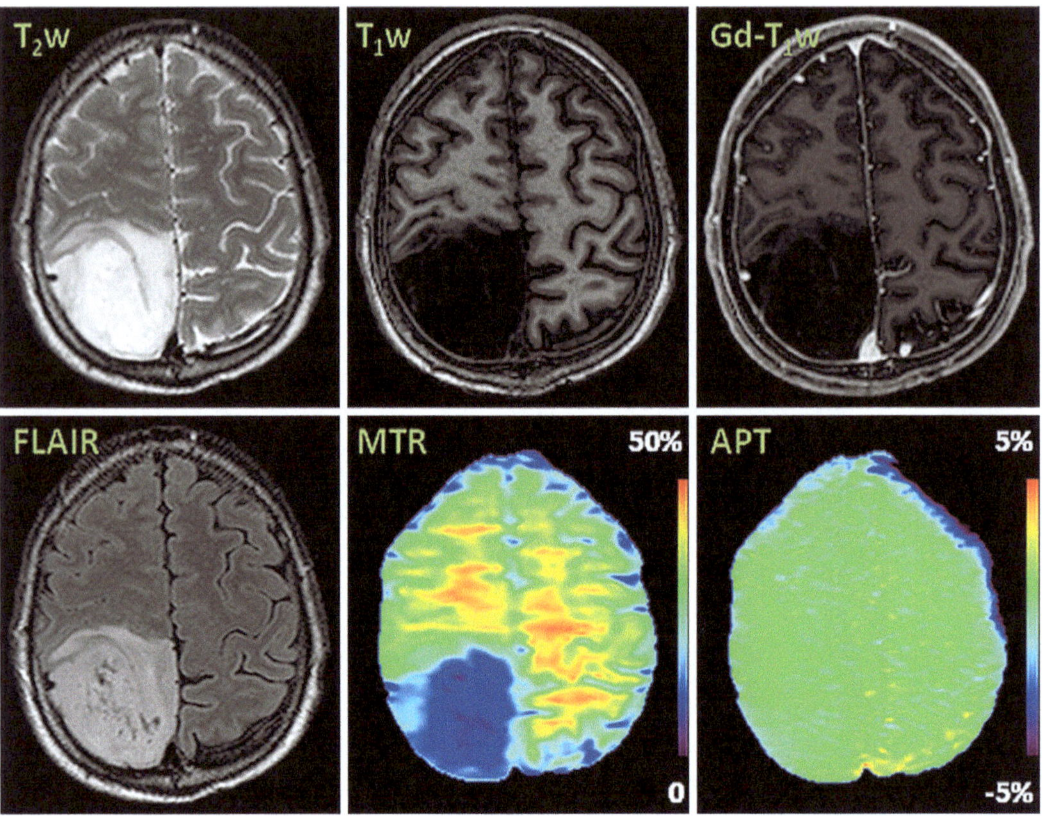

Fig. 10.3 Example of APT imaging of low-grade glioma (grade II). APT image shows isointensity in the lesion with respect to the contralateral normal brain

man with a glioblastoma in the left frontal lobe. Both the Gd-enhancing tumor core (red arrow) and the cystic cavity (black arrow) have hyperintense signal characters on APT imaging. The mean APT signal intensities in the tumor core are significantly higher than in the necrotic regions (3.8 % ± 0.5 % vs. 2.9 % ± 0.6 %, $p = 0.004$). In this example, peritumoral edema and adjacent normal-appearing white matter have isointense APT signal intensities compared to contralateral normal brain, and can be easily distinguished from the hyperintense tumor core. Quantitative analysis of the APT signal intensities in a cohort of high-grade gliomas ($n = 12$) are shown in Fig. 10.2b. The results indicate that APT signal intensities in the tumor core are significantly higher than those in the necrosis ($p = 0.004$), peritumoral edema ($p < 0.001$), and ipsilateral and contralateral normal-appearing white matter (both $p < 0.001$) [11]. APT imaging in combination with standard MRI techniques may help to determine the heterogeneous pathological components in malignant brain tumors, which may provide valuable information for preoperative planning and treatment guidance.

Another important clinical application of brain tumor imaging is tumor grading. A suite of MR methods, such as T_1-weighted image, T_2-weighted image, and Gd-T_1-weighted image, are applied as a mainstay for glioma grading. However, Gd enhancement is not always specific for tumor grading as some low-grade gliomas enhance occasionally, such as pilocytic astrocytomas [4], whereas approximately 10–30 % of high-grade gliomas have no Gd enhancement [2, 3]. Pilot clinical studies show that APT imaging provides quantitative information that may assist in the grading of gliomas [10–12]. Figure 10.3 shows MR images for a patient with low-grade glioma (grade II) in the left frontal lobe. The mass has typical MRI features of hyperintensity on T_2-weighted and FLAIR images, hypointensity on T_1-weighted and MTR images, and no enhancement on the Gd-T_1-weighted image. On the APT image, the tumor core is isointense when compared to the contralateral normal brain, which is distinctly different from the typical high-grade glioma appearance (Fig. 10.2). Zhou et al. quantitatively analyzed the APT signal intensities in the tumor core between high-grade gliomas ($n=6$) and low-grade gliomas ($n=3$) [12]. APT signal intensities of high-grade gliomas were significantly higher than in the contralateral normal-appearing white matter ($p=0.008$), while they were similar to contralateral normal-appearing white matter ($p=0.8$) in low-grade gliomas. There were significantly positive correlations between signal intensities of APT imaging and tumor grade ($p=0.004$).

Differentiation Between Radiation Necrosis and Gliomas in Preclinical Animal Models

Radiotherapy is frequently recommended as a part of standard care for the management of malignant gliomas [25]. The efficacy of radiotherapy is limited by the fact that it not only kills the tumor cells, but it also frequently injures normal brain tissue. The incidence of biopsy-proven radiation necrosis has been reported to be as high as 24 % [29]. Radiation necrosis and tumor recurrence cannot be reliably differentiated by conventional MRI because both are associated with edema, contrast enhancement due to the BBB disruption, and mass effects [30, 31]. There are numerous ongoing investigations into the ability of functional and molecular imaging techniques to assess tumor tissue properties and treatment effects [32–35]. The cardinal pathological features of radiation necrosis include coagulative necrosis with loss of normal brain tissue, and vascular hyalinization or fibrinoid deposition [29, 36, 37], leading to loss of mobile proteins and peptides. On the contrary, active gliomas typically consist of a solid tumor mass with high cellular density, as well as highly aggressive tumor cells infiltrating into adjacent brain tissue [38], resulting in higher expression of mobile proteins and peptides [39, 40]. APT imaging, thus, may have advantages to resolve this diagnostic dilemma in neuro-oncology.

Figure 10.4 shows MR images and H&E-stained histopathological sections of radiation necrosis, SF188/V+human glioma, and 9L gliosarcoma in a rat model [41]. The radiation necrosis was produced using a small animal radiation research platform [42]. These animals received a single, well-collimated X-ray beam in the left hemisphere (single dose of 40 Gy; 10×10 mm^2 region) under the planar fluoroscopic image guidance. Radiation necrosis was confirmed with the enhancement on the Gd-T_1-weighted image (Fig. 10.4a, black solid arrow). On the APT image, the lesion was isointense to hypointense compared to contralateral normal brain. Histological evaluation revealed coagulative necrosis with loss of normal brain tissue in the necrotic center as well as dilated vessels (white arrows) in the peri-necrotic regions. Both SF188/V+(Fig. 10.4b, pink open arrow) and 9L gliosarcomas (Fig. 10.4c, red open arrow) showed obvious Gd enhancement, which was indistinguishable from radiation necrosis (Fig. 10.4a). On the APT images, both tumors showed hyperintense tumor cores. Quantitative analysis of APT signal intensities on radiation necrosis and experimental gliomas is shown in Fig. 10.4d, where APT signal intensities of SF188/V+human gliomas and 9L gliosarcomas are significantly higher than those for the radiation necrosis and contralateral brain tissue (all $p<0.001$). It can be concluded that APT imaging shows a distinct imaging pattern that can be used to distinguish between these two pathologies.

Assessment of Brain Cancer Treatment Response

The most widely adopted criterion for response assessment in gliomas is the Macdonald criterion, by which the treatment response is defined as complete response (complete disappearance of all enhancing lesions), partial response (more than 50 % reduction of maximum diameter), progression (more than 25 % increase of maximum diameter), and stable disease (not qualified for complete and partial response, or progression) [43]. However, this criterion is not sufficiently specific and

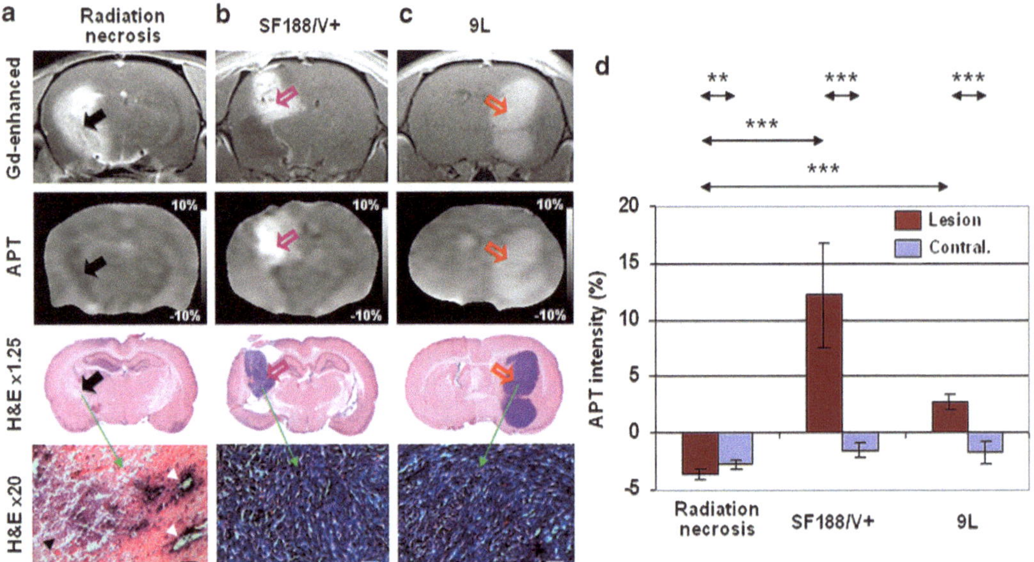

Fig. 10.4 APT imaging differentiation of radiation necrosis and glioma in a rat tumor model. (**a**) Radiation necrosis has isointense to hypointense signal characters on the APT image. Histology confirms that coagulative necrosis and vacuolation changes (*black arrowhead*), as well as dilated damaged vessels (*white arrowhead*), are the major pathological changes for this necrosis. On the contrary, SF188/V+human glioma (**b**) and 9L gliosarcoma (**c**) have hyperintense ATP signals, which can be distinguished from radiation necrosis. (**d**) There are opposite APT signal intensities between the radiation necrosis and gliomas ($n=9$ each group) (reproduced, with permission, from Zhou J, et al. Nature Med. 2011;17:130–134)

primarily reflects passage of contrast agents across a disrupted BBB, while it does not provide information regarding tumor cell apoptosis or necrosis.

Using APT imaging, Zhou and coworkers assessed the brain cancer response to radiation using the U87MG glioma animal model [41]. The data showed that the mean APT intensities of the U87MG tumors were significantly decreased at 3 days post radiotherapy (40 Gy treatment dose), compared to baseline (3.1 % ± 0.3 % vs. 2.1 % ± 0.5 %, $p<0.05$). The APT signal intensities further reduced to 0.6 % ± 1.1 % at 6 days post radiation ($p<0.001$). On the other hand, several commonly used MRI parameters (T_1, T_2, ADC, and MTR) did not show significant changes after radiation. The earlier reduction of APT signal intensities after radiotherapy may be associated with irradiation-induced glioma tumor cell apoptosis or necrosis, leading to reduction of the mobile proton and peptide content. It is still unclear whether the early reduction of APT signal intensities after radiotherapy can provide a reliable prognosis, but the preliminary data support that APT can potentially provide early information to evaluate brain cancer treatment response.

Limitations and Future Development

The primary limitations of APT-MRI are that the effect is relatively small and that its magnitude depends highly on the acquisition parameters used. APT effects of about 2–4% have been reported in animal models [7, 22] and in high-grade human gliomas [10–12]. Therefore, the spatial resolution and quality of APT images are generally worse than those of conventional MRI due to the limited signal-to-noise ratio. Second, the APT effects are affected by several factors, including tissue water content, pH, mobile protein and peptide concentration, and T_1 time of water. Finally, it is possible that the APT signal is associated with many proteins and peptides.

Table 10.1 Typical APT imaging protocols

	Animal experiment [24]	Clinical experiment [11, 12]
MRI scanner	4.7 T animal MRI scanner	3 T clinical MRI scanner
Coil	4 cm volume coil	8-channel phased-array coil
RF saturation power	1.3 μT	2–4 μT
Saturation time	4,000 ms	500 ms
Time of repetition	10 s	3 s
Time of echo	30 ms	30 ms
Sensitivity-encoding factor	N.A.	2
Matrix	64 × 64	128 × 64
Field of view	32 × 32 mm^2	200 × 200 mm^2
Slice thickness	Single 2 mm	Single 5 mm
APT data acquisition	Offsets of ±3.5 ppm; 16 averages	±3, ±3.5, ±4 ppm; 8 averages
Unsaturated image	One (without RF, same TR)	One (without RF, same TR)
Image acquisition	Single-shot, spin-echo echo planar imaging	Turbo spin-echo readout
Total scanning time	10 min	4 min

Currently, it is still unknown which specific proteins and peptides actually generate APT contrast. Fortunately, knowledge of the specific molecular species involved is not needed to allow the APT approach to be useful as a contrast mechanism in the clinic.

Table 10.1 summarizes the currently used APT imaging scanning protocols in experimental and clinical practice. MRI physicists have recognized that the successful clinical translation of APT imaging requires the continued development of new pulse sequences that enable a more rapid acquisition as well as improve the APT imaging quality [44–46]. Recent research efforts are focused on the design of the fast and whole-brain APT methodology for more easy use in the clinic. Particularly, based on the high-performance multichannel coil, Zhu et al. [45] and Jones et al. [44] designed three-dimensional (3D) fast APT imaging sequences, which have a great potential in clinical applications. Importantly, based on a time-interleaved, parallel transmission approach, Keupp et al. recently demonstrated that long saturation pulses (several sec) are feasible on human MRI scanners. This technique could significantly increase the magnitude of the APT imaging signal. Finally, it seems that the use of ultrahigh magnetic field MRI scanners should significantly improve the signal-to-noise ratio of APT imaging [44, 47].

Conclusions

Molecular imaging is developing as a new subspecialty in radiological science in the near further. APT imaging provides a noninvasive molecular imaging contrast at the protein level, which could provide clinicians extra biological information of brain tumors. APT imaging contrast is endogenous and can thus already be applied on standard MRI platforms. With the optimizing of scanning protocols, this specific MRI modality is expected to contribute significantly to clinical brain tumor imaging.

Acknowledgements This study was supported in part by grants from NIH (EB009112, EB009731, EB015032, and RR015241).

References

1. Kelly PJ, Daumas-Duport C, Kispert DB, Kall BA, Scheithauer BW, Illig JJ. Imaging-based stereotaxic serial biopsies in untreated intracranial glial neoplasms. J Neurosurg. 1987;66(6):865–74.
2. Scott JN, Brasher PM, Sevick RJ, Rewcastle NB, Forsyth PA. How often are nonenhancing supratentorial gliomas malignant? A population study. Neurology. 2002;59:947–9.
3. Segall HD, Destian S, Nelson MD. CT and MR imaging in malignant gliomas. In: Apuzzo MLJ, editor.

Malignant cerebral glioma. Park Ridge, IL: American Association of Neurological Surgeons; 1990. p. 63–78.
4. Knopp EA, Cha S, Johnson G, et al. Glial neoplasms: dynamic contrast-enhanced T2*-weighted MR imaging. Radiology. 1999;211(3):791–8.
5. Hasebroock KM, Serkova NJ. Toxicity of MRI and CT contrast agents. Expert Opin Drug Metab Toxicol. 2009;5(4):403–16.
6. Ersoy H, Rybicki FJ. Biochemical safety profiles of gadolinium-based extracellular contrast agents and nephrogenic systemic fibrosis. J Magn Reson Imaging. 2007;26(5):1190–7.
7. Zhou J, Payen J, Wilson DA, Traystman RJ, van Zijl PCM. Using the amide proton signals of intracellular proteins and peptides to detect pH effects in MRI. Nat Med. 2003;9:1085–90.
8. Zhou J, Lal B, Wilson DA, Laterra J, van Zijl PC. Amide proton transfer (APT) contrast for imaging of brain tumors. Magn Reson Med. 2003;50(6):1120–6.
9. Jia G, Abaza R, Williams JD, et al. Amide proton transfer MR imaging of prostate cancer: a preliminary study. J Magn Reson Imaging. 2011;33(3):647–54.
10. Jones CK, Schlosser MJ, van Zijl PC, Pomper MG, Golay X, Zhou J. Amide proton transfer imaging of human brain tumors at 3T. Magn Reson Med. 2006;56(3):585–92.
11. Wen Z, Hu S, Huang F, et al. MR imaging of high-grade brain tumors using endogenous protein and peptide-based contrast. Neuroimage. 2010;51(2):616–22.
12. Zhou J, Blakeley JO, Hua J, et al. Practical data acquisition method for human brain tumor amide proton transfer (APT) imaging. Magn Reson Med. 2008;60(4):842–9.
13. Sun PZ, Zhou J, Sun W, Huang J, van Zijl PCM. Detection of the ischemic penumbra using pH-weighted MRI. J Cereb Blood Flow Metab. 2007;27:1129–36.
14. Zhao X, Wen Z, Huang F, et al. Saturation power dependence of amide proton transfer image contrasts in human brain tumors and strokes at 3 T. Magn Reson Med. 2011;66:1033–41.
15. Forsen S, Hoffman RA. Study of moderately rapid chemical exchange reactions by means of nuclear magnetic double resonance. J Chem Phys. 1963;39:2892–901.
16. Ward KM, Aletras AH, Balaban RS. A new class of contrast agents for MRI based on proton chemical exchange dependent saturation transfer (CEST). J Magn Reson. 2000;143(1):79–87.
17. Sherry AD, Woods M. Chemical exchange saturation transfer contrast agents for magnetic resonance imaging. Annu Rev Biomed Eng. 2008;10:391–411.
18. Terreno E, Castelli DD, Aime S. Encoding the frequency dependence in MRI contrast media: the emerging class of CEST agents. Contrast Media Mol Imaging. 2010;5(2):78–98.
19. van Zijl PCM, Yadav NN. Chemical exchange saturation transfer (CEST): what is in a name and what isn't? Magn Reson Med. 2011;65:927–48.
20. Zhou J, van Zijl PC. Chemical exchange saturation transfer imaging and spectroscopy. Prog NMR Spectsc. 2006;48:109–36.
21. Hua J, Jones CK, Blakeley J, Smith SA, van Zijl PC, Zhou J. Quantitative description of the asymmetry in magnetization transfer effects around the water resonance in the human brain. Magn Reson Med. 2007;58(4):786–93.
22. Goplen D, Wang J, Enger PO, et al. Protein disulfide isomerase expression is related to the invasive properties of malignant glioma. Cancer Res. 2006;66(20): 9895–902.
23. Niclou SP, Fack F, Rajcevic U. Glioma proteomics: status and perspectives. J Proteomics. 2010;73(10): 1823–38.
24. Salhotra A, Lal B, Laterra J, Sun PZ, van Zijl PCM, Zhou J. Amide proton transfer imaging of 9L gliosarcoma and human glioblastoma xenografts. NMR Biomed. 2008;21:489–97.
25. Stupp R, Mason WP, van den Bent MJ, et al. Radiotherapy plus concomitant and adjuvant temozolomide for glioblastoma. N Engl J Med. 2005;352(10):987–96.
26. Maier SE, Sun Y, Mulkern RV. Diffusion imaging of brain tumors. NMR Biomed. 2010;23(7):849–64.
27. Wippold 2nd FJ, Lammle M, Anatelli F, Lennerz J, Perry A. Neuropathology for the neuroradiologist: palisades and pseudopalisades. AJNR Am J Neuroradiol. 2006;27(10):2037–41.
28. Xu Z, Marko NF, Angelov L, et al. Impact of preexisting tumor necrosis on the efficacy of stereotactic radiosurgery in the treatment of brain metastases in women with breast cancer. Cancer. 2011;118(5): 1323–33.
29. Kumar AJ, Leeds NE, Fuller GN, et al. Malignant gliomas: MR imaging spectrum of radiation therapy- and chemotherapy-induced necrosis of the brain after treatment. Radiology. 2000;217(2):377–84.
30. Brandsma D, Stalpers L, Taal W, Sminia P, van den Bent MJ. Clinical features, mechanisms, and management of pseudoprogression in malignant gliomas. Lancet Oncol. 2008;9(5):453–61.
31. Yaman E, Buyukberber S, Benekli M, et al. Radiation induced early necrosis in patients with malignant gliomas receiving temozolomide. Clin Neurol Neurosurg. 2010;112(8):662–7.
32. Graves EE, Nelson SJ, Vigneron DB, et al. Serial proton MR spectroscopic imaging of recurrent malignant gliomas after gamma knife radiosurgery. AJNR Am J Neuroradiol. 2001;22:613–24.
33. Sugahara T, Korogi Y, Tomiguchi S, et al. Posttherapeutic intraaxial brain tumor: The value of perfusion-sensitive contrast-enhanced MR imaging for differentiating tumor recurrence from nonneoplastic contrast-enhancing tissue. AJNR Am J Neuroradiol. 2000;21:901–9.
34. Galban CJ, Chenevert TL, Meyer CR, et al. The parametric response map is an imaging biomarker for

early cancer treatment outcome. Nat Med. 2009;15: 572–6.
35. Wang S, Chen Y, Lal B, et al. Evaluation of radiation necrosis and malignant glioma in rat models using diffusion tensor MR imaging. J Neurooncol. 2011;107(1):51–60. doi:10.1007/s11060-011-0719-x.
36. Yang I, Aghi MK. New advances that enable identification of glioblastoma recurrence. Nat Rev Clin Oncol. 2009;6:648–57.
37. Wang SL, Wu EX, Qiu DQ, Leung LHT, Lau HF, Khong PL. Longitudinal diffusion tensor magnetic resonance imaging study of radiation-induced white matter damage in a rat model. Cancer Res. 2009;69:1190–8.
38. Burger PC, Dubois PJ, Schold Jr SC, et al. Computerized tomographic and pathologic studies of the untreated, quiescent, and recurrent glioblastoma multiforme. J Neurosurg. 1983;58(2):159–69.
39. Howe FA, Barton SJ, Cudlip SA, et al. Metabolic profiles of human brain tumors using quantitative in vivo 1H magnetic resonance spectroscopy. Magn Reson Med. 2003;49(2):223–32.
40. Hobbs SK, Shi G, Homer R, Harsh G, Atlas SW, Bednarski MD. Magnetic resonance image-guided proteomics of human glioblastoma multiforme. J Magn Reson Imaging. 2003;18(5):530–6.
41. Zhou J, Tryggestad E, Wen Z, et al. Differentiation between glioma and radiation necrosis using molecular magnetic resonance imaging of endogenous proteins and peptides. Nat Med. 2011;17(1):130–4.
42. Wong J, Armour E, Kazanzides P, et al. High-resolution, small animal radiation research platform with X-ray tomographic guidance capabilities. Int J Radiant Oncol Biol Phys. 2008;71:1591–9.
43. Macdonald DR, Cascino TL, Schold Jr SC, Cairncross JG. Response criteria for phase II studies of supratentorial malignant glioma. J Clin Oncol. 1990;8(7):1277–80.
44. Jones CK, Polders D, Hua J, et al. In vivo 3D whole-brain pulsed steady state chemical exchange saturation transfer at 7T. Magn Reson Med. 2012;67(6):1579–89.
45. Zhu H, Jones CK, van Zijl PC, Barker PB, Zhou J. Fast 3D chemical exchange saturation transfer (CEST) imaging of the human brain. Magn Reson Med. 2010;64(3):638–44.
46. Keupp J, Baltes C, Harvey PR, van den Brink J. Parallel RF transmission based MRI technique for highly sensitive detection of amide proton transfer in the human brain. Paper presented at: Proceedings of the 19th annual meeting ISMRM 2011; Montreal.
47. Mougin OE, Coxon RC, Pitiot A, Gowland PA. Magnetization transfer phenomenon in the human brain at 7 T. Neuroimage. 2010;49(1):272–81.

Advanced Diffusion MR Tractography for Surgical Planning

11

Jeffrey I. Berman

Introduction

A goal of neurosurgery is to preserve both functionally important cortices and the underlying white matter tracts. Damage to either portion of a pathway may cause postoperative functional deficit. Diffusion MR tractography remains the only noninvasive method of determining the subcortical course of white matter tracts. Tractography based upon diffusion MR can follow a specific white matter tract from voxel to voxel in 3D through the brain. Diffusion MR tractography complements other surgical mapping techniques which are restricted to the grey matter. However, the quality and clinical utility of diffusion tractography is dependent on the type of MRI acquisition and post-processing algorithm used. Traditional diffusion tensor imaging (DTI) is widely used for surgical planning, but fails to accurately represent the microstructure of crossing white matter tracts. The insufficiencies of DTI have motivated the development of advanced diffusion MR techniques capable of accurately describing the microstructure and connectivity of complex white matter tracts. This chapter describes how advanced diffusion MR improves white matter tract localization and enhances surgical planning.

It is critical that the capabilities and limitations of advanced diffusion MR be understood so the technique can be safely used for surgical planning. The first section of this chapter describes the motivation for translating advanced diffusion MR into a tool for surgical planning. The second section reviews the acquisition and reconstruction of various advanced diffusion MR techniques. The final section describes how high angular resolution diffusion imaging (HARDI) tractography has been translated into a routinely used tool for surgical planning.

Part 1: Complex White Matter and the Insufficiency of DTI

The goal of diffusion MR is to infer the microstructure of brain tissue from the measured pattern of water diffusion [1]. Water is used as a probe to assess the organization of structures such as membranes and myelin. The underlying assumption is that water is relatively free to diffuse along axonal bundles and more restricted perpendicular to axons [2]. Where axonal bundles cross, water is free to move along the direction of each component fiber population, creating a complex pattern of diffusion. Millions of axons may pass through a single MR voxel within the white matter. If the brain's white matter were randomly structured, axons of every orientation would be present within this voxel. The pattern of

J.I. Berman, Ph.D. (✉)
Children's Hospital of Philadelphia, and University of Pennsylvania Perelman School of Medicine, Philadelphia, 19104-4399, PA, USA
e-mail: bermanj@email.chop.edu

J.J. Pillai (ed.), *Functional Brain Tumor Imaging*, DOI 10.1007/978-1-4419-5858-7_11,

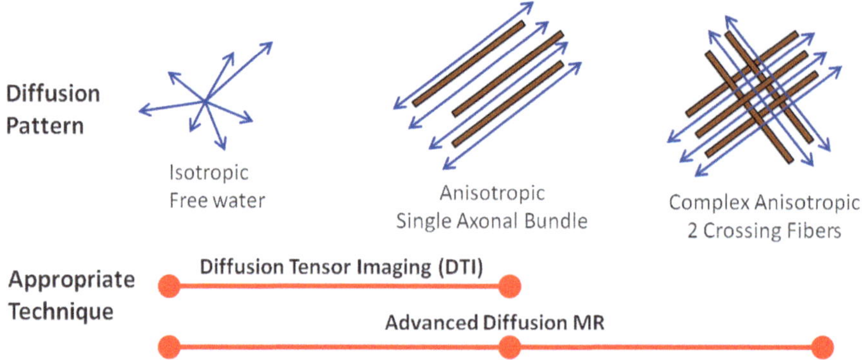

Fig. 11.1 Three modes of water diffusion within brain tissue are shown. The isotropic and single fiber anisotropic patterns are relatively simple and can be accurately characterized with diffusion tensor imaging and advanced diffusion MR. Complex white matter with two or more crossing fiber populations requires an advanced diffusion MR approach to discriminate the orientation and properties of each fiber population. It is important to note that advanced diffusion MR can also be used to depict the isotropic and single fiber anisotropic architectures

diffusion from this random arrangement of axons would appear isotropic. Fortunately, the brain is highly organized into white matter bundles with common grey matter origins and destinations. Some regions of the brain contain only a single axonal bundle that spans the entire dimension of the imaged voxel. A large portion of voxels in the brain's white matter contain multiple axonal bundles with different orientations [3]. These axonal bundles may interdigitate and cross at the axonal level. Or the axonal bundles can be adjacent to each other and only appear to cross because of spatial resolution limitations. A voxel which overlaps the border between two tracts will contain both axonal bundles. Diffusion-weighted imaging cannot distinguish between these two arrangements because of volume averaging over all structures within a voxel.

DTI has rapidly become a familiar component of clinical MR exams and surgical planning protocols. DTI pulse sequences and analysis software are available on all current-generation MRI systems. Many surgical navigation systems provide DTI analysis, tractography, and visualization software. DTI can be acquired on the order of several minutes and tractography can then be generated in seconds. However, the fast imaging and analysis times of DTI are achievable because of the technique's limitations. DTI applies only a single fiber model to the pattern of diffusion within a voxel [1]. The diffusion tensor model assumes a 3D Gaussian pattern of diffusion which can be visualized with the diffusion ellipsoid. The primary eigenvector of the diffusion tensor is assumed to indicate the orientation of least restricted diffusion along a single axonal bundle. Complex or crossing white matter architectures cannot be accurately modeled with the DTI approach [4].

The inadequacies of DTI have motivated the development of advanced diffusion MR methods for the characterization of complex white matter architecture (Fig. 11.1). Advanced diffusion MR extends our ability to accurately describe the microstructure of the brain. HARDI with the q-ball reconstruction is one such advanced diffusion method which can discriminate multiple crossing white matter fibers [5]. The fundamental concepts underlying HARDI will be presented later in this chapter. Figure 11.2 illustrates the difference between DTI and HARDI representations of the callosal tracts. The genu of the corpus callosum contains a large bundle of parallel axons. Both DTI and HARDI accurately identify the orientation of the axons within the genu. The models produced by DTI and HARDI can detect the highly anisotropic diffusion within the genu and are elongated in the orientation of least restricted diffusion. However, the callosal fibers emerge from the genu and intersect, cross, or interdigitate with

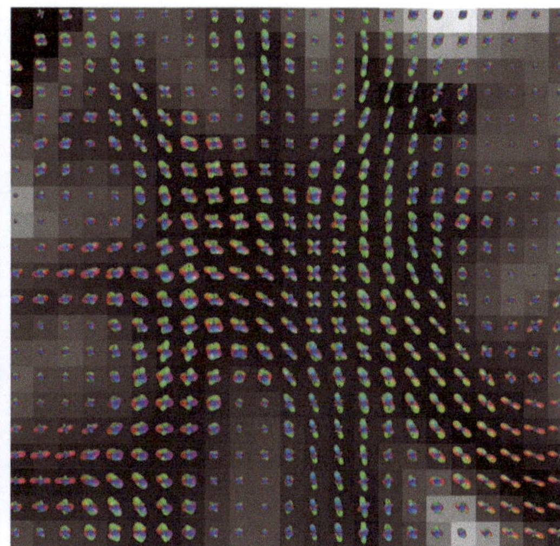

Fig. 11.2 A section of the frontal lobe at the intersection of the corpus callosum with other deep white matter tracts. DTI (*left*) and q-ball HARDI (*right*) reconstructions of the same data are shown. Within the corpus callosum (*bottom right* of each panel) both DTI and HARDI accurately identify the single fiber population. However, in the center of each panel, the callosal fibers intersect, cross, or interdigitate with other white matter tracts. The DTI model fails to accurately portray the complex architecture. The q-ball reconstructions indicate the presence of multiple crossing fibers with different orientations and patterns of connectivity. Each peak of the q-ball HARDI glyph represents an axonal bundle

other white matter tracts within the frontal lobe. The DTI model fails to accurately portray this complex architecture. The 3D Gaussian diffusion tensor model produces an oblate or spherical ellipsoid indicating an isotropic pattern of diffusion. The orientation of the primary eigenvector is not reliable and most likely will not indicate the correct orientation of any of the component fiber populations. The q-ball reconstructions have multiple sharp peaks which distinguish fibers of different orientations and patterns of connectivity.

All major commissural and projection brain tracts have architectures which vary from simple to complex along their length. DTI can successful depict white matter architecture where there exists a single or dominant fiber population. Advanced diffusion MR technique development has been a priority for many research groups because it is one of the only noninvasive methods of studying white matter architecture and connectivity through all regions of the brain. The improvements gained with advanced diffusion MR strongly motivate rapid translation of clinical applications.

Part 2: Overview of Advanced Diffusion MR Techniques

This section provides an overview of the different advanced diffusion methods capable of detecting multiple crossing fiber populations. All diffusion MR experiments have both a data MR acquisition component and a software post-processing component. Diffusion MR can characterize tissue microstructure at a level of detail ultimately dictated by the quality and length of the data acquisition. The type of data acquired during a diffusion MR scan determines which post-processing fiber crossing techniques can be chosen.

The diffusion-weighted images acquired for DTI and advanced diffusion MR methods are very similar. Multiple diffusion-weighted volumes are acquired which have image intensity sensitive to the Brownian motion in a particular direction. The two parameters of diffusion-weighted imaging that dictate which post-processing methods can be used are the number of diffusion gradient directions and the level of diffusion sensitivity. DTI only requires a minimum of six directions of diffusion weighting for its single fiber model [6]. Advanced diffusion methods require dozens or hundreds of gradient directions to provide angular resolution between multiple fibers. The level of diffusion sensitivity, termed the *b*-value, can be increased to improve angular resolution between fibers. DTI typically uses a *b*-value of 1,000 s/mm^2 while advanced diffusion MR may use much higher *b*-values.

For simplicity, post-processing techniques can be categorized into diffusion spectrum imaging (DSI) and HARDI methods. Unlike DTI, the software for DSI and HARDI post-processing cannot typically be found on commercial MR or surgical navigation systems. The following sections outline the fundamental concepts of how advanced diffusion MR infers tissue structure.

Diffusion Spectrum Imaging

DSI does not rely on any predefined models of water diffusion and does not assume a Gaussian pattern of diffusion. DSI attempts to measure the entire 3D probability density function (PDF) of water diffusion [7]. The PDF describes how likely it is for a water molecule to move a particular distance and orientation from its starting point during a diffusion experiment. This level of detailed information on tissue microstructure requires long imaging times. The acquisition includes hundreds of diffusion-weighted images that probe diffusion in hundreds of different directions and at many levels of diffusion sensitivity (*b*-values).

The fundamental relationship between the PDF($\mathbf{r}$) and the diffusion-weighted data $S(\mathbf{q})$ from a single voxel is

$$S(\mathbf{q}) = S_0 \int PDF(\mathbf{r}) e^{i\mathbf{q}\mathbf{r}} d\mathbf{r}.$$

S_0 is the signal intensity without diffusion weighting, $\mathbf{r}$ is a position vector, and $\mathbf{q}$ is the diffusion gradient vector. PDF($\mathbf{r}$) can be solved for by performing a 3D Fourier transform on S($\mathbf{q}$).

Validation studies for DSI have been performed in manganese-enhanced rat optic tracts [8]. Kuo et al. determined which DSI parameters optimize the accuracy and precision of measured fiber orientation on a 3T clinical scanner [9]. The study found that a maximum *b*-value of 6,500 s/mm^2 was optimal for DSI with 515 sampling points and a maximum *b*-values of 4,000 s/mm^2 was optimal for DSI with 203 sampling points. It was also determined that DSI with 203 sampling points could be acquired in about 30 min and produce results with a similar accuracy to DSI with 515 sampling points. Further studies have used a simultaneous image refocusing echo planar pulse sequence to significantly decrease the imaging time by acquiring two adjacent slices during each readout [10]. Decreased MR acquisition times may improve the feasibility of including DSI in a surgical planning protocol.

HARDI

For applications such as fiber tractography, it is not necessary to measure all of q-space and calculate a detailed PDF. Only the orientation of the axonal bundles is necessary to conduct fiber tractography. The 3D PDF can be mathematically collapsed into a 2D orientation distribution function, ODF ($\mathbf{u}$). The ODF describes the probability of water molecules diffusing in a direction described by unit vector $\mathbf{u}$. HARDI methods estimate the ODF or fiber orientations without the time intensive acquisition of DSI.

As with DSI, HARDI probes diffusion in many more directions than DTI. Unlike DSI, HARDI only requires diffusion-weighted images at a single *b*-value. Thus, HARDI scan times are much more feasible for research or clinical use. Figure 11.3 compares the acquisition requirements of a typical HARDI experiment to that of DTI. There are a number of post-processing algorithms described in the literature which can take raw HARDI data and calculate the orientation of multiple fiber populations. All are based upon the underlying principal that diffusion along axonal bundles is less restricted than diffusion transverse to diffusion bundles.

The q-ball reconstruction of HARDI data is a model-free method of estimating the ODF [11–13].

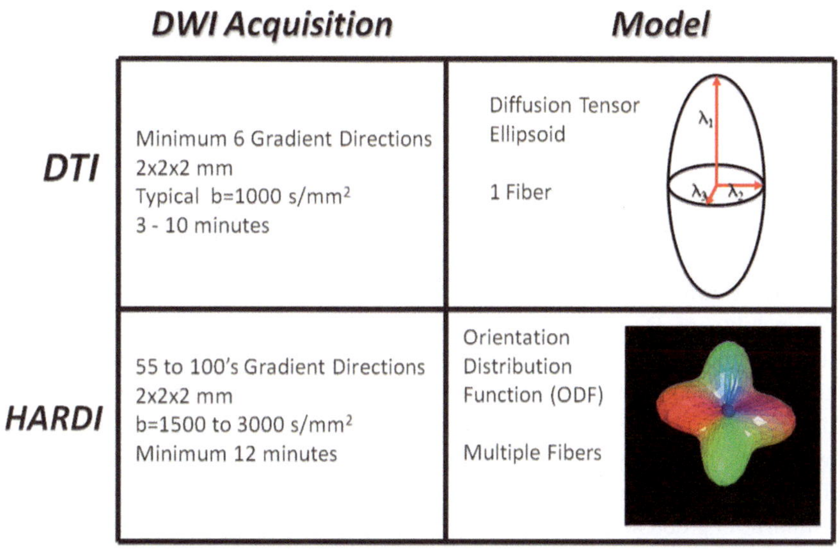

	DWI Acquisition	Model
DTI	Minimum 6 Gradient Directions 2x2x2 mm Typical b=1000 s/mm^2 3 - 10 minutes	Diffusion Tensor Ellipsoid 1 Fiber λ_1 λ_2 λ_3
HARDI	55 to 100's Gradient Directions 2x2x2 mm b=1500 to 3000 s/mm^2 Minimum 12 minutes	Orientation Distribution Function (ODF) Multiple Fibers

Fig. 11.3 Comparison of DTI and HARDI acquisitions and the models which are produced. The parameters of the diffusion-weighted acquisitions are typical of sequences used in diagnostic MR exams or clinical research

The ODF can be directly estimated from a single spherical shell in **q**-space with the Funk-Radon transform as follows:

$$ODF(\mathbf{u}) = \int_{\mathbf{q}\cdot\mathbf{u}=0} S(\mathbf{q})d\mathbf{q}.$$

To evaluate the ODF in direction **u**, the diffusion-weighted signals $S(\mathbf{q})$ are integrated along an equator perpendicular to **u**. The Funk-Radon transform can be challenging to directly implement, because $S(\mathbf{q})$ is limited to the finite number of diffusion-weighted images acquired. Spherical harmonics can be used to model $S(\mathbf{q})$ and analytically compute the Funk-Radon transform without additional interpolation to estimate the ODF [14].

The spherical deconvolution technique generates a fiber orientation distribution from HARDI data [15]. This technique is model-based as it assumes a particular response function for each component fiber population. The diffusion-weighted signal from a voxel with multiple fiber bundles is modeled as a linear combination of multiple response functions. This combined signal can be deconvolved to determine the number and orientation of the fiber populations. Spherical deconvolution can be combined with linear regularization to remove spurious peaks on the fiber orientation distribution [16]. Spherical convolution achieves high angular resolution; however the method is susceptible to errors in regions of the brain where neuronal tissue does not conform to the assumed response function.

Numerous other methods have been proposed to analyze complex diffusion patterns with HARDI. The apparent diffusion coefficient profile can also be represented with spherical harmonic basic functions to detect multiple fiber populations [4]. Diffusion can be modeled with multiple tensors [17] or as multiple axially symmetric tensors [18]. The diffusion orientation transform is a method of estimating the displacement probability function directly from the HARDI data [19].

Hybrid diffusion imaging (HYDI) is an acquisition strategy that allows DTI, DSI, and q-ball post-processing techniques to be performed on the same limited data set [20]. Multiple concentric q-space shells are acquired with approximately 100 points spanning *b*-values from about 375 to 9,500 s/mm^2. The diffusion tensor can be calculated from the data with diffusion weighting of under 2,000 s/mm^2. The q-ball ODF is constructed with data from a single shell with high diffusion weighting. DSI can be performed with all the acquired q-space data.

Part 3: Clinical Translation of HARDI

Fiber Tracking with Multiple Fibers

DTI tractography has become a standard of care for the presurgical localization of functionally important white matter tracts [21–26]. However, the limitations of the diffusion tensor model translate into the inability of DTI fiber tracking to robustly traverse regions of complex white matter [3]. Many tractography algorithms have been proposed to take advantage of multiple propagators provided by advanced diffusion MR [3, 27–33]. Much like DTI tractography, these new algorithms can be deterministic or probabilistic. Deterministic algorithms typically propagate fiber trajectories along the best estimate of axonal orientation. Probabilistic algorithms propagate trajectories in multiple alternative directions by incorporating an estimate of fiber orientation uncertainty. All tractography algorithms are ultimately based upon the fundamental assumption that water diffusion is correlated with axon orientation.

Figure 11.4 demonstrates the ability of probabilistic q-ball HARDI tractography to delineate a larger portion of the motor tract than DTI tractography. This HARDI algorithm uses the residual bootstrap to estimate uncertainty in the orientation of the q-ball ODFs [28]. Both DTI and HARDI tractography are able to connect the superior-medial section of the motor cortex to the midbrain. However, HARDI tractography improves the ability to identify the portion of the motor system connected to the inferior-lateral portion of the motor cortex. The lateral sections of the motor cortex controls head and face motions. These cortices are functionally important and mouth motor is critical for speaking and language function. The white matter carrying these functions can be visualized with HARDI tractography in relation to the subcortical lesion borders. Figure 11.5 shows another comparison between DTI motor tractography and HARDI tractography. In this case, the HARDI tractography passes through the lesion and delineates connections to the lateral motor cortex. The DTI fiber tractography remains in the core of motor pathway and does not turn off to connect to the lateral motor cortex.

The motor tract, like other major white matter tracts, has heterogeneous microstructure. The main trunk of the motor track, within the cerebral peduncle and internal capsule, is a large bundle of axons with no major crossing fibers. DTI and HARDI tractography can both easily follow the tract through

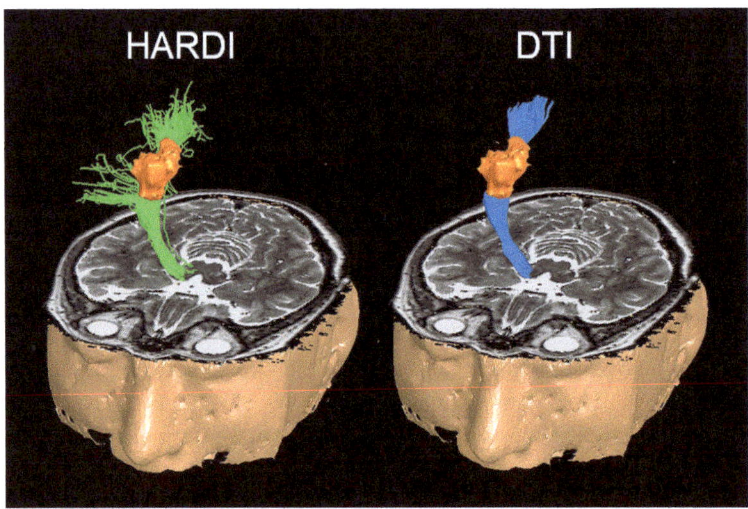

Fig. 11.4 HARDI tracrography of the motor system (*green streamlines* on *left*) is compared to DTI tractography (*blue streamlines* on *right*). The lesion is in orange. (Figure adapted from Berman 2009 [45])

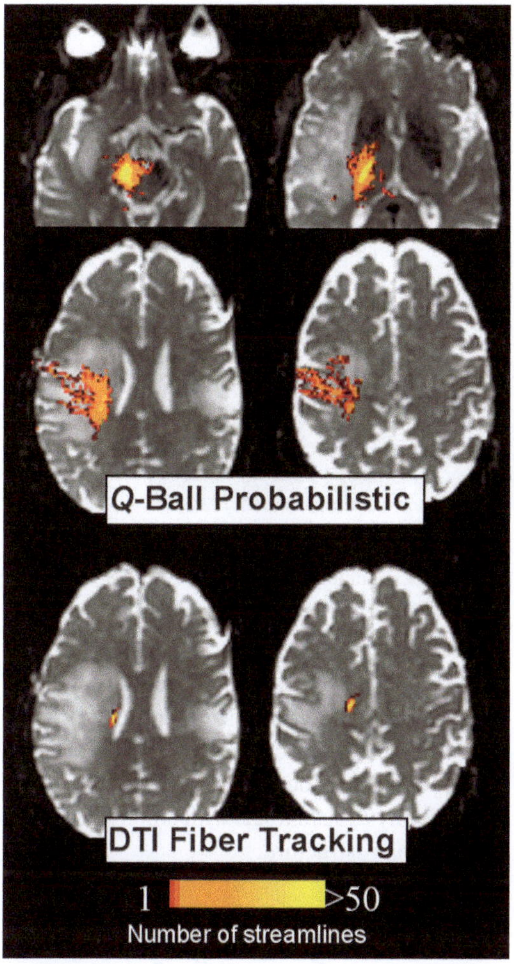

Q-Ball Probabilistic

DTI Fiber Tracking

1 >50

Number of streamlines

Fig. 11.5 Comparison between HARDI (q-ball) probabilistic tractography and DTI fiber tracking of the motor pathway in an adult brain tumor patient. HARDI tractography courses laterally through the centrum semiovale through the lesion to the lateral motor cortex

the internal capsule, to the centrum semiovale. The portion of the motor pathway connecting the superior-medial motor cortex to the internal capsule is still a dominant pathway and can be visualized with DTI tractography. However, the centrum semiovale contains multiple crossing white matter tracts including the motor pathway, superior longitudinal fasciculus, and the corpus callosum. DTI cannot consistently traverse the motor pathway laterally within this region of complex architecture. This shortcoming of DTI within the centrum semiovale explains the improvements gained with HARDI motor tractography. Figure 11.6 exhibits in detail the performance of DTI and HARDI at this point along the motor pathway.

Combination with Functional Mapping

Diffusion MR tractography is not sensitive to neuronal activation and provides no information on brain function. Tractography is strictly a structural method which cannot inherently distinguish different white matter tracts. Functional information must be added to create a starting region of interest within a specific white matter tract. This functional information can simply come from a textbook or atlas describing the brain's organization. Alternatively, subject-specific mapping techniques such as fMRI, magnetoencephalography, or electrocorticography can be used to locate specific cortices [34–40]. These noninvasive functional mapping techniques are restricted to the brain's grey matter and complement the subcortical localization provided by diffusion MR tractography.

The introduction of subject-specific functional mapping technique such as magnetoencephalography (MEG) improves the ability of diffusion MR tractography to delineate the full extent of a specific pathway. Figure 11.7 displays the success rate of tractography between the midbrain and hand motor cortex with and without the introduction of subject-specific functional mapping. Seeding the tractrography with MEG defined hand motor regions improved the success rate of motor system tractography. In many brain tumor cases it is difficult to visually define the exact boundary of the motor, sensory, or language cortex. By using functional mapping to define the cortical area, we achieve better specificity and an indication that the pathway is functioning.

During surgery, diffusion tractography should never be completely relied upon to determine resection extent. Diffusion tractography is tool which produces results which must be combined with complementary imaging and clinical experience. In many brain tumor cases, the lesion has shifted or infiltrated the surrounding tissue, altering the shape and architecture of white matter

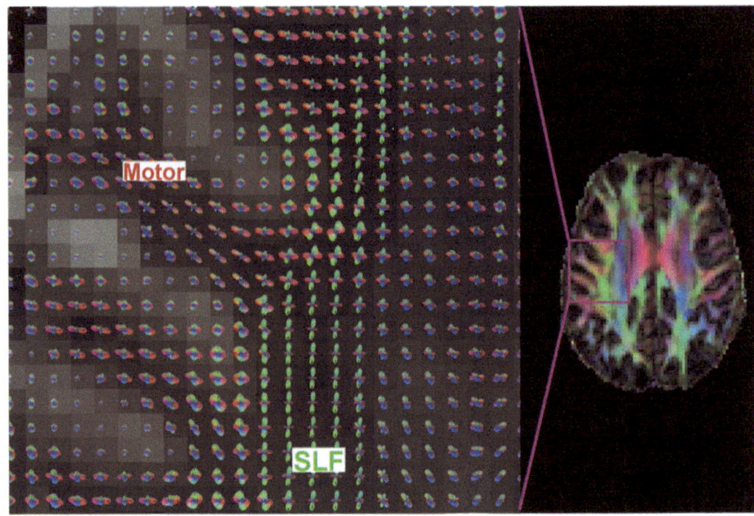

Fig. 11.6 Close-up of the centrum semiovale with HARDI (*left*) and DTI color overlay (*right*). The DTI image shows only a single dominant fiber pathway per voxel. However, the q-ball HARDI reconstruction shows the intersection of the superior longitudinal fasciculus (SLF, *green*) and motor tract (*red* in gyrus, *blue* in internal capsule)

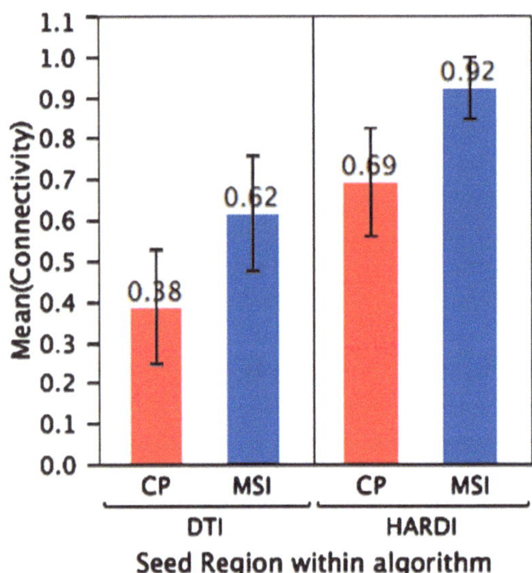

Fig. 11.7 Comparison of HARDI and DTI tractography abilities to successfully delineate the motor tract between the cerebral peduncle (CP) and the hand motor cortex. Data represents results from 11 surgical patients. The mean connectivity is the percent of patients where connectivity was revealed between the CP and the hand motor cortex. *Red* bars indicate tractography was launched from manually drawn regions of interest in the cerebral peduncle. *Blue* bars indicate tractography was launched from the hand motor cortex as defined by magnetic source imaging (MSI) hand dipoles. Success of tractography improves with HARDI tractography and the introduction of subject-specific functional mapping. Courtesy of Roland Henry, Monica Bucci, and Marisa Luisa Mandelli

tracts [41, 42]. In these cases, functional mapping should be used to define tractography starting and target regions. Advanced diffusion MR tractography may also provide an advantage in performing tractography in such tracts with unfamiliar geometry and microstructure.

HARDI Presurgical Imaging and Tractography Protocol

This section serves as a practical guide for implementing HARDI as a clinical tool for surgical planning. The procedures describes here are based upon the protocol routinely used at the University of California San Francisco. Figure 11.8 provides a flowchart view of the interactions between the MRI system, laboratory computer, picture archiving and communication system (PACS), and the surgical navigation system.

HARDI acquisitions are performed on a 3T GE EXCITE scanner with a parallel imaging factor of 2, TR/TE = 12.4 s/73 ms, 2.2 mm isotropic voxels, field of view = 280 × 280 mm, and a 128 × 128 matrix zero filled to a 256 × 256 matrix. A similar diffusion acquisition is readily available on all MR manufactures' platforms. A total of 55 diffusion gradient directions are measured at $b = 2{,}000$ s/mm^2. The imaging time is approximately 13 min.

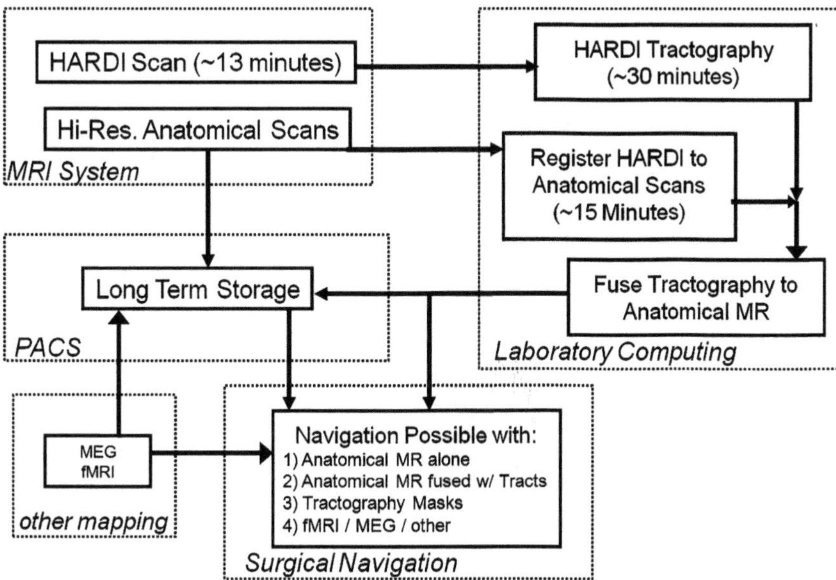

Fig. 11.8 This flowchart shows tractography work flow and communication between various medical center platforms and computers

During the MR exam, other high resolution T1- and T2-weighted anatomical images are acquired. The contrast and resolution of these volumes are independent of the HARDI acquisition and determined by the preferences of the clinicians and requirements of the intraoperative neuronavigation system.

The raw HARDI images are removed from the PACS system and placed on a laboratory computer system. The q-ball reconstruction of HARDI is used in conjunction with a probabilistic tractography algorithm using the residual bootstrap to estimate uncertainties in the q-ball ODF's [28]. The algorithm is run in Interactive Data Language (ITT Visual Systems) on a Linux workstation. The procedure for drawing starting and target regions of interest is similar to methods used to generate deterministic DTI fiber tracks. A starting region is placed in the cerebral peduncle of the midbrain, encompassing the entire motor tract at that level. A target region of interest is drawn surrounding the posterior limb of the internal capsule. Fiber trajectories passing through both regions of interest are retained. Additional target regions of interest may be place in the precentral gyrus based upon anatomical knowledge or patient-specific fMRI or MEG cortical mapping. Approximately 30 min is required for region of interest setup, tractography computation, and quality assessment. This time requirement will vary with computer speed.

After HARDI fiber tractography is complete, the results are fused with the high resolution anatomical MR volumes. Diffusion MR volumes typically have much poorer resolution than the anatomical MR and cannot be used alone for surgical navigation. The echo planar diffusion images without diffusion weighting ($b=0$) are registered to one or more anatomical volumes [43, 44]. The registration is then applied to a binary mask of the HARDI tractography to transform it to the coordinate space of the anatomical volume. The registered binary mask is then added to the anatomical images and the tracks appear as bright white voxels. The fused images are then pushed onto the PACS system or to the surgical navigation system. The fused volume can be viewed in any orientation and allows the surgeon to intraoperatively view the relation between the scalpel, tumor, and white matter tract. The images with tractography can also be made available on the PACS system for all clinicians in the medical center. The registered binary mask can also be independently loaded onto a surgical navigation

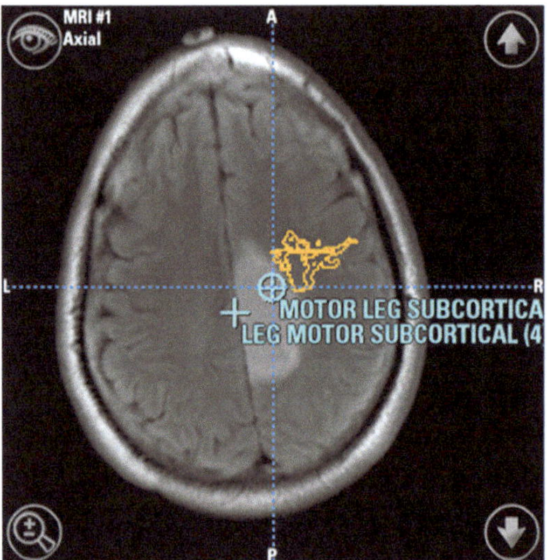

Fig. 11.9 Screen capture from a surgical navigation system. The *blue circle* in the crosshairs indicates the location of a subcortical stimulation of leg motor on the slice shown. The *blue cross* is the projected location of a leg motor subcortical stimulation site from another slice. The *orange outline* indicates the borders of the HARDI tractography mask

system (Fig. 11.9). Some navigation systems can perform the image fusion and registration steps and visualize the tractography with color overlays. Tractography from different white matter pathways can be viewed in unique colors and each can be made invisible to reveal anatomy obscured by the tractography.

Conclusions

The need for improved surgical planning is a primary driving force for the development of advanced diffusion MR. It is expected that advanced diffusion MR tractography for surgical planning will become the standard of care in the near future. Many medical centers already have the infrastructure and protocols in place to acquire DTI, process tractography, and visualize white matter tracts in conjunction with other functional mapping on a surgical navigation system. This established framework can be easily altered to include improved or additional functional mapping techniques. The DTI acquisition and post-processing can be swapped out and replaced with advanced diffusion MR methods. It is important to remember that diffusion MR is only a tool that must be used in conjunction with other functional mapping techniques and can never be relied upon alone.

References

1. Basser PJ, Mattiello J, LeBihan D. Estimation of the effective self-diffusion tensor from the NMR spin echo. J Magn Reson B. 1994;103(3):247–54.
2. Beaulieu C. The basis of anisotropic water diffusion in the nervous system—a technical review. NMR Biomed. 2002;15(7–8):435–55.
3. Behrens TE, Berg HJ, Jbabdi S, Rushworth MF, Woolrich MW. Probabilistic diffusion tractography with multiple fibre orientations: what can we gain? Neuroimage. 2007;34(1):144–55.
4. Frank LR. Anisotropy in high angular resolution diffusion-weighted MRI. Magn Reson Med. 2001;45(6):935–9.
5. Tuch DS, Reese TG, Wiegell MR, Wedeen VJ. Diffusion MRI of complex neural architecture. Neuron. 2003;40(5):885–95.
6. Basser PJ, Pierpaoli C. A simplified method to measure the diffusion tensor from seven MR images. Magn Reson Med. 1998;39(6):928–34.
7. Wedeen VJ, Hagmann P, Tseng WI, Reese TG, Weisskoff RM. Mapping complex tissue architecture with diffusion spectrum magnetic resonance imaging. Magn Reson Med. 2005;54(6):1377–86.
8. Lin C, Wedeen VJ, Chen J, Yao C, Tseng WI. Validation of diffusion spectrum magnetic resonance imaging with manganese-enhanced rat optic tracts and ex vivo phantoms. Neuroimage. 2003;19(3): 482–95.
9. Kuo L, Chen J, Wedeen VJ, Tseng WI. Optimization of diffusion spectrum imaging and q-ball imaging on clinical MRI system. Neuroimage. 2008;41(1):7–18.
10. Reese TG, Benner T, Wang R, Feinberg DA, Wedeen VJ. Halving imaging time of whole brain diffusion spectrum imaging and diffusion tractography using simultaneous image refocusing in EPI. J Magn Reson Imaging. 2009;29(3):517–22.
11. Aganj I, Lenglet C, Sapiro G, Yacoub E, Ugurbil K, Harel N. Reconstruction of the orientation distribution function in single- and multiple-shell q-ball imaging within constant solid angle. Magn Reson Med. 2010;64(2):554–66. PMCID: PMC2911516.
12. Fritzsche KH, Laun FB, Meinzer H, Stieltjes B. Opportunities and pitfalls in the quantification of fiber integrity: what can we gain from Q-ball imaging? Neuroimage. 2010;51(1):242–51.
13. Tuch DS. Q-ball imaging. Magn Reson Med. 2004;52(6):1358–72.
14. Hess CP, Mukherjee P, Han ET, Xu D, Vigneron DB. Q-ball reconstruction of multimodal fiber orientations

using the spherical harmonic basis. Magn Reson Med. 2006;56(1):104–17.

15. Tournier JD, Calamante F, Gadian DG, Connelly A. Direct estimation of the fiber orientation density function from diffusion-weighted MRI data using spherical deconvolution. Neuroimage. 2004;23(3):1176–85.
16. Sakaie KE, Lowe MJ. An objective method for regularization of fiber orientation distributions derived from diffusion-weighted MRI. Neuroimage. 2007;34(1):169–76.
17. Tuch DS, Reese TG, Wiegell MR, Makris N, Belliveau JW, Wedeen VJ. High angular resolution diffusion imaging reveals intravoxel white matter fiber heterogeneity. Magn Reson Med. 2002;48(4):577–82.
18. Anderson AW. Measurement of fiber orientation distributions using high angular resolution diffusion imaging. Magn Reson Med. 2005;54(5):1194–206.
19. Özarslan E, Shepherd TM, Vemuri BC, Blackband SJ, Mareci TH. Resolution of complex tissue microarchitecture using the diffusion orientation transform (DOT). Neuroimage. 2006;31(3):1086–103.
20. Wu Y, Alexander AL. Hybrid diffusion imaging. Neuroimage. 2007;36(3):617–29.
21. Berman JI, Berger MS, Mukherjee P, Henry RG. Diffusion-tensor imaging—guided tracking of fibers of the pyramidal tract combined with intraoperative cortical stimulation mapping in patients with gliomas. J Neurosurg Pediatr. 2004;101(1):66–72.
22. Mikuni N, Okada T, Enatsu R, Miki Y, Hanakawa T, Urayama S, Kikuta K, Takahashi JA, Nozaki K, Fukuyama H, Hashimoto N. Clinical impact of integrated functional neuronavigation and subcortical electrical stimulation to preserve motor function during resection of brain tumors. J Neurosurg. 2007;106(4):593–8.
23. Mikuni N, Okada T, Nishida N, Taki J, Enatsu R, Ikeda A, Miki Y, Hanakawa T, Fukuyama H, Hashimoto N. Comparison between motor evoked potential recording and fiber tracking for estimating pyramidal tracts near brain tumors. J Neurosurg. 2007;106(1):128–33.
24. Bello L, Gambini A, Castellano A, Carrabba G, Acerbi F, Fava E, Giussani C, Cadioli M, Blasi V, Casarotti A, Papagno C, Gupta AK, Gaini S, Scotti G, Falini A. Motor and language DTI fiber tracking combined with intraoperative subcortical mapping for surgical removal of gliomas. Neuroimage. 2008;39(1):369–82.
25. Holodny AI, Schwartz TH, Ollenschleger M, Liu WC, Schulder M. Tumor involvement of the corticospinal tract: diffusion magnetic resonance tractography with intraoperative correlation. J Neurosurg. 2001;95(6):1082.
26. Kamada K, Todo T, Masutani Y, Aoki S, Ino K, Takano T, Kirino T, Kawahara N, Morita A. Combined use of tractography-integrated functional neuronavigation and direct fiber stimulation. J Neurosurg. 2005;102(4):664–72.
27. Campbell JS, Siddiqi K, Rymar VV, Sadikot AF, Pike GB. Flow-based fiber tracking with diffusion tensor and q-ball data: validation and comparison to principal diffusion direction techniques. Neuroimage. 2005; 27(4):725–36.
28. Berman JI, Chung S, Mukherjee P, Hess CP, Han ET, Henry RG. Probabilistic streamline q-ball tractography using the residual bootstrap. Neuroimage. 2008;39(1):215–22.
29. Perrin M, Poupon C, Cointepas Y, Rieul B, Golestani N, Pallier C, Riviere D, Constantinesco A, Le Bihan D, Mangin JF. Fiber tracking in q-ball fields using regularized particle trajectories. Inf Process Med Imaging. 2005;19:52–63.
30. Descoteaux M, Deriche R, Knosche TR, Anwander A. Deterministic and probabilistic tractography based on complex fibre orientation distributions. IEEE Trans Med Imaging. 2009;28(2):269–86.
31. Parker GJM, Alexander DC. Probabilistic anatomical connectivity derived from the microscopic persistent angular structure of cerebral tissue. Philos Trans R Soc Lond B Biol Sci. 2005;360(1457):893–902.
32. Wedeen VJ, Wang RP, Schmahmann JD, Benner T, Tseng WY, Dai G, Pandya DN, Hagmann P, D'Arceuil H, de Crespigny AJ. Diffusion spectrum magnetic resonance imaging (DSI) tractography of crossing fibers. Neuroimage. 2008;41(4):1267–77.
33. Jeurissen B, Leemans A, Jones DK, Tournier J, Sijbers J. Probabilistic fiber tracking using the residual bootstrap with constrained spherical deconvolution. Hum Brain Mapp. 2011;32(3):461–79.
34. Guye M, Parker GJ, Symms M, Boulby P, Wheeler-Kingshott CA, Salek-Haddadi A, Barker GJ, Duncan JS. Combined functional MRI and tractography to demonstrate the connectivity of the human primary motor cortex in vivo. Neuroimage. 2003;19(4):1349–60.
35. Krishnan R, Raabe A, Hattingen E, Szelenyi A, Yahya H, Hermann E, Zimmermann M, Seifert V. Functional magnetic resonance imaging-integrated neuronavigation: correlation between lesion-to-motor cortex distance and outcome. Neurosurgery. 2004;55(4):904–14. discusssion 914-5; 904–14; discusssion 914–5.
36. Schulder M, Maldjian JA, Liu WC, Holodny AI, Kalnin AT, Mun IK, Carmel PW. Functional image-guided surgery of intracranial tumors located in or near the sensorimotor cortex. J Neurosurg. 1998;89(3):412–8.
37. Ganslandt O, Buchfelder M, Hastreiter P, Grummich R, Fahlbusch R, Nimsky C. Magnetic source imaging supports clinical decision making in glioma patients. Clin Neurol Neurosurg. 2004;107(1):20–6.
38. Nagarajan S, Kirsch H, Lin P, Findlay A, Honma S, Berger MS. Preoperative localization of hand motor cortex by adaptive spatial filtering of magnetoencephalography data. J Neurosurg. 2008;109(2):228–37.
39. Schiffbauer H, Berger MS, Ferrari P, Freudenstein D, Rowley HA, Roberts TP. Preoperative magnetic source imaging for brain tumor surgery: a quantitative comparison with intraoperative sensory and motor mapping. J Neurosurg. 2002;97(6):1333–42.
40. Engel AK, Moll CK, Fried I, Ojemann GA. Invasive recordings from the human brain: clinical insights and beyond. Nat Rev Neurosci. 2005;6(1):35–47.

41. Wieshmann UC, Symms MR, Parker GJ, Clark CA, Lemieux L, Barker GJ, Shorvon SD. Diffusion tensor imaging demonstrates deviation of fibres in normal appearing white matter adjacent to a brain tumour. J Neurol Neurosurg Psychiatry. 2000;68(4):501–3.
42. Nimsky C, Ganslandt O, Hastreiter P, Wang RP, Benner T, Sorensen AG, Fahlbusch R. Intraoperative diffusion-tensor MR imaging: shifting of white matter tracts during neurosurgical procedures—initial experience. Radiology. 2005;234(1):218–25.
43. Woods RP, Grafton ST, Holmes CJ, Cherry SR, Mazziotta JC. Automated image registration: I. General methods and intrasubject, intramodality validation. J Comput Assist Tomogr. 1998;22(1):139–52.
44. Jenkinson M, Smith S. A global optimisation method for robust affine registration of brain images. Med Image Anal. 2001;5(2):143–56.
45. Berman J. Diffusion MR tractography as a tool for surgical planning. Magn Reson Imaging Clin N Am. 2009;17(2):205–14.

Ultra-High Field MRSI (7T and Beyond)

12

Peter B. Barker

Introduction

Both magnetic resonance imaging (MRI) and spectroscopy (MRS) are expected to improve with increasing magnetic field strengths (B_0). For MRI, theoretical considerations suggest that signal-to-noise ratios (SNR) should improve approximately linearly with increasing field strength [1]; improved SNR can be used either to shorten scan times while maintaining comparable image quality, or alternatively to improve spatial resolution for a similar scan time. For MRS, in addition to increasing SNR, higher B_0 also has an additional advantage in that the spectral resolution (i.e., chemical shift dispersion, measured in Hz) also increases linearly with B_0. However, not all of the many factors that effect the quality of MRI and MRS change favorably as B_0 increases. Factors which may unfavorably influence SNR and resolution as B_0 increases include changes in relaxation times (particularly shortening of T_2 and T_2* relaxation times [2]), and increased magnetic susceptibility effects which will broaden resonances in MRS (causing both reduced spectral resolution and decreased SNR). Other technical factors include increased problems with slice selection chemical shift displacement (CSD) effects (i.e., the phenomenon that each metabolite originates from a slightly difference slice location) and increased radiofrequency power deposition (specific absorption rate (SAR)) at higher fields. Finally, as the operating resonance frequency (ω_0) increases ($\omega_0 = \gamma B_0$, where γ is the nuclear gyromagnetic ratio), the homogeneity of the transmit and receive radiofrequency fields (B_1) increases due to wavelength (often termed "dielectric") effects [3], which causes a reduction in image homogeneity and may also alter image contrast. Therefore, it is not guaranteed that high-field MRI or MRS will always offer improvements over lower field measurements; rather, techniques have to be developed and optimized in order to address these issues in order to demonstrate improved performance at higher magnetic field strengths. This chapter reviews recent technical advances in high-field MRS and touches on clinical applications; however, to date, there have been very few 7 T MRS studies reported in pathological conditions.

Field Dependence of MRS

MRS of the human brain has been performed at a number of different field strengths, ranging from 0.5 T [4], 1.0 T [5], 1.5 T [6], 2.0 T [7], 3.0 T [8], 4.0 T [9], 7.0 T [10], and 9.4 T [11]. In general, MRS is preferred to be performed at higher field because of the higher SNR associated with the increased field strength and increased chemical shift dispersion. Theoretical considerations suggest

P.B. Barker, D.Phil. (✉)
Department of Radiology, Johns Hopkins University School of Medicine, 600 N. Wolfe Street, Baltimore, MD 21287, USA
e-mail: pbarker2@jhmi.edu

J.J. Pillai (ed.), *Functional Brain Tumor Imaging*, DOI 10.1007/978-1-4419-5858-7_12,

that SNR should increase approximately linearly with increasing field [1] for biological samples in vivo, since the signal is predicted to have a B_0^2 dependence, while noise in the receiver coil is predicted to increase linearly when dominated by "tissue loading," therefore leading to the prediction that MRS at 3 T should have double the SNR of MRS 1.5 T:

$$S / N \propto B_0^2 / B_0 = B_0 \qquad (12.1)$$

In addition, spectral resolution is expected to improve since the frequency difference (chemical shift, σ) between different metabolites (measured in Hz) also increases linearly

$$\omega = \omega_0 \times (1-\sigma) = \gamma B_0 \times (1-\sigma) \qquad (12.2)$$

However, some factors adversely affect SNR and resolution as field strength increases, in particular in vivo T_2 and T_2* relaxation times are shorter, and in fact an almost linear increase in metabolite line widths (=1/T_2*) occurs with increasing field strength [12, 13]. The decrease in metabolite T_2 was considered "anomalous" when first observed, as "classically" in MR spectroscopy, T_2 is expected to not change with resonance frequency [2]. However, both metabolite T_2 (as measured using single-echo, rather than Carr-Purcell-Meiboom-Gill (CPMG) sequences) and T_2* relaxation times in brain are shortened by the presence of paramagnetic deoxyhemoglobin in the brain's microvasculature (a microscopic susceptibility effect) which causes field-dependent linewidth increases [14]. Therefore, while spectral quality at 3 T is superior to that at 1.5 T, improvements in both SNR and spectral resolution are somewhat less than predicted by simple theoretical considerations [8, 15]. For instance, one study found a 28 % improvement in SNR for NAA in short TE spectra, less than the "simple" prediction of 100 % [8]. Since for compounds such as *N*-acetyl aspartate (NAA), choline (Cho), or creatine (Cr) the improvements in SNR are quite small, it is perhaps not surprising that studies based on these resonances did not find any improvement in "diagnostic quality" at 3.0 T compared to 1.5 T [16]. However, probably the biggest improvements at higher field strengths are for metabolites which are "harder to detect," i.e., those with relatively lower signal intensities and those which overlap with signals from other compounds—some examples include γ-aminobutyric acid (GABA), glutamate (Glu), and glutamine (Gln). Figure 12.1 shows representative spectra from normal human brain at 1.5, 3.0, and 7.0 T, recorded under similar (but not identical) conditions. It can be seen that the 7 T spectrum shows the best SNR, and that the fine detail in the regions of the spectra containing Glu, Gln, and other resonances (e.g. 2.1–2.6 ppm, 3.5–3.9 ppm) has greater fine detail at 7 T. Figure 12.2 shows simulations of Glu and Gln as a function of field strength ranging from 1.5 to 9.4 T—it can be seen at 1.5 T there is almost complete overlap of the C3 and C4 multiplets of Glu and Gln, but that as the field strength increases the C4 resonances start to separate, and that by 7 T there is almost complete separation of the two.

The fair comparison of spectra between different field strengths is a difficult undertaking, as it is quite rare for MR systems to be "identical" other than the strength of the magnetic field. For instance, similar RF coils, preamplifiers, and receiver electronics, as well as pulse sequences, slice selective pulses, and data processing methods should be used at both field strengths. Indeed, a "philosophical" question is whether identical methods should be in fact be used at both field strengths, or whether different (i.e., optimal) methods are used at each field strength.

Relatively few studies have systematically compared 7 T MRS to lower fields [12, 13, 17]. One study compared 3 and 7 T MRS using very similar methodology at both field strengths, including the use of the same pulse sequence (very short echo time (TE—6 ms) "SPECIAL," see below) and quadrature transmit-receive surface coils which provided coverage of posterior brain regions [17]. This study found an increased sensitivity by a factor of 1.7 (per unit time) at 7 T compared to 3 T, and improved accuracy of determination for 12 different metabolites. Figure 12.3 shows an example of 3 and 7 T spectra from the anterior cingulate cortex recorded with 32-channel head coils using the semi-LASER (sLASER, see below) in the same subject; while the spectra look

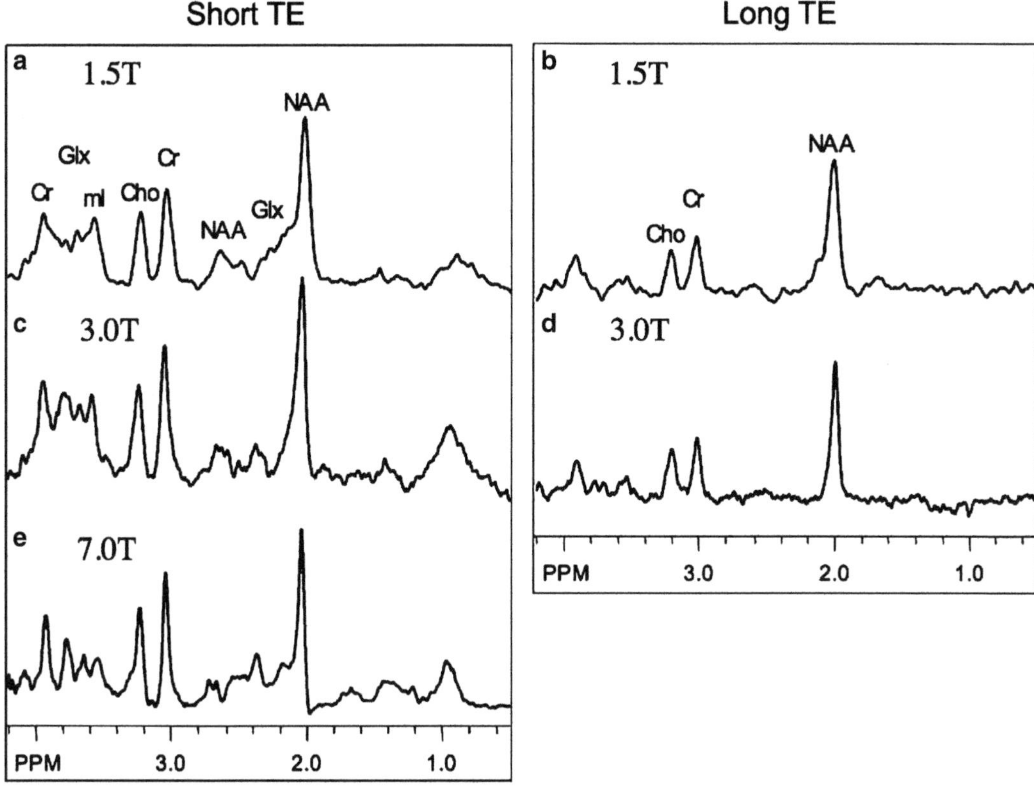

Fig. 12.1 Representative spectra at short (~35 ms) and long (~280 ms) TE from centrum semiovale white matter at 1.5 T (**a**, **b**), 3.0 T (**c**, **d**), and 7.0 T (**e**). (**a**–**d**) are taken from [8], (**e**) courtesy of Dr Murdoch

quite similar on initial inspection, the 7 T spectra have about a 48 % improvement in SNR compared to 3 T in this example.

Pulse Sequences for High-Field MRS

General Considerations

As already mentioned above, magnetic susceptibility effects (both microscopic and macroscopic) increase linearly with increasing magnetic field strength. Therefore, in order to achieve expected improvements in spectral resolution, it is important that the magnetic field homogeneity is fully optimized at high-field strengths. Automated shimming routines using field maps and high-order shim (second and third) corrections have been shown to give the best results [18, 19] provided that strong enough shim currents are available.

Radiofrequency (RF) coil design is also important for studies at high field. RF head coils that give uniform B_1 fields at 1.5 or 3.0 T (such as "birdcage" or other resonator coils [20]) have appreciable inhomogeneities at 7.0 T [21], which can result in significant spatial variations in image intensity and contrast, and in the context of MRS, can result in reduced sensitivity, suboptimal water or lipid suppression, or quantification errors. This may particularly be a problem if the scanner flip angle optimization routine is performed on a different (and/or larger) volume than the localized MRS experiment; therefore it is important to make sure that the flip angle is correctly optimized on a volume that closely matches the MRS region of interest [22].

There is also currently interest in multiple coil/amplifier systems to overcome the problem of transmit B_1 inhomogeneity [23, 24]; also, as discussed below, it is possible to use pulse sequence

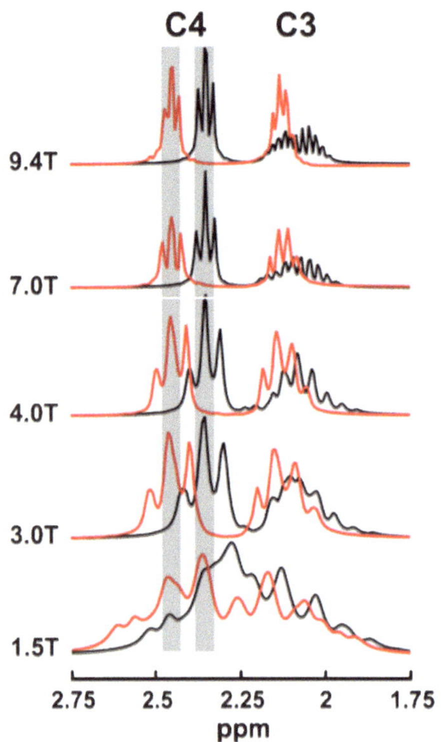

Fig. 12.2 Simulations of the C4 and C3 proton resonances of glutamate (Glu) and glutamine (Gln) as a function of field strength ranging from 1.5 to 9.4 T. The C2 protons which resonate around ~3.75 ppm are not shown. It can be seen that the C4 protons of Glu and Gln become increasingly well resolved with increasing field strength. Adapted with permission from [56]

design to minimize the effects of these transmit B_1 inhomogeneities. Similar to lower field strengths, best SNR is obtained (both for MRI and MRS) using multiple, phased-array receiver coils with optimal channel combination [25].

Single Voxel (SV) MRS

Similar pulse sequences as used at 1.5 or 3.0 T can also be used for 7.0 T, such as the commonly used STEAM [6] or PRESS [26] sequences (Fig. 12.4). However, results may not always be optimal if directly using a 1.5 or 3.0 T protocol at 7.0 T. Various issues may arise: first of all, use of long echo times (e.g., TE 140 or 280 ms) is generally not advised because of the shorter metabolite T_2s at higher field. In addition, the sequence should be designed to be as insensitive as possible to variations in the transmit B_1 field, and, in addition, slice selective RF pulses should be used with high bandwidths in order to minimize "chemical shift displacement" CSD effects [27]. The magnitude of the CSD is given by

$$\mathrm{CSD} = \gamma B_0 \times (\sigma - \sigma_0) \times \mathrm{ST} / \mathrm{BW}(\mathrm{mm}) \quad (12.3)$$

where ST is the slice thickness in mm, BW is the bandwidth of the slice selective pulse (Hz), and σ_0 is the chemical shift corresponding to the scanner transmitter ("center") frequency (usually the water chemical shift (4.7 ppm) for MRI, but for MRS should be applied in the middle of the spectral region of interest (e.g., ~2.5 ppm if desired to cover metabolites from ~4 to ~1 ppm)). For instance, if the RF pulse has a bandwidth of 430 Hz, for a 15 mm slice thickness the CSD is 10.4 mm/ppm, since 1 ppm = 298 Hz at 7 T. Therefore, in this example, the resonances of myo-inositol (mI at 3.56 ppm) and NAA (2.02 ppm) in the spectrum will originate from totally different slice locations (1.56 ppm ≡ 16.2 mm, i.e., more than 1 slice thickness) (Fig. 12.5). Solutions to this problem include using higher transmit B_1 fields to increase the pulse bandwidth, or using alternative RF pulse waveforms with higher bandwidths. Figure 12.6a shows an example of a frequency modulated 90° excitation pulse [28] which has a duration of 8.7 ms, maximum amplitude of 13.5 μT, and a bandwidth of 4.7 kHz. Use of such a high bandwidth pulse minimizes the chemical shift dispersion problem (the mI-NAA displacement drops to ~10 % of the slice thickness (Fig. 12.6b)). However, these pulses are typically longer and require more RF power than lower bandwidth pulses, thereby increasing the SAR of the sequence. SAR is a significant concern for high-field MRS, since the SAR is predicted to increase with approximately the square of the Larmor frequency ($\omega_0 = \gamma B_0$) [21].

While frequency modulated pulses can be incorporated into sequences such as PRESS and STEAM, their increased duration limits the shortest echo times (TE) that can be used. STEAM is arguably favorable to PRESS at high fields in that 90° pulses are somewhat easier to

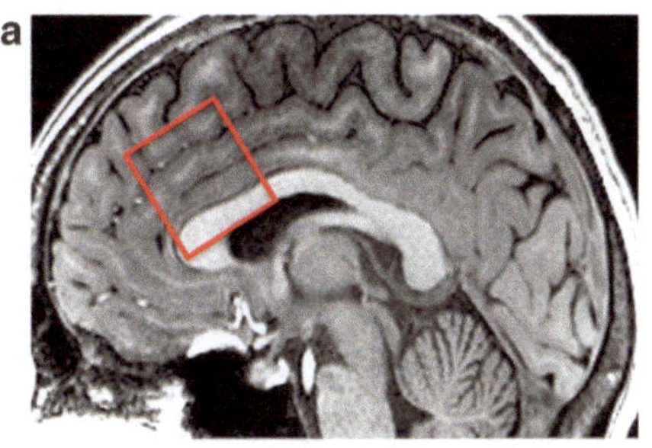

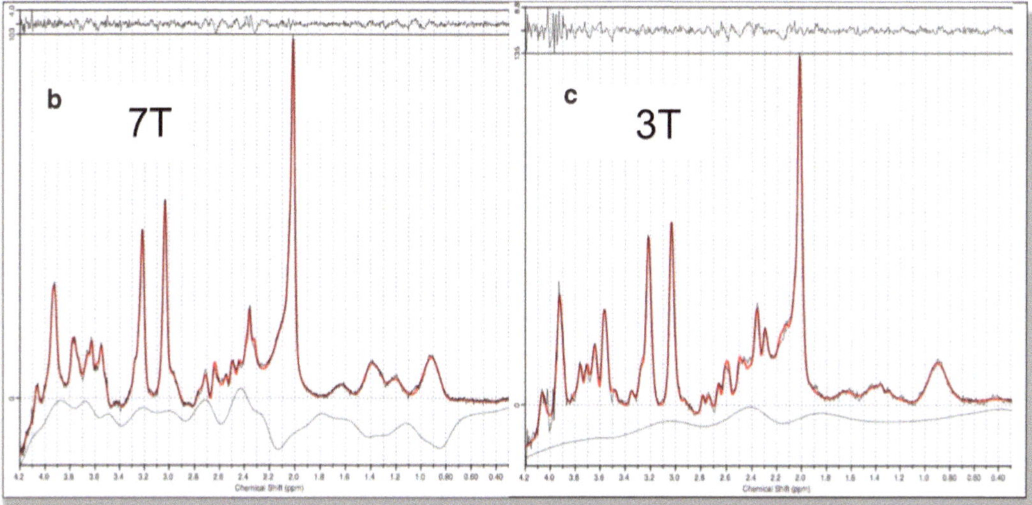

Fig. 12.3 (**a**) Sagittal MRI showing the 3×3×3 cm voxel location in the anterior cingulate cortex (ACC) in one subject scanned under identical conditions at both (**b**) 7 T and (**c**) 3 T, using 32-channel head coils and the sLASER pulse sequence. Scan parameters were TR/TE 3,000/32 ms, 32 averages, 1 min 36 s scan time. Average SNR in four subjects was 50.1 at 7 T and 33.8 at 3 T (i.e., 48 % improvement at 7 T). *Spectral line* widths were 0.030 ppm (8.9 Hz) at 7 T and 0.035 ppm (4.5 Hz) at 3 T. Spectra are fit using LCModel software (*red line*—fit results, *gray line* estimated spectral baseline, and the top trace is the difference between the experimental data and the fit)

design than 180° pulses, in terms of bandwidth, slice profile and SAR, and relatively short TEs can be obtain (due to the TM time period during which the magnetization is on the *Z*-axis). However, STEAM only detects the stimulated echo created by the three 90° pulses, which has half of the full signal magnitude. Therefore an alternative approach, dubbed "SPECIAL" [17], was designed to detect the full signal while still maintaining short TE, but using a slice selective inversion pulse (turned on and off on alternating scans) to achieve spatial localization in one direction (Fig. 12.7). SPECIAL works well, but does have the potential for subtraction artifacts since it is a localization method based on subtracting two scans. SPECIAL can be implemented with a frequency swept adiabatic inversion pulse, not only providing a high bandwidth but also to provide full inversion even in the presence of an inhomogeneous transmit field (provided that the minimum transmit B_1 is above the "adiabatic threshold" of the pulse used).

Pulse sequences may be made fully adiabatic (i.e., theoretically giving the full signal, even if the transmit B_1 is inhomogeneous, or not properly calibrated) by replacing all the pulses in the sequence with adiabatic pulses [29]; this type of sequence was dubbed "LASER" [30]; since frequency swept adiabatic pulses induce a strong, frequency-dependent phase error when used as refocusing pulses, they have to be used in pairs (the phase error of the second pulse reverses (i.e., cancels out) the phase error associated with the first). The LASER sequence is fully adiabatic, but

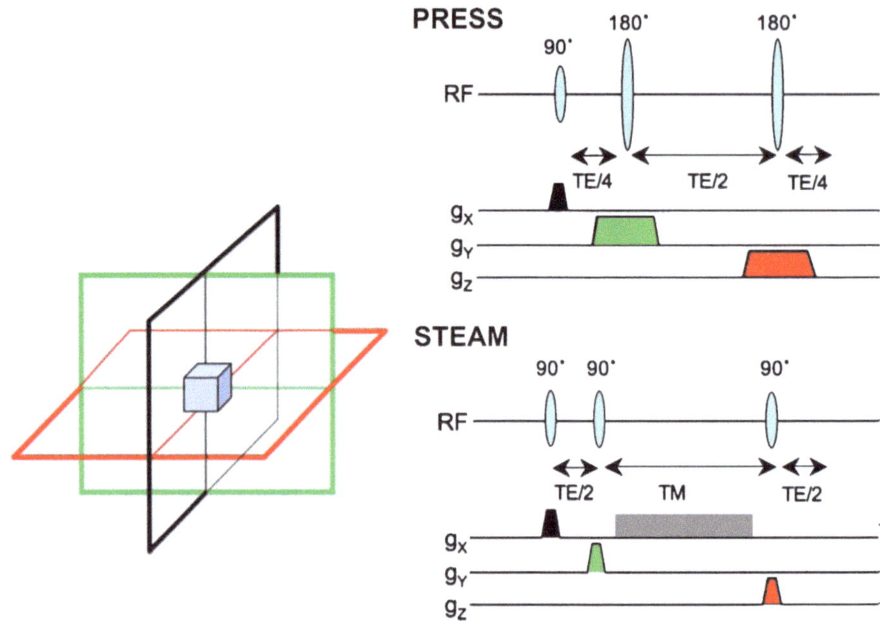

Fig. 12.4 Schematic illustration (note; not all gradients shown, graphic illustration only) of conventional pulse sequences for single voxel MRS; STEAM and PRESS. Both sequences involve the application of three slice selective pulses with field gradients applied in orthogonal directions

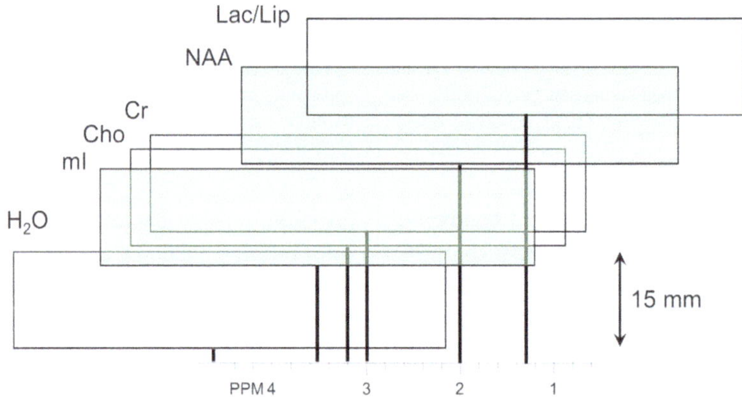

Fig. 12.5 Graphic illustration of the chemical shift displacement effect; the slice location for each metabolite is displayed as a function of its chemical shift. Slice locations are displayed for a 15 mm thick slice at 7 T (298 Hz/ppm) for a slice selective pulse with a bandwidth of 430 Hz (≈10 μT). It can be seen the resonances of mI and NAA (*shaded green*) originate from entirely different (non-overlapping) slice locations (mI-NAA CSD = 1.54 ppm = 458 Hz, CSD = 458/430 = 106 %)

does have quite a long minimum TE because six adiabatic 180° pulses are required, in addition to a non-slice selective adiabatic 90° excitation pulse (Fig. 12.7); because of the 7 RF pulses, the SAR of the sequence is also quite high. A "compromise" sequence that has become quite popular at high fields (e.g., 3 and 7 T) is the "semi-LASER" (sLASER) sequence which retains a non-adiabatic

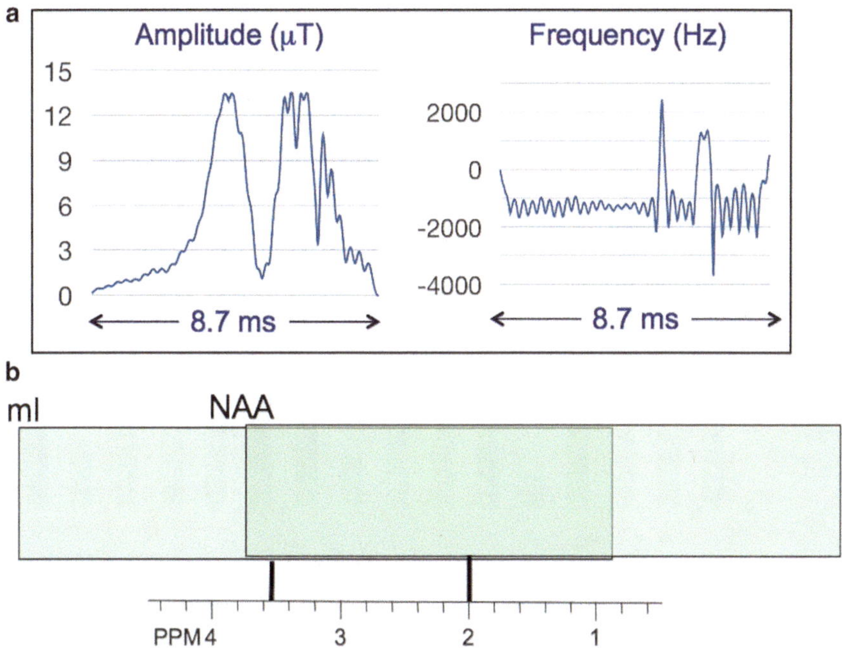

Fig. 12.6 (a) An example of a high bandwidth amplitude and frequency modulated excitation pulse ("fremex05," courtesy of Dr James Murdoch, [57]) with a duration of 8.7 ms, a maximum B_1 amplitude of 13.5, and a frequency-sweep (bandwidth) of 4.7 kHz. The pulse has been numerically optimized to give a rectangular excitation profile and uniform flip angle over a range of B_1 values. (b) Illustration of the large reduction (compared to Fig. 12.5) of the chemical shift displacement artifact at 7 T using this pulse; with a bandwidth of 4.7 kHz, the mI-NAA CSD is now only ≈10 % (1.5 mm for a 15 mm slice thickness)

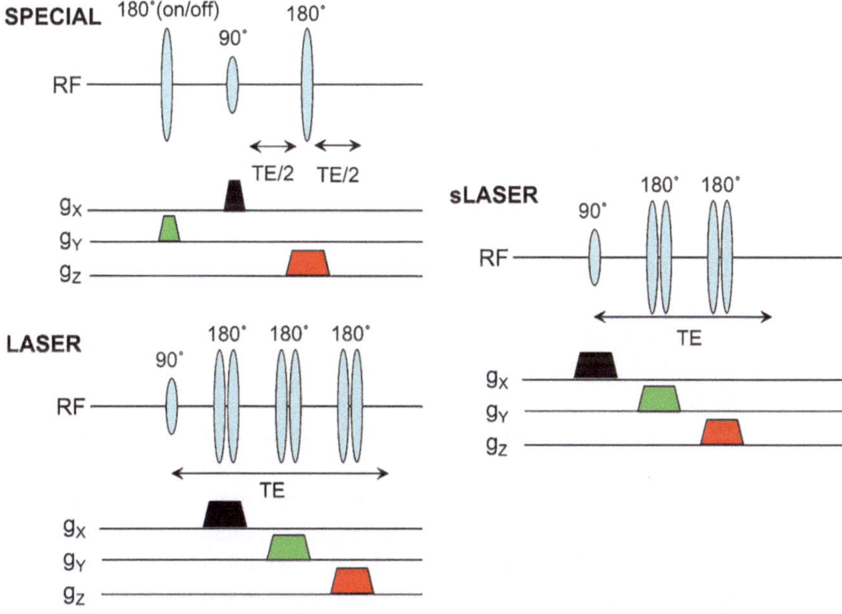

Fig. 12.7 Alternative pulse sequences for SV MRS which may be preferable at high magnetic field strengths: SPECIAL, LASER, and semi-LASER (sLASER). All three sequences make use of adiabatic RF pulses; only LASER is fully adiabatic, however

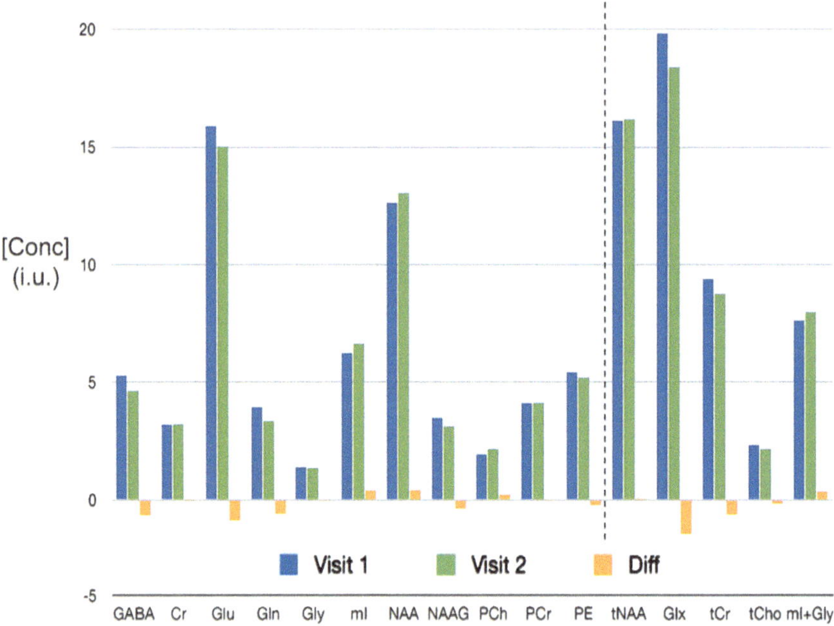

Fig. 12.8 An example of a 7 T MRS reproducibility study; short TE STEAM spectra recorded at 7 T from the anterior cingulate cortex were analyzed with LCModel software to yield concentration values (institutional units—i.u.). Metabolite concentrations ($N=5$) are shown for 11 different compounds (and the composite signals tNAA (NAAG+NAA), Glx (Glu+Gln), tCr (Cr+PCr), tCho (PCh+PE), (mI+Gly)) recorded in the same subjects 1 week apart. The average coefficient of variation (CV) was approximately 6 %. Data from [58]

slice selective excitation pulse and uses two pairs of adiabatic refocusing pulses [31, 32] (Fig. 12.7). This sequence is adiabatic in two dimensions, with a somewhat shorter minimum TE and lower SAR than the full LASER sequence. Figure 12.3 shows example spectra from the human brain (anterior cingulate gyrus) recorded at 3 and 7 T user the sLASER sequence. Because of the higher spectral resolution and signal-to-noise ratios available at 7 T, more compounds can be accurately determined compared to lower field strengths; using the "LCModel" analysis method, it has been shown that up to 17 compounds can be estimated [13]. Figure 12.8 shows reproducibility for 7 T STEAM MRS anterior cingulate data from five subjects; in this study, the average coefficient of variation was ~6 %, and in addition to the reliable determination of compounds readily detected at lower fields (tNAA, tCt, tCho, Glx, and mI) it is noteworthy that reliable estimates of glutamate (Glu), glutamine (Gn), γ-aminobutyric acid (GABA), and *N*-acetylaspartyl glutamate (NAAG) are obtained, among others.

All SV-MRS sequences are generally also performed with water suppression pulses, some of which are optimized specifically for use at 7 T [33]; also, outer-volume suppression (OVS) [34] and phase-cycling [35] are typically used to remove residual signals from outside the target region of interest. Frequency-selective lipid suppression may also be applied [27], particular in conjunction with MR spectroscopic imaging (MRSI) sequences (see below).

MRSI

A wide variety of methods exist for MRSI [36]. MRSI may be performed in one, two, or three spatial dimensions and combined with many of the sequences mentioned above to limit the spatial extent of excitation. A commonly used MRSI sequence at 1.5 or 3.0 T in clinical applications is the 2D-PRESS-MRSI sequence [37], which combines PRESS excitation (limited to one-slice) with two-dimensional phase-encoding.

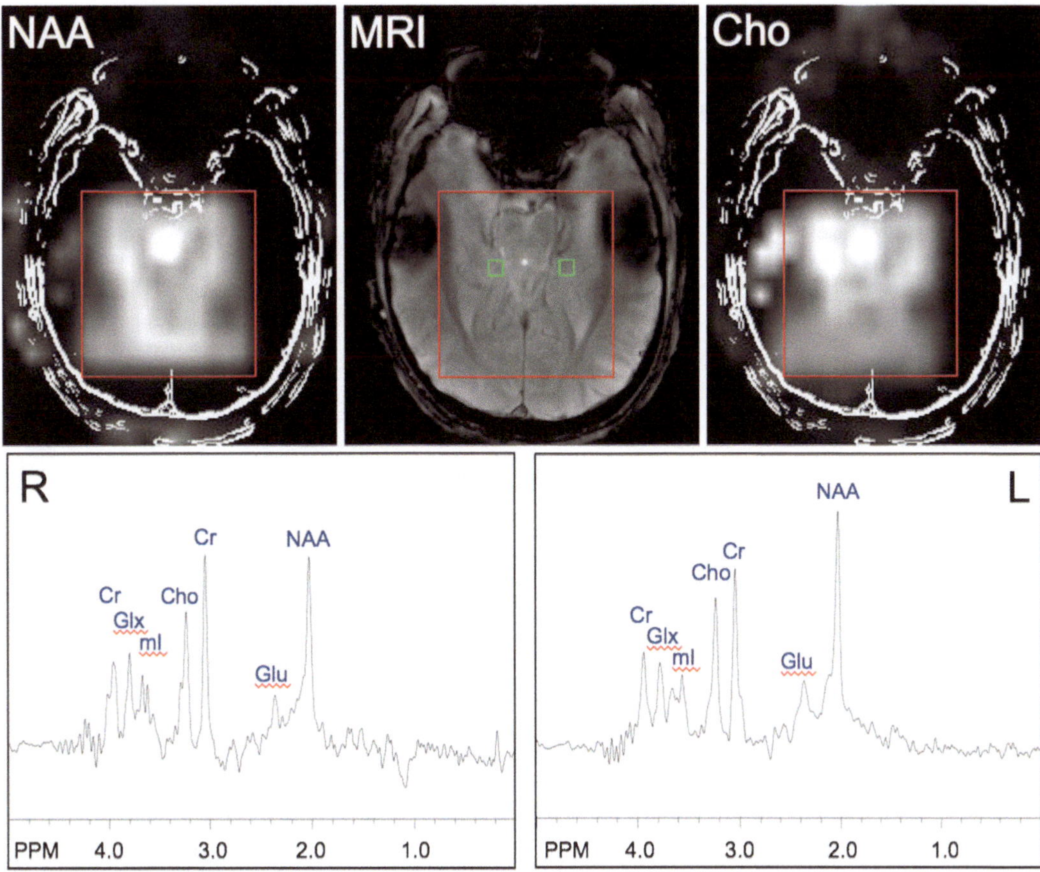

Fig. 12.9 An example of a 7 T 2D-MRSI scan performed using STEAM localization in a patient with seizures of *right* mesial temporal onset on intracranial EEG. Reconstructed images of NAA and Cho are shown, as well as the corresponding localizer MRI scan, and selected spectra from the body of the *right* and *left* hippocampus (voxel locations indicated on MRI). The voxel size was $10 \times 7 \times 7$ mm ≈ 0.5 cm^3, and the scan time 12 min 25 s with a TR of 2.5 s and a TE of 22.5 ms, and a SENSE-acceleration factor of $1.5 \times 1.5 = 2.25$ (matrix size 32×26, FOV 220×178 mm, circular k-space sampling). High bandwidth slice selective pulses were used as well as dual band water and lipid suppression. It can be seen that the ratio of NAA/Cho and NAA/Cr are lower in the *right* hippocampus than the *left*, particularly apparent as an increased signal on the Cho image. The patient subsequently had a *right* temporal lobectomy and was subsequently seizure free

The PRESS volume is chosen to excite as much of the slice as possible while at the same time avoiding exciting the subcutaneous lipid signals in the scalp. The PRESS sequence can also be used with a thicker slice and 3D phase-encoding (3D-PRESS-MRSI) to extend coverage to three dimensions. While 3D-PRESS-MRSI has been demonstrated at 7 T [38], it does have appreciable problems. First, coverage is incomplete because the rectangular PRESS voxel cannot be placed close to the surface of the brain without also including lipids. In addition, voxels near the edges cannot be reliably interpreted because of the pulse profile of the slice selective pulses (particularly the 180° pulses) and chemical shift dispersion effects. If a STEAM sequence is used, the slice profiles are somewhat better since all the slices are defined by 90° pulses, and SAR is also lower; however, SNR will be lower than in PRESS (as discussed above, STEAM has about 50 % of the signal compared to PRESS).

Figure 12.9 shows an example of a 2D-STEAM-MRSI scan of a patient with right-sided mesial temporal lobe epilepsy recorded at 7 T. It can be seen that the body of the right hippocampal body has a lower ratio of NAA/Cho and NAA/Cr than

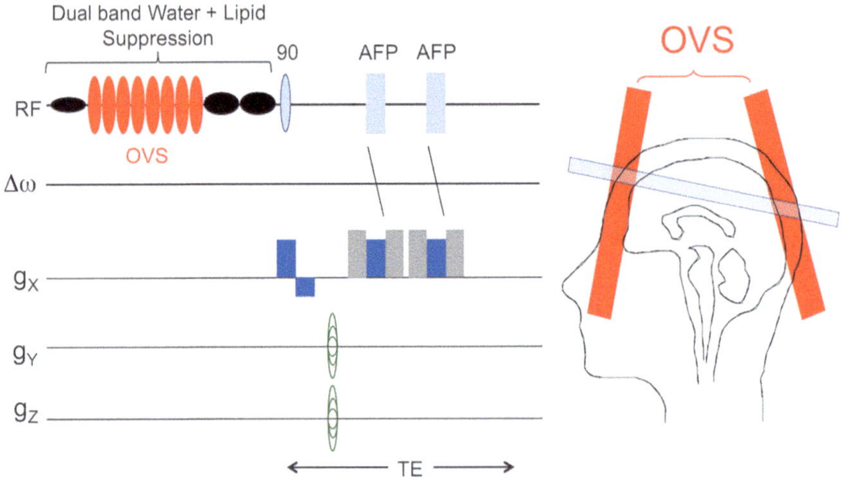

Fig. 12.10 Schematic illustration of a pulse sequence for slice-selective MRSI at 7 T, using dual band water and lipid suppression, outer-volume suppression (OVS) for lipid suppression in the scalp, 2D-phase encoding, and a paid of adiabatic fast passage (AFP) refocusing pulses

the left, in spite of the fact that the conventional MRI was considered normal in this case.

In mesial temporal lobe epilepsy, the regions of interest are primarily the bilateral hippocampi, so the lack of cortical coverage is not particularly a problem. However, in other pathologies, cortical coverage may be essential. Therefore, there have been many attempts to increase coverage or MRSI using whole-slice (and multiple whole-slice) acquisition methods, many of which were pioneered at lower field strengths [39–41]. One approach used a multi (whole) slice acquisition, with OVS pulses used for lipid suppression [39]. Translating this method to high field is challenging for several reasons, including obtaining sufficient magnet homogeneity (B_0) over the volume of tissue, dealing with inhomogeneities in the transmit B_1 field (which cause uneven excitation and suboptimal water and lipid suppression), and high SAR due to the use of high-bandwidth pulses. Solutions to some of these issues include the use of field-map-based high-order shimming [18], including dynamic slice-by-slice shimming [41], use of adiabatic pulses which are insensitive to variations in the B_1 field [31], improved transmit RF coil design (including the use of multiple-transmit coils [23]), or the use of fewer RF pulses [42] to lower SAR. One sequence just uses a single excitation pulse (with water and OVS lipid suppression) followed by phase-encoding ("FIDLOVS" [42]), which is both low SAR and also allows a very short TE to be used. The drawback to this sequence is that spectral analysis (fitting) may be more difficult because of the resulting first-order phase error (since a spin echo is not formed), and the substantial presence of macromolecule resonances and other baseline effects at very short TEs. Since long TRs often have to be used to lower SAR, the use of fast-encoding techniques (e.g., SENSE-encoding [27, 43] or echo-planar spectroscopic imaging (EPSI) [12]) is important to keep scan time within reasonable limits.

Figure 12.10 shows a pulse sequence for one implementation of MRSI at 7 T: water and lipids are suppressed by a dual band pre-saturation sequence which also includes eight spatial OVS pulses for additional lipid suppression in the scalp, followed by a high bandwidth excitation pulse, phase encoding in two directions, and then a pair of high-bandwidth, adiabatic refocusing pulses [27]. When performed with a 32-channel head coil, high SENSE-encoding factors can be used to keep scan time within clinically reasonable limits. Figure 12.11 shows an example of the use of this sequence in a patient with HIV infection treated with highly active anti-retroviral therapy (HAART). Scan time was just over 10 min using a SENSE-acceleration factor of 4.

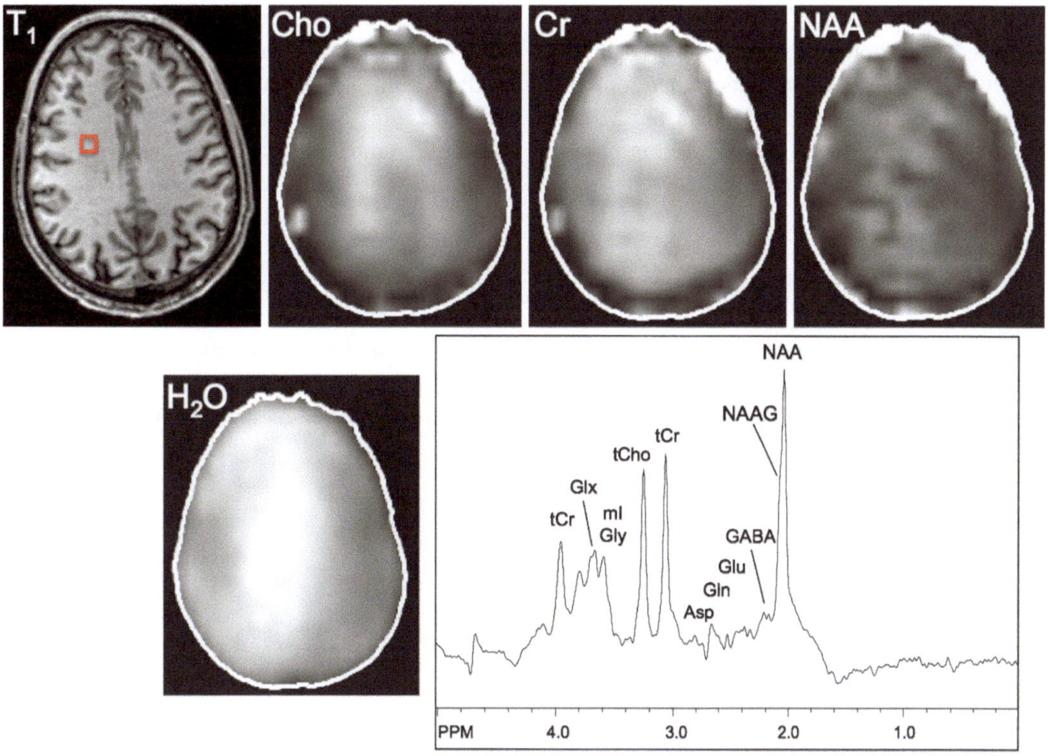

Fig. 12.11 Single slice MRSI data in a patient with HIV infection recorded using the pulse sequence of Fig. 12.10 at 7 T with a 32-channel head coil. Scan parameters include TR 4.3 s, TE 29 ms, voxel size 8×8×15 mm, SENSE factor 4 (2×2), scan time 10 min 19 s. The AFP pulses were of 7 ms duration and had a bandwidth of 4.7 kHz. A T_1 localizer image, as well as reconstructed images of H_2O, Cho, Cr, and NAA are shown, as well as a selected spectrum from the *right* centrum semiovale white matter

Coupled Spin Systems: Spectral Editing and Chemical Shift Displacement Effects

As can be seen in Fig. 12.2, spectral patterns for coupled molecules (in this case glutamate and glutamine) change as field strength increases. Whereas the chemical shift between different functional groups in the spectra (e.g., the C3 and C4 protons of Glu and Gln, Fig. 12.2) measured in Hz increases linearly with field, the scalar couplings (J) remain constant (in Hz). Therefore, the relative separation between groups increases with field, and the spectral multiplets transition from "strongly-coupled" to "weakly-coupled." This improves the ability to measure and discriminate between different compounds.

However, the increased CSD effect at high fields can also lead to problems. For instance, the modulation (inversion) of the lactate signal in a spin-echo experiment with an echo times of $1/J$ (i.e., ~140 ms, $J \approx 7$ Hz) is a well-known method for helping distinguish lactate from lipid. However, this modulation occurs only if both the CH (4.1 ppm) and CH_3 (1.3 ppm) resonances both experience the same refocusing pulses [44]. As can be seen in Fig. 12.5, with weak slice selective pulses, this is unlikely to be the case, and the lactate signal may be positive, negative, or disappear altogether, depending on the bandwidth of the pulses used at TE 140 ms. Therefore, if detection of lactate is important, careful consideration of the experimental protocol is required; either high bandwidth refocusing pulses should be used (TE 140 ms), and/or either short (TE < 35 ms) or long (TE 280 ms) echo times used. Finally, the same considerations also apply if using spectral editing techniques (such as the MEGA-PRESS sequence [45]) to observe lower concentration compounds such as GABA or glutathione (GSH)

[46]; the spectral editing sequence only works as expected when both coupled spins experience the refocusing pulses in the sequence; therefore, high bandwidth pulses (such as used in the MEGA-sLASER sequence [47]) are required in order to achieve good editing efficiency at high field.

7 T MRS of Brain Pathology

To date, much of the published work on MRS or MRSI at 7 T has focused on technique development, rather than clinical applications. However, studies of pathological conditions are now beginning to appear. For instance, one study of patients with preclinical Huntington's disease found that decreases in NAA and especially glutamate occurred compared to age-matched control subjects, and correlated with cognitive assessment (Fig. 12.12), most likely indicating early neuronal loss or dysfunction [48]. Glutamate seems to be a good marker of neuronal health [49] and is difficult to measure accurately (i.e., separate for glutamine) at lower field strengths [50]. Other studies of 7 T MRS have been published on demyelinating diseases such as multiple sclerosis

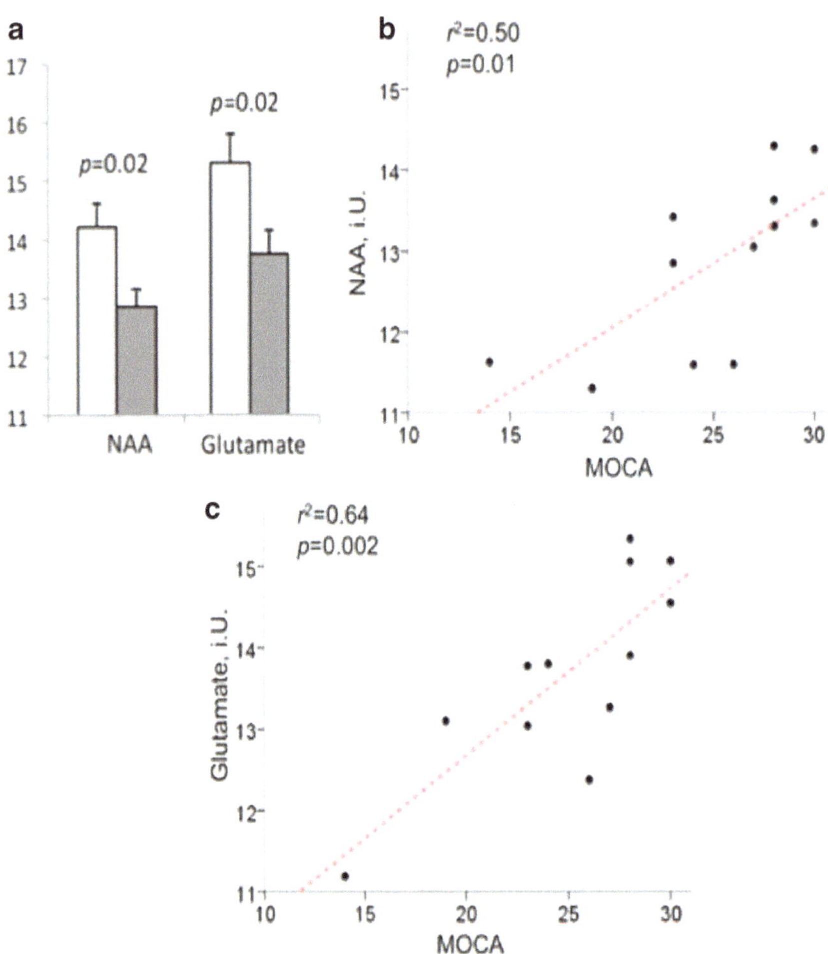

Fig. 12.12 7 T MRS data in a study of patients with early (prodromal) Huntington's disease (HD, $n=12$). (**a**) Compared to age-matched control subjects ($n=12$), early HD patients had lower levels of both NAA and glutamate in the posterior cingulate cortex (PCC), suggestive of early neuronal loss or dysfunction, which correlated with the Montreal Cognitive Assessment score (MOCA) both for (**b**) NAA ($p=0.01$) and (**c**) glutamate ($p=0.002$). Adapted from [48]

(MS) [51] and adrenoleukodystrophy (ALD) [52], as well as in Parkinson's disease [53]. However, to the best of our knowledge, no studies of human brain tumors have yet been published at 7 T. No doubt as time goes by and techniques evolve, 7 T MRSI studies of brain tumors will emerge, most likely making use of both the higher sensitivity (and hence higher spatial resolution) of 7 T MRSI, as well as the access to more compounds that can be measured at the current clinical field strengths of 1.5 and 3.0 T.

Safety and Physiological Effects of High Magnetic Fields

Patient safety is an absolute requirement for all magnetic resonance studies. Conventional MRI is generally considered a nonsignificant risk, so long as appropriate subject screening (e.g., to avoid patients with magnetic implants or other contra-indications) and procedures (no untrained personnel in the scanner magnet room, scanner operating within approved SAR, gradient switching, and sound pressure level limits) are used. The United States Food and Drug Administration (FDA) have approved magnet systems up to 8 T as nonsignificant risk, although since, to date, only 1.5 and 3.0 T systems are approved for marketing, studies in systems >3.0 T are required to be performed under local institutional review board (IRB) approval. Whereas the risks associated with implanted devices patient implants (e.g., pacemakers, deep brain stimulators, aneurysm clips, cranial fixation plates, other prostheses) are very well known at 1.5 and 3.0 T, almost no testing has been done above these field strengths. Devices considered completely safe at 3 T are also likely to be safe at higher magnetic fields (and vice versa—i.e., those unsafe at 3 T are also unsafe above 3 T), but every device must be considered on a case-by-case basis and in vitro tested for forces and heating effects in the magnet prior to assuming that it is safe.

Motion within magnetic fields is known to cause some perturbation of the vestibular system through its effects on the inner ear, and for this reason care should be taken in high-field systems that subjects (or scan operators) do not move too rapidly around, or in or out, of high-field magnet systems. Temporary mild vertigo, disequilibrium, and nausea are not uncommon in subjects undergoing high-field MRI scans [54]. The risk of this can be minimized by moving the subject slowly in and out of the magnetic field. Recently it has also been discovered that transient nystagmus may also occur during motion in the magnetic field [55], as a results of stimulation of the rotational sensors in the brain.

Conclusions: 7 T and Beyond?

MRS and MRSI undoubtedly benefit from being performed at high magnetic field strengths such as 7 T, in particular for the more accurate determination of more compounds than can be done at lower field strength. However, a number of technical challenges need to be overcome in order to fully achieve the predicted advantages, particularly for MRSI. One of the biggest challenges remains dealing with the inhomogeneities of the transmit B_1 field, and B_0, when trying to perform MRSI with large spatial coverage. As mentioned above, hardware advances including multiple-transmit coils and dynamic (e.g., slice-by-slice) high-order shimming have been shown to have the potential to address these problems.

The scientific and clinical benefits of high-field MRI and MRS have to be balanced against the considerable added expense of high-field MR systems (both in terms of installation and operation), particularly in the current economic climate, and with rising costs of commodities such as liquid helium and niobium superconducting wire. To date, the majority of high-field MRS studies have focused on technique development, rather than clinical applications, and more studies in pathological conditions are therefore needed to establish their value in specific disorders, in particular brain tumors. However, it appears likely that high-field MR systems will be at the forefront of MR research studies in academic medical centers in upcoming years.

Magnets large enough for scanning the human brain in vivo can also be manufactured at field strengths even higher than 7 T—systems at 8 and 9.4 T have been built and used in humans [11]. However, to date, little in vivo MRS has been performed in these systems. The technical challenges described above in moving from 1.5 or 3.0 T to 7.0 T of course continue to be even more important at these higher field strengths, so many logistic and developmental factors will need to be addressed to successfully demonstrate improvements beyond 7 T. In addition, human subject safety issues need to be carefully addressed as field strengths progress ever higher.

Acknowledgments This work supported in part by NIH P41EB015909. I would like to thank Mr Joseph Gillen and Drs He (Henry) Zhu, Susanne Bonekamp, Andrew Wijtenburg, Laura Rowland, Mona Mohamed, and Jim Murdoch for their contributions to the work presented here.

References

1. Hoult DI, Lauterbur PC. The sensitivity of the zeugmatographic experiment involving human samples. J Magn Reson. 1979;34:425–33.
2. Posse S, Cuenod CA, Risinger R, Le Bihan D, Balaban RS. Anomalous transverse relaxation in 1H spectroscopy in human brain at 4 Tesla. Magn Reson Med. 1995;33:246–52.
3. Van de Moortele PF, Akgun C, Adriany G, et al. B(1) destructive interferences and spatial phase patterns at 7 T with a head transceiver array coil. Magn Reson Med. 2005;54:1503–18.
4. Prost RW, Mark L, Mewissen M, Li SJ. Detection of glutamate/glutamine resonances by 1H magnetic resonance spectroscopy at 0.5 tesla. Magn Reson Med. 1997;37:615–8.
5. Sauter R, Loeffler W, Bruhn H, Frahm J. The human brain: localized H-1 MR spectroscopy at 1.0 T. Radiology. 1990;176:221–4.
6. Frahm J, Bruhn H, Gyngell ML, Merboldt KD, Hanicke W, Sauter R. Localized high-resolution proton NMR spectroscopy using stimulated echoes: initial applications to human brain in vivo. Magn Reson Med. 1989;9:79–93.
7. Michaelis T, Merboldt KD, Bruhn H, Hanicke W, Frahm J. Absolute concentrations of metabolites in the adult human brain in vivo: quantification of localized proton MR spectra. Radiology. 1993;187:219–27.
8. Barker PB, Hearshen DO, Boska MD. Single-voxel proton MRS of the human brain at 1.5T and 3.0T. Magn Reson Med. 2001;45:765–9.
9. Gruetter R, Garwood M, Ugurbil K, Seaquist ER. Observation of resolved glucose signals in 1H NMR spectra of the human brain at 4 Tesla. Magn Reson Med. 1996;36:1–6.
10. Tkac I, Andersen P, Adriany G, Merkle H, Ugurbil K, Gruetter R. In vivo 1H NMR spectroscopy of the human brain at 7 T. Magn Reson Med. 2001;46:451–6.
11. Deelchand DK, Van de Moortele PF, Adriany G, et al. In vivo 1H NMR spectroscopy of the human brain at 9.4 T: initial results. J Magn Reson. 2010;206:74–80.
12. Otazo R, Mueller B, Ugurbil K, Wald L, Posse S. Signal-to-noise ratio and spectral linewidth improvements between 1.5 and 7 Tesla in proton echo-planar spectroscopic imaging. Magn Reson Med. 2006;56:1200–10.
13. Tkac I, Oz G, Adriany G, Ugurbil K, Gruetter R. In vivo 1H NMR spectroscopy of the human brain at high magnetic fields: metabolite quantification at 4T vs. 7T. Magn Reson Med. 2009;62:868–79.
14. Michaeli S, Garwood M, Zhu XH, et al. Proton T2 relaxation study of water, N-acetylaspartate, and creatine in human brain using Hahn and Carr-Purcell spin echoes at 4T and 7T. Magn Reson Med. 2002;47:629–33.
15. Gonen O, Gruber S, Li BS, Mlynarik V, Moser E. Multivoxel 3D proton spectroscopy in the brain at 1.5 versus 3.0 T: signal-to-noise ratio and resolution comparison. AJNR. Am J Neuroradiol. 2001;22:1727–31.
16. Kantarci K, Reynolds G, Petersen RC, et al. Proton MR spectroscopy in mild cognitive impairment and Alzheimer disease: comparison of 1.5 and 3 T. AJNR. Am J Neuroradiol. 2003;24:843–9.
17. Mekle R, Mlynarik V, Gambarota G, Hergt M, Krueger G, Gruetter R. MR spectroscopy of the human brain with enhanced signal intensity at ultrashort echo times on a clinical platform at 3T and 7T. Magn Reson Med. 2009;61:1279–85.
18. Pan JW, Lo KM, Hetherington HP. Role of very high order and degree B(0) shimming for spectroscopic imaging of the human brain at 7 tesla. Magn Reson Med. 2012;68(4):1007–17.
19. Tkac I, Gruetter R. Methodology of H NMR spectroscopy of the human brain at very high magnetic fields. Appl Magn Reson. 2005;29:139–57.
20. Mekle R, van der Zwaag W, Joosten A, Gruetter R. Comparison of three commercially available radio frequency coils for human brain imaging at 3 Tesla. MAGMA. 2008;21:53–61.
21. Vaughan JT, Garwood M, Collins CM, et al. 7T vs. 4T: RF power, homogeneity, and signal-to-noise comparison in head images. Magn Reson Med. 2001;46:24–30.
22. Versluis MJ, Kan HE, van Buchem MA, Webb AG. Improved signal to noise in proton spectroscopy of the human calf muscle at 7 T using localized B1 calibration. Magn Reson Med. 2010;63:207–11.
23. Avdievich NI, Oh S, Hetherington HP, Collins CM. Improved homogeneity of the transmit field by simultaneous transmission with phased array and volume coil. J Magn Reson Imaging. 2010;32:476–81.
24. Adriany G, Van de Moortele PF, Wiesinger F, et al. Transmit and receive transmission line arrays for 7 Tesla parallel imaging. Magn Reson Med. 2005;53:434–45.

25. Brown MA. Time-domain combination of MR spectroscopy data acquired using phased-array coils. Magn Reson Med. 2004;52:1207–13.
26. Bottomley PA. Spatial localization in NMR spectroscopy in vivo. Ann N Y Acad Sci. 1987;508:333–48.
27. Zhu H, Soher BJ, Ouwerkerk R, Schar M, Barker PB. Spin-echo magnetic resonance spectroscopic imaging at 7 T with frequency-modulated refocusing pulses. Magn Reson Med. 2013;69(5):1217–25.
28. Murdoch JB. 10th ISMRM Scientific Meeting. Hawai'i; 2002;923
29. Slotboom JB, Bovée WMMJ. Adiabatic slice-selective RF pulses and a single-shot adiabatic localization pulse sequence. Concept Magnetic Res. 1995;7:193–217.
30. Garwood M, DelaBarre L. The return of the frequency sweep: designing adiabatic pulses for contemporary NMR. J Magn Reson. 2001;153:155–77.
31. Scheenen TW, Heerschap A, Klomp DW. Towards 1H-MRSI of the human brain at 7T with slice-selective adiabatic refocusing pulses. MAGMA. 2008;21:95–101.
32. Scheenen TW, Klomp DW, Wijnen JP, Heerschap A. Short echo time 1H-MRSI of the human brain at 3T with minimal chemical shift displacement errors using adiabatic refocusing pulses. Magn Reson Med. 2008;59:1–6.
33. Tkac I, Starcuk Z, Choi IY, Gruetter R. In vivo 1H NMR spectroscopy of rat brain at 1 ms echo time. Magn Reson Med. 1999;41:649–56.
34. Zhu H, Ouwerkerk R, Barker PB. Dual-band water and lipid suppression for MR spectroscopic imaging at 3 Tesla. Magn Reson Med. 2010;63:1486–92.
35. Wijtenburg SA, Knight-Scott J. Reconstructing very short TE phase rotation spectral data collected with multichannel phased-array coils at 3 T. Magn Reson Imaging. 2011;29:937–42.
36. Zhu H, Barker PB. MR spectroscopy and spectroscopic imaging of the brain. Methods Mol Biol. 2011;711:203–26.
37. Moonen CT, Sobering G, van Zijl PCM, Gillen J, von Kienlin M, Bizzi A. Proton spectroscopic imaging of human brain. J Magn Reson. 1992;98:556–75.
38. Xu D, Cunningham CH, Chen AP, et al. Phased array 3D MR spectroscopic imaging of the brain at 7 T. Magn Reson Imaging. 2008;26:1201–6.
39. Duyn JH, Gillen J, Sobering G, van Zijl PC, Moonen CT. Multisection proton MR spectroscopic imaging of the brain. Radiology. 1993;188:277–82.
40. Schuster C, Dreher W, Geppert C, Leibfritz D. Fast 3D 1H spectroscopic imaging at 3 Tesla using spectroscopic missing-pulse SSFP with 3D spatial preselection. Magn Reson Med. 2007;57:82–9.
41. Boer VO, Klomp DW, Juchem C, Luijten PR, de Graaf RA. Multislice (1) H MRSI of the human brain at 7 T using dynamic B(0) and B(1) shimming. Magn Reson Med. 2012;68:662–70.
42. Henning A, Fuchs A, Murdoch JB, Boesiger P. Slice-selective FID acquisition, localized by outer volume suppression (FIDLOVS) for (1)H-MRSI of the human brain at 7 T with minimal signal loss. NMR Biomed. 2009;22:683–96.
43. Dydak U, Weiger M, Pruessmann KP, Meier D, Boesiger P. Sensitivity-encoded spectroscopic imaging. Magn Reson Med. 2001;46:713–22.
44. Edden RA, Schar M, Hillis AE, Barker PB. Optimized detection of lactate at high fields using inner volume saturation. Magn Reson Med. 2006;56:912–7.
45. Edden RA, Barker PB. Spatial effects in the detection of gamma-aminobutyric acid: improved sensitivity at high fields using inner volume saturation. Magn Reson Med. 2007;58:1276–82.
46. Terpstra M, Marjanska M, Henry PG, Tkac I, Gruetter R. Detection of an antioxidant profile in the human brain in vivo via double editing with MEGA-PRESS. Magn Reson Med. 2006;56:1192–9.
47. Andreychenko A, Boer VO, Arteaga de Castro CS, Luijten PR, Klomp DW. Efficient spectral editing at 7 T: GABA detection with MEGA-sLASER. Magn Reson Med. 2012;68:1018–25.
48. Unschuld PG, Edden RA, Carass A, et al. Brain metabolite alterations and cognitive dysfunction in early Huntington's disease. Mov Disord. 2012;27: 895–902.
49. Eid T, Williamson A, Lee TS, Petroff OA, de Lanerolle NC. Glutamate and astrocytes–key players in human mesial temporal lobe epilepsy? Epilepsia. 2008;49 Suppl 2:42–52.
50. Ross B, Kreis R, Ernst T. Clinical tools for the 90s: magnetic resonance spectroscopy and metabolite imaging. Eur J Radiol. 1992;14:128–40.
51. Wood ET, Ronen I, Techawiboonwong A, et al. Investigating axonal damage in multiple sclerosis by diffusion tensor spectroscopy. J Neurosci. 2012;32:6665–9.
52. Ratai E, Kok T, Wiggins C, et al. Seven-Tesla proton magnetic resonance spectroscopic imaging in adult X-linked adrenoleukodystrophy. Arch Neurol. 2008; 65:1488–94.
53. Emir UE, Tuite PJ, Oz G. Elevated pontine and putamenal GABA levels in mild-moderate Parkinson disease detected by 7 tesla proton MRS. PLoS One. 2012;7:e30918.
54. Versluis MJ, Teeuwisse WM, Kan HE, van Buchem MA, Webb AG, van Osch MJ. Subject tolerance of 7 T MRI examinations. JMRI: Journal of magnetic resonance imaging; 2012.
55. Roberts DC, Marcelli V, Gillen JS, Carey JP, Della Santina CC, Zee DS. MRI magnetic field stimulates rotational sensors of the brain. Curr Biol. 2011;21:1635–40.
56. Yang S, Hu J, Kou Z, Yang Y. Spectral simplification for resolved glutamate and glutamine measurement using a standard STEAM sequence with optimized timing parameters at 3, 4, 4.7, 7, and 9.4T. Magn Reson Med. 2008;59:236–44.
57. Murdoch J. Still iterating… and iterating … to solve pulse design problems. In: Proceedings of the 10th ISMRM Scientific Meeting. Hawai'i. 2002:923.
58. Wijtenburg SA, Rowland LM, Edden RA, Barker PB. Reproducibility of brain spectroscopy at 7T using conventional localization and spectral editing techniques. J Magn Reson Imaging. 2013 Jan 4. doi: 10.1002/jmri.23997. [Epub ahead of print].

13 Sodium Magnetic Resonance Imaging in the Management of Human High-Grade Brain Tumors

Keith R. Thulborn, Ian C. Atkinson, Andrew Shon, Neil A. Das Gupta, John L. Villano, Tamir Y. Hersonskey, and Aiming Lu

Introduction

The standard of care for treatment of brain tumors varies with grade and histology. For high-grade tumors (World Health Organization classification grades III and IV), treatment often involves surgical resection (removing as much visible tumor as possible without compromising neurological function), fractionated radiation treatment (e.g., ~60 G total in ~2 G fractions for ~30 doses for 5 out of 7 days over 6 weeks) with concurrent chemotherapy (daily temozolomide, 75 mg/m^2), and follow-up cycles of chemotherapy (e.g., temozolomide, 150 mg/m^2 on days 1–5 of a 28-day cycle for the first cycle and 200 mg/m^2 for cycles 2–6) [1]. Greater than 98 % surgical resection of the contrast-enhancing mass is believed to be required to have any impact on prognosis for high-grade tumors [2]. Intraoperative imaging procedures and technologies have been developed to aid in achieving this goal. There is evidence that these advances achieve cost-effectiveness through reducing the number of repeat resections of recurrences and the length of hospital stays [3]. The survival at 5 years (considered long-term survival for this disease) varies from less than 10–32 %, depending on tumor grade and location and the health and age of the patient. The overall prognosis has improved slightly over proceeding decades to about 35 % for the period from 1995 to 2006 [4]. However, the most common brain tumor remains the glioblastoma that also has the worst prognosis with a 5-year survival for young adults of only 16–20 % and for older adults of even less at 1–6 % [4]. Unlike most other tumors in the rest of the body, patients with tumors of the central nervous system (CNS) die from local tumor recurrence rather than metastatic disease. The high frequency of local recurrence, often at a higher tumor grade, suggests that the current multimodal standard of care is failing to control the remaining tumor cells infiltrating the brain parenchyma extending away from the surgical bed. The current treatments may even be selecting for more malignant cell lines, including possibly pluripotent malignant stem cells, by

K.R. Thulborn • I.C. Atkinson (✉) • A. Lu
Center for Magnetic Resonance Research, University of Illinois Medical Center, 1801 West Taylor Street, Room 1307, CMRR M/C 707, Chicago, IL 60612, USA
e-mail: kthulbor@uic.edu; ian@uic.edu

A. Shon
Department of Radiology, Physiology and Biophysics, Center for Magnetic Resonance Research, University of Illinois Medical Center, 1801 West Taylor Street, M/C 707, Chicago, IL, USA

N.A.D. Gupta
Department of Radiation Oncology, Fox Valley Radiation Oncology, Naperville, IL, USA

J.L. Villano
Neuro-Oncology Program, University of Illinois, Chicago, IL, USA

T.Y. Hersonskey
Provena St. Joseph Medical Center, Joliet, IL, USA

J.J. Pillai (ed.), *Functional Brain Tumor Imaging*, DOI 10.1007/978-1-4419-5858-7_13,

removing competition for resources from the more vulnerable cells that respond to the chemotherapy and radiation treatment.

As local recurrence apparently can be expected, it seems reasonable to seek ways to measure prospectively the regional effectiveness of each treatment session across the brain. Since these tumors are heterogeneous, treatment responsiveness can be also expected to be heterogeneous. For example, responsiveness to radiation is compromised in regions of reduced oxygen content. Variable perfusion of residual tumor and of tissue at the margins of a surgical resection can result in such variable responsiveness to radiation treatment. Regions of reduced treatment effectiveness may be predictive of future local recurrence. If unresponsive regions can be identified and appropriately sensitive surveillance strategies introduced for early detection of recurrence, minimal time would be lost until retreatment. Reducing the time before retreatment would prevent malignant cells from multiplying into larger masses that become more difficult to treat. The surveillance frequency of follow-up MR imaging studies can then be adjusted to reflect the risk of recurrence. More frequent surveillance would seem appropriate for tumors of higher grade and limited resection and especially for tumors with reduced responsiveness. However, even given the statistics that show, for example, that adults over the age of 55 years have a death rate from recurrence within 1 year of diagnosis of over 60 % for glioblastoma but under 17 % for oligodendroglioma, the same surveillance schedules are used. Although variable across institutions and among physicians, follow-up MR imaging examinations are routinely scheduled at fixed intervals, irrespective of tumor grade and type, extent of surgical resection, or patient age.

There is a perception that conventional MR imaging lacks sensitivity and specificity with ambiguity as to recurrence, pseudo-progression, pseudo-responsiveness, and radiation necrosis. This may have been true for anatomical imaging but more recent advances with perfusion and permeability MR imaging are addressing such concerns [5, 6]. Inevitably, the perceived high cost of imaging is cited to justify infrequent surveillance imaging. This is an untenable position given that a single contrast-enhanced MR examination is less than 1 % of the high cost of surgery, radiation therapy, and chemotherapy. A more reasonable rationale for not looking more frequently for recurrence in patients at high risk for recurrence, given the statistics for this disease, is that there are few alternatives for successful treatment of recurrence. Given this handicap, less interference with the patient's remaining life may be an acceptable reason.

The poor prognosis of high-grade brain tumors from local recurrence shows that the current standard of care is inadequate. Rather than performing inadequate retrospective surveillance for treatment failure, there is a need for real-time surveillance of the treatments to measure tumor response. The purpose of therapy is the selective killing of tumor cells with minimum collateral damage to normal brain cells. Tumors are masses of abnormal cells that, unlike normal brain, have an expanded interstitial space that further increases as tumor cells are destroyed by successful treatments. As tissue biopsies are not adequate or feasible, imaging methods can be used to measure changes in the interstitial space of tumors during and following treatment.

This chapter describes the potential role of quantitative sodium MRI for measuring the tissue sodium concentration (TSC) and the derived interstitial volume fraction (IVF) based on a simple metabolic model of sodium ion homeostasis. Such parameters have been termed bioscales to imply that these quantitative and spatially resolved parameters are directly interpretable in terms of tissue biochemistry [7]. The term bioscale is to be distinguished from biomarker that conveys the notion of a risk factor without spatial information or a quantitative relationship to the biological process to be detected. The method has been published [8] and is currently being used in an NIH-funded investigation to test the hypothesis that tumor cell kill can be monitored as an expanding interstitial space with increasing sodium concentration during the course of fractionated radiation treatment. Early results suggest that treatment response can be measured. Whether the treatment response is predictive of the location of recurrence will require longer follow-up studies. Although diffusion-weighted imaging with apparent diffusion coefficient maps has also been correlated with treatment response, the inference is likely to be related to many structural features within a treated tumor [9]. Although such imaging based on water diffusion is easy to perform on a clinical scanner, quantitative sodium imaging may be a more sensitive method for quantitatively measuring changes in the interstitial volume fraction to reflect tumor response to treatment.

A Model for Measuring Cell Density

The ionic environment of the brain is tightly controlled by a very large number of sodium–potassium ion pumps (Na^+–K^+ ATPase) in the endothelium of the capillary bed and at the cell membranes of the neurons and glial cells that make up brain tissue. The interstitial compartment outside cell membranes is small, representing only about 20 % of the total brain tissue volume. It has a high sodium concentration (~145 mM) and a low potassium concentration (~3 mM). In contrast, the intracellular environment maintains a high potassium concentration (~145 mM) and a low sodium concentration (~12 mM) [10]. As the cell membranes are semipermeable, the resultant ion concentration gradients must be actively maintained using the energy-consuming Na^+–K^+ ATPase pumps. Loss of ion homeostasis results in cell swelling via cytotoxic edema as water passively follows the osmotic pressure established by the ionic distributions. Adenosine triphosphate (ATP) is the metabolic energy currency that is consumed by the Na^+–K^+ ATPase. A continuous and sufficient supply of ATP is produced by oxidative phosphorylation in the mitochondria of normal brain tissue. This requires a continuous supply of oxygen delivered by the blood. As much as 70 % of the energy produced in normal brain tissue is used by the Na^+–K^+ ATPases. The resting electrical potential and sodium ion gradients across the cell membrane are then coupled to the many other membrane transport and metabolic processes of the cell that drive cell function including action potentials and the transport of neurotransmitters.

Given the importance of sodium ion homeostasis, a model can be proposed to use tissue sodium concentration to measure the interstitial space. Brain tissue can be considered as having two compartments of free water, termed the interstitial (V_i) and intracellular (V_c) volumes with sodium concentrations of C_i and C_c, respectively. As the blood volume of the brain is less than 3 % of brain tissue volume and has a comparable ionic composition, the capillary bed can be incorporated into the interstitial compartment. A third compartment is defined for the volume that is occupied by macromolecules and bound water that may contain bound sodium ions. Such bound sodium ions will not be observed by sodium MR imaging performed in the manner described in this chapter. This third compartment is deliberately an ill-defined volume as these solid components are suspended in solution and this volume does not directly reflect the mass of these components.

The model assumes, in the first instant, that the imaging voxel samples only brain tissue (thereby ignoring partial volume averaging with the cerebrospinal fluid, CSF). Sodium MR imaging only observes the sodium ions in the free solution state and so the model is concerned only with the free water compartments and can ignore any sodium ions bound to macromolecules in the third compartment that do not contribute to the MR signal. The IVF of the tissue free water outside the cells can be defined as the fraction of the voxel volume V_v that is outside the cells:

$$\mathrm{IVF} = \mathrm{V_i} / \mathrm{V_v}. \tag{13.1}$$

This approximation of ignoring the ill-defined volume of the third compartment limits the meaning on the term IVF to mean the fraction of free water outside the cells. The tissue concentration TSC_m of sodium ions in solution from the model becomes the number of moles of sodium M_m in free solution divided by the voxel volume which is approximately equivalent to the sum of the volume fraction-weighted sodium concentrations in the two compartments of free water:

$$\mathrm{TSC_m} = \mathrm{M_m} / \mathrm{V_v} \approx \left\{ \mathrm{C_c} \cdot (1 - \mathrm{IVF}) + \mathrm{C_i} . \mathrm{IVF} \right\}. \tag{13.2}$$

However, the unit of concentration for TSC_m in this equation refers to moles of sodium ions per liter of tissue. In practice, tissue volume is an awkward parameter to measure and so the usual biochemical parameter of concentration in tissue is expressed in terms of mass of wet tissue in grams. However, as the voxel volume also contains the third compartment of solids, these hydrated macromolecules contribute to the overall wet weight of tissue. Thus, the concentration from (13.2) can be re-expressed in the more convenient biochemical unit by correcting for the tissue density. The tissue density, TD, shows very little variation in normal tissue, being about 1.02–1.04 g/mL [11]. Thus, as the wet weight of a voxel of tissue is the product of the tissue density and that volume, (13.2) can be rearranged to more conventional units (moles/g wet weight) as

$$TSC_m = \{C_c.(1 - IVF) + C_i.IVF\} / TD. \quad (13.3)$$

This model allows the TSC to be calculated from known literature values. The literature values for C_c and C_i are expressed in terms of the free water within each compartment in normal tissue as about 12 and 145 mM, respectively. The IVF has been reported in human brain as 0.2 [11, 12]. Using these literature values, the model predicts a TSC as about 37 mM.

The experimental tissue sodium concentration (TSC_e) measured by sodium MR imaging is determined by calibrating the arbitrary signal intensity, SI, scale that reflects the number of moles, m, of free sodium ions within the imaging voxel volume V_v such that $TSC_e = m/V_v$. The calibration of the sodium MR signal intensity is made by comparing the tissue SI_t to the signal intensities SI_c of sodium salt solutions at different concentrations, C_p, in a phantom under the same imaging conditions and, specifically, the same voxel dimensions. The calibration curve can be fitted with a linear calibration equation:

$$SI_c = m / V_v = A \times C_p + B, \quad (13.4)$$

where A and B are fitting coefficients for the two variables SI_c and C_p. The experimental TSC for a signal intensity SI_t measured in tissue is computed using A and B as

$$TSC_e = (SI_t - B) / A. \quad (13.5)$$

However, the implicit assumption that the transverse relaxation signal losses are the same in brain tissue and the calibration solutions introduces a quantification bias [13]. The different rapid T2 relaxations during spatial encoding for imaging and the use of projection k-space trajectories also contribute to this quantification bias. As the in vivo and in vitro T2 values can be measured, this quantification bias, Q, can be calculated and corrected [12]. The value of Q found from simulations is 0.93 such that

$$TSC_e = Q \times C_t, \quad (13.6)$$

where C_t is the actual free sodium concentration in brain tissue.

The complete derivation of Q and the impact of the rapid transverse relaxation of the sodium signal are beyond the scope of this chapter but it is important to note that the dimensions of the voxel element overestimate the spatial resolution of sodium MR images. Furthermore, the MR measurement of TSC can be obtained in units of tissue wet weight, as used by the model above, by converting the voxel volume to mass (wet weight) using the TD. As the mass of tissue in a voxel is V_v.TD, the TSC_e in units of moles per gram of wet weight is given by

$$TSC_e = (SI_t - B) / (A \times TD) = Q \times C_t / TD. \quad (13.7)$$

If the TSC unit is required in terms of tissue water content rather than wet weight, (7) could be further divided by the tissue water content, usually reported as around 0.8 [11, 12].

There is good agreement between TSC_e and TSC_m for normal human brain tissue [8]. As tumors lack cell adhesion, the interstitial space of tumors is expanded and TSC is much higher than in normal brain tissue. Although the pathologist, seeing the abundance of stained nuclei in histological sections of tumor, will describe the high cellularity of tumors, this description is not a comparison to normal brain tissue which is the most densely packed tissue in the body. Tumors have expanded interstitial space.

Given the agreement between the experimental and model estimates of TSC, the model can be used to calculate IVF for tumors from the measured TSC_e values and literature values of C_c, C_i, and TD by rearranging (13.3):

$$\text{IVF} = (\text{TSC} \times \text{TD} - C_c)/(C_i - C_c). \quad (13.8)$$

When the voxel of interest contains CSF as well as tissue, the measured TSC must be corrected for the volume of CSF before a value of IVF can be derived accurately. This can be readily done using co-registered proton images that can be obtained at much higher spatial resolution and with high CSF–tissue contrast. Thus, sodium voxels obtained at 5 mm isotropic dimensions can be segmented into tissue and CSF fractions with great accuracy. Even better corrections may be possible using a mixture modeling approach for signal intensities for tissue and CSF [14]. As the CSF sodium concentration is known from the sodium MR measurement in voxels containing only CSF, voxels can be corrected for partial volume averaging effects to obtain IVF in such voxels. For simplicity, this discussion has used the nominal voxel as the unit of spatial resolution. In fact, the appropriate unit to use is the point spread function that is slightly larger than a voxel [13]. This difference arises from the short transverse relaxation of the sodium signal and the use of a projection acquisition that samples a sphere of k-space [13]. However the same principle applies to allow the partial volume correction to be made.

The concept of using sodium MRI to examine brain tumors is not new but dates back to the early development of MR imaging in the 1980s [15]. The technology at that time was insufficient to provide adequate SNR to compete with the development of the more sensitive proton MRI techniques. More recently, quantitative sodium imaging has been applied to human brain tumors but without consideration for monitoring therapeutic responses [16].

Quantitative Sodium MR Imaging Methodology

Conventional clinical MR imaging is based on spatially encoding the MR signal that arises from the nuclei of hydrogen atoms (protons) bound to water and fat. For brain imaging, only protons covalently bound to oxygen in water, at a concentration of approximately 80 M as the brain tissue is about 80 % water, need to be considered. Although the MR phenomenon produces very weak signals, the high concentration of protons and the development of superconducting wide-bore high-field magnets have allowed MR imaging to evolve into a practical medical tool. Clinical MR scanners currently use magnetic fields up to 3.0 T. The proton has the highest intrinsic sensitivity of all the elements of the periodic table and is four times more sensitive than the sodium nucleus. Meanwhile, the sodium ion concentration in brain parenchyma is only about 30–40 mM and, as a quadrupolar nucleus, the rapid biexponential relaxation behavior of the nuclear signal of sodium in tissue is challenging to image. The sensitivity challenge can be met by higher field magnets such as on current 3.0 T clinical scanners and improved still further with 7.0 and 9.4 T scanners designed for human MR imaging. Results from 3.0 and 9.4 T scanners are presented in this chapter.

Because the nuclear relaxation properties of sodium are very different from those of protons, different imaging strategies must be used. Most clinical MR imaging is qualitative and relies only on signal contrast between different anatomical structures and distortions of normal patterns of anatomy to detect pathology. Although sodium MR imaging cannot, as yet, hope to compete with proton imaging for spatial resolution, quantitative sodium imaging does provide highly reproducible values for TSC [8]. The small biological variation in the distribution of TSC for brain tissue reflects the tightly controlled sodium ion homeostasis that is essential for normal function. The small variance of this metabolic parameter is why quantitative sodium MR imaging yields new

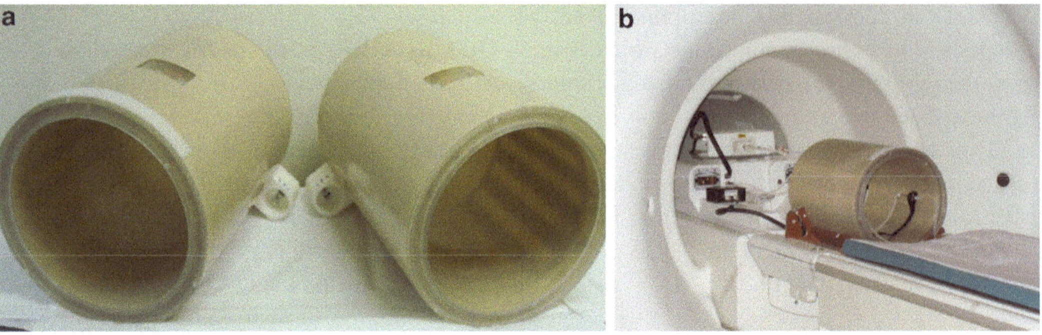

Fig. 13.1 Pictures of (**a**) the near-identical ^{1}H and ^{23}Na birdcage RF coils and (**b**) RF coil positioned on the sled that has the cantilevered head holder on the patient table at entrance to the 3.0 T magnet. Similar sodium coils are used at 9.4 T

information that justifies its development for clinical applications.

The steps required to perform quantitative sodium MR imaging are presented only briefly as the details have been published elsewhere in the cited articles. The MR scanner should be at or above 3 T and have a broadband capability to operate at frequencies other than the proton frequency specified by the field strength. For example, a 3.0 T scanner operates at 128 MHz for proton imaging but at 34 MHz for sodium imaging. This usually requires the use of a separate multinuclear spectroscopy package (MNS module) that can be supplied by the scanner manufacturers. A head volume radio-frequency (RF) coil tuned to the sodium frequency with corresponding transmit and receive switch and preamplifier must also be purchased. The pulse sequences for the sodium and proton acquisitions must also be obtained along with the image reconstruction software. Proton imaging is required as a part of the sodium signal quantification process to optimize the B0 static magnetic field. The 3.0 T scanner (HDx, CMR gradients, GE Healthcare, WI) used by the Center for Magnetic Resonance Research at the University of Illinois at Chicago has the MNS package with two customized single-tuned head birdcage RF coils for each of the sodium and proton frequencies. The patient lies on the patient table with their head located in a cantilevered head holder that allows the RF coils to be swapped without moving the patient (Fig. 13.1). The proton imaging provides the anatomical imaging and allows very rapid automated linear shimming that is maintained for the sodium imaging and mapping of the B0 inhomogeneities. As the proton and sodium coil are made from the same materials and have identical geometries, the assumption that swapping the RF coils does not alter the B0 homogeneity is reasonable and has been demonstrated [8]. The sodium pulse sequence is the flexible twisted projection imaging sequence (flexTPI) that provides an efficient projection acquisition starting at the center of k-space to minimize signal loss due to the short transverse relaxation times of the biexponentially decaying sodium signal [8]. The k-space trajectories cover a set of nested cones such that, once having moved away from the oversampled center of k-space by a specified radial fraction, the trajectory twists on the surface of a cone to acquire the equivalent of several radial projections at once. This twisting enhances the efficiency while also being constrained to avoid violation of the slew rate limits of the gradient set. Examples of the k-space trajectories are shown in Fig. 13.2. The sodium imaging is performed at different power levels to obtain a B1 map to correct for nonuniform sensitivity of the RF coil across the three-dimensional (3D) field of view (FOV). The quantitative sodium imaging is done in just over 8 min with short TE (0.31 ms), and long repeat times (160 ms or approximately five times the tissue sodium longitudinal relaxation time, T1 = 30 ms), thereby avoiding signal loss from rapid transverse relaxation and saturation effects from incomplete longitudinal relaxation. The proton and sodium imaging are then repeated

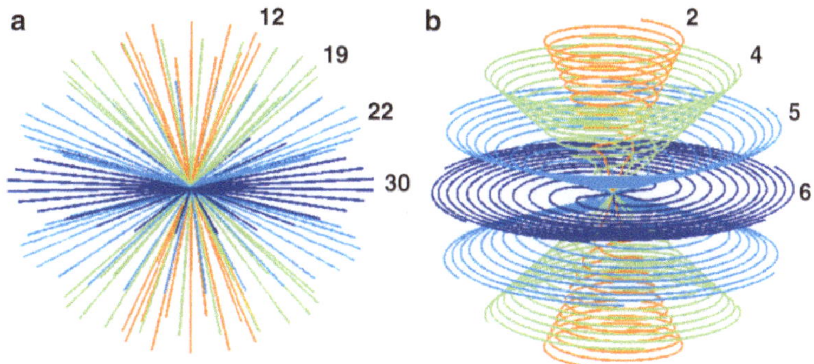

Fig. 13.2 Schematic of the different k-space trajectories for (**a**) conventional radial projection imaging and (**b**) flexible twisted projection imaging (flexTPI) showing that the twisted trajectory requires fewer projections and so is more efficient in covering the same volume of k-space

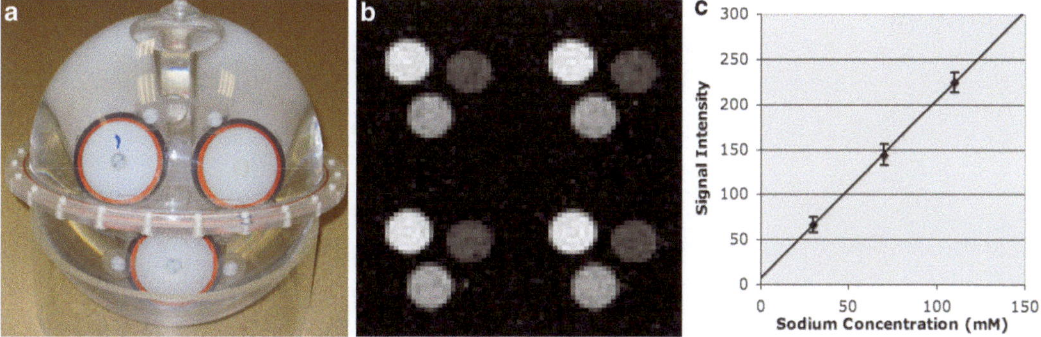

Fig. 13.3 Quantification of the ^{23}Na MR signal into concentration units uses (**a**) a spheric phantom with three compartments at different sodium concentrations (30, 70, and 110 mM) in 3 % agar surrounded by potassium chloride solution (60 mM). This gives an electrical loading similar to a human head for the RF coil. (**b**) Four axial partitions from the 3D sodium image dataset through the phantom. (**c**) The linear calibration curve over the biological range of interest

using a calibration phantom under the same conditions (excitation power and receiver gains) as the patient. The calibration phantom and calibration curve are shown in Fig. 13.3. The calibration phantom is designed to have the same electrical loading of the RF coils as a human head. It contains three separate compartments of different sodium concentrations (30, 70, 110 mM NaCl) in agar gel (3 %) surrounded by a spherical compartment of potassium chloride (60 mM). Although the signal-to-noise ratio of the sodium imaging is sufficient to use a two-point calibration, a three-point calibration confirms the linearity of this step. The only difference between 3.0 and 9.4 T is that the increased sensitivity permits shimming and B0 field mapping to be done directly with the sodium signal saving the time by avoiding the need to exchange the RF coils.

Patient tolerance and their ability to maintain stationary head position limit practical imaging times to less than 10 min. As a TR value (160 ms) equal to about five times the T1 value of brain parenchyma is used to avoid T1 saturation, there is a fixed number of twisted projections that can be acquired in this total acquisition time. The spatial resolution of sodium imaging becomes a balance between the length of the k-space trajectory and the rapid T2 relaxation that occurs during this spatial encoding. Simulations of this balance indicate that optimal resolution comes with longer encoding times than conventionally expected [13]. However, it is important to

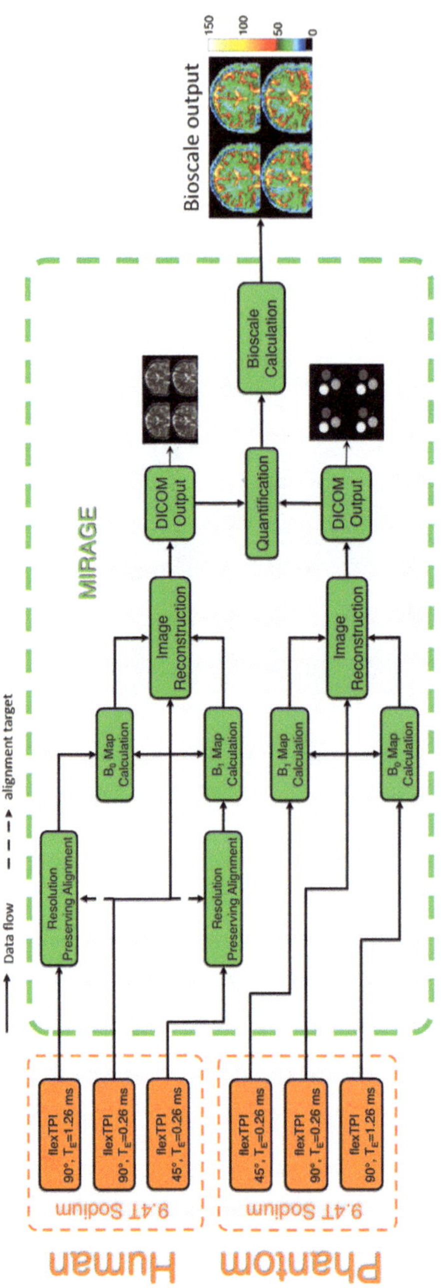

Fig. 13.4 The quantification of the sodium MR signal into a TSC bioscale is achieved algorithmically by combining data from sodium imaging of the human brain and calibration phantom after correction of B0 and B1 inhomogeneities. At 3.0 T, the B0 corrections use proton imaging to minimize data acquisition time. At 9.4 T, the SNR is sufficient to require only sodium images for both the B0 and B1 corrections. The software pipeline is termed metabolic image reconstruction analysis and graphics engine (MIRAGE)

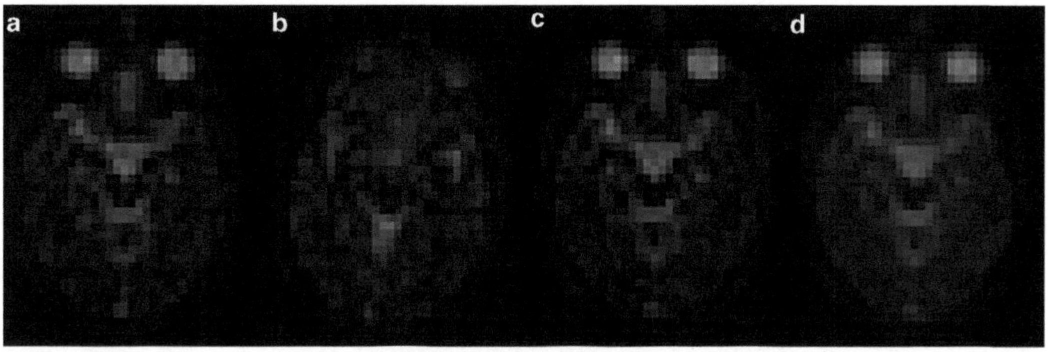

Fig. 13.5 Demonstration that image alignment in k-space avoids image blurring. (**a**) Sodium MR image of human head in (**a**) position A, and then rotated to (**b**) position B. The transformations required to align the images from positions A and B were found in image space and then applied to the k-space data from position B to yield (**c**) aligned image to position A. If the transformation is aligned in image space for position B, the resultant (**d**) image is blurred compared to (**a**)

recognize that the nominal voxel size is smaller than the actual resolution. The typical resolution at 3.0 T is 8.7 mm isotropic for a voxel size of 5 mm isotropic while at 9.4 T, an actual resolution of 5.7 mm isotropic can be achieved within 10 min with sufficient SNR for quantification. The use of phase array coils may further improve SNR to allow higher resolution if uniform sensitivity can be obtained for quantification.

The image reconstruction from the k-space data and quantification steps are performed offline from the scanner and have been described elsewhere [8]. The processing has been reduced to an automated pipeline so that the TSC maps can be produced in less than 60 min for the larger datasets from 9.4 T and less than 30 min for 3.0 T on a desktop computer. This time includes image alignment to account for any small head movement over the multiple acquisitions and is certainly adequate for clinical applications. It is certainly no more complex than analogous analyses for clinical functional MRI. The processing algorithm is summarized in Fig. 13.4. An important feature for following tumor response over time is the alignment of TSC bioscales across time. The projection method of data acquisition uses gridding of the radial and twisted k-space data samples onto a Cartesian reference frame to which a 3D Fourier transformation is applied to generate the image. Once the alignment transform between the reference TSC image and the subsequent TSC image has been determined for two difference imaging sessions in image space, these same transforms can be applied to the k-space data during gridding to avoid blurring of the realigned image data (Fig. 13.5). By avoiding such blurring, comparison of TSC values for single voxels to determine the magnitude of the response is straightforward.

Because it is important to know the treatment dose for each voxel to understand tumor response to radiation, the computed tomography (CT) of the head from which the radiation treatment was planned is aligned with the proton MR images. This radiation plan is usually produced as a DICOM image that can then be superimposed over the co-aligned sodium and proton MR images to which the CT images have been registered. As all of the sodium and proton MR images can be developed from projection acquisitions and the transformation can be applied to the k-space data, no loss of spatial resolution is incurred (Fig. 13.5) during this alignment process. These strategies ensure that the measurement of temporal changes in the TSC bioscale has the highest accuracy possible.

Application of Quantitative Sodium MRI to Brain Tumors: Early Results

The application of the TSC bioscale for measuring primary brain tumor response to radiation treatment has been under investigation in humans

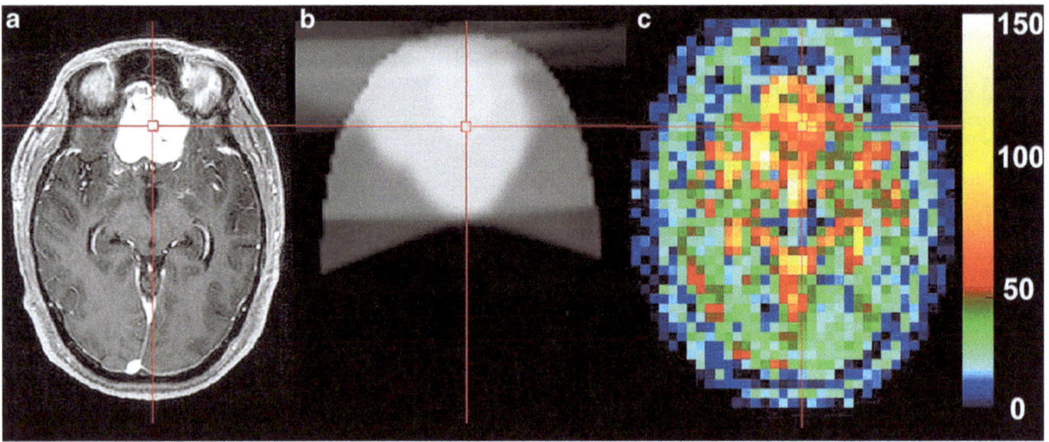

Fig. 13.6 Case #1: Alignment of (**a**) an axial contrast-enhanced high-resolution 3D ^{1}H image from 3.0 T showing the contrast-enhancing mass in the medial frontal region, (**b**) dosimetry treatment plan for proton beam radiation derived from computed tomography (CT) imaging, and (**c**) one axial partition from the 3D bioscale of tissue sodium concentration with color scale in mM concentration units, also obtained at 3.0 T. The *red reference lines* show the same tissue sample across the three maps

for only a few years at one institution that does not specialize in treatment of this type of pathology. The technology for quantitative sodium imaging has now been migrated to another institution specializing in brain tumor treatment and hopefully the results of a larger clinical trial will become available. The early results from the first patients for whom there have been up to a 2-year follow-up are consistent with TSC being sensitive to an expanding interstitial space in tumors that respond to radiation treatment as predicted by earlier studies in animal models of brain tumor [17]. This result is illustrated in the following case.

Case #1 is a 38-year-old man with a history of a grade II oligoastrocytoma treated by surgical resection 7 years ago without further treatment. He presented again with a large recurrent bifrontal mass that, on biopsy, was confirmed as recurrent grade III oligoastrocytoma. Because of its location in close proximity to the eyes and visual pathways, the lesion was referred for proton beam radiation treatment, as shown in Fig. 13.6. Consistent with the new classification of grade III, this tumor showed markedly increased relative cerebral blood volume by dynamic susceptibility contrast (DSC) perfusion MRI and increased permeability by dynamic contrast enhancement (DCE) permeability MRI. Sodium MR imaging was performed weekly during proton beam radiation treatment and TSC bioscales were calculated and aligned. Voxels throughout the brain were divided into three groups: untreated tissue away from the irradiated region (dose <34 Gy, TSC <35 mM, 633 total ^{23}Na voxels), treated margins within the radiation portal but outside the enhancement including areas of edema (dose >54 Gy, 55<TSC<80 mM, 436 total ^{23}Na voxels), and tumor showing contrast enhancement and increased blood volume by perfusion MRI (dose >54 Gy, 186 total ^{23}Na voxels). These divisions excluded CSF. These regions were examined statistically at a 95 % confidence limit for voxel-wise TSC changes between weeks 0–2 and 4–6. The weeks were grouped together to obtain the means and variances for each voxel in the aligned TSC bioscales. Each group was then divided into subgroups of voxels for which TSC increased, decreased, or remained unchanged and the proportions of voxels in these subgroups were calculated. The results are summarized in Fig. 13.7. Increased TSC values were observed in only 3 % of voxels in the untreated regions, 7 % of voxels in treated margins outside the enhancing regions, and 22 % of voxels within the enhancing tumor. The percentage in the untreated area is within the number expected for the 95 % statistical confidence level. However, the margins and tumor showed significantly TSC increases consistent

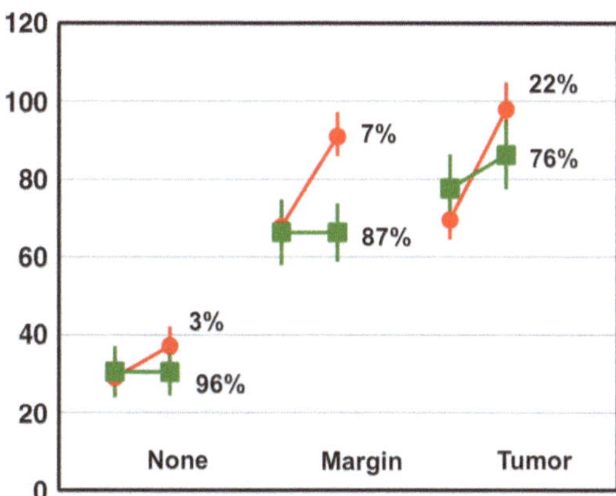

Fig. 13.7 Case #1 TSC responses to proton beam radiation from weeks 0–2 to 4–6 for different brain regions. Responses for voxels in regions not treated with high-dose radiation are labeled "None," responses for voxels in the radiation portal but outside the enhancing tumor are labeled "Margin," and responses for voxels within the enhancing tumor are labeled "Tumor." The TSC responses are measured in mM units. The percentage of voxels showing increases in TSC (*red lines with circles*) or no change in TSC (*green lines with squares*) are shown. The small percentage of voxels showing responses with decreasing TSC values are not shown. Changes in voxel percentage below 5 % is expected to be by chance for the 95 % confidence limit used to detect statistical significance changes in TSC

with expanded interstitial space from cell kill. This tumor also showed reduction in relative blood volume by MR perfusion over the weeks following radiation. The voxels displaying these increases in TSC and corresponding expansion of IVF are consistent with the desired tumor response to treatment. This patient continues to show decreases in lesion volume and vascularity months after completing radiation.

In contrast, case #2 is a 40-year old man who presented with a seizure and was found to have a grade IV glioblastoma in the medial aspect of the right frontal lobe. He underwent surgical resection followed by 6 weeks of fractionated radiation therapy with low-dose chemotherapy. Sodium MR imaging was performed weekly during radiation treatment. Figure 13.8 shows the surgical resection of the medial superior portion of the right frontal lobe and the radiation portal used. Voxels throughout the brain were divided into two groups: untreated (dose <34 Gy, TSC <35 mM, 1,248 ^{23}Na voxels) and treated (34<dose<54 Gy, 55<TSC<80 mM, 274 ^{23}Na voxels) volumes. This division also excluded CSF. These regions were also examined statistically at a 95 % confidence limit on a voxel-wise basis for TSC changes between weeks 0–2 and 4–6. Each division was then divided into subgroups of voxels in which TSC increased, decreased, or remained unchanged and the proportions of these voxels in these subgroups were calculated. Most of the voxels in the untreated tissue (95 %) maintained TSC values of around 30 mM with only 3.5 % of voxels showing an increase to 37 mM (Fig. 13.9). Unlike case #1, the treated brain tissue showed no significant changes in TSC for 91 % of voxels which maintained the same elevated TSC values in the 60–70 mM range with only 8 % of voxels showing an increase to 75 mM. This increase is only slightly above the confidence level. This result suggested that the tissue around the surgical margin had little change in IVF in response to radiation during the treatment. Following radiation, tissue edema increased rapidly and a recurrence was detected in the surgical bed within 12 weeks of ending radiation. Recurrence was proven by a repeat surgical resection. Retrospective examination to characterize the TSC response during radiation in the region of the recurrence showed the same behavior in that these TSC values did not change in response to radiation (Fig. 13.9). This single case suggests that a lack of TSC response during radiation in a region of elevated TSC values may portend a region of recurrence. This patient had a second recurrence at 7 months when the patient had to stop chemotherapy due to complications from the surgical incision in his scalp following the second surgery. An initial tiny area of enhancement increased in size over 4 weeks on the contrast-enhanced MR imaging and showed increased blood volume by perfusion imaging. The two imaging MR examinations separated by 4 weeks allowed an estimation of the tumor doubling time as about 20 days. This case supports the view that high-grade tumors should be imaged more frequently than every 3 months if early detection is the goal. This would be particularly important when changes are made to the treatment protocol.

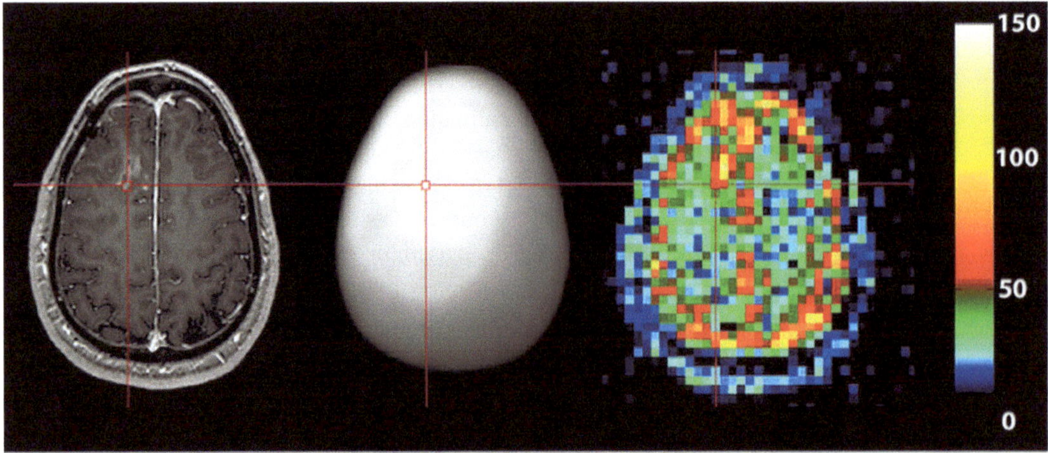

Fig. 13.8 Case #2 showing (*left*) an axial contrast-enhanced proton T1-weighetd image, (*middle*) axial radiation distribution, and (*right*) axial partition of the 3D TSC bioscale in mM units as shown on the *vertical color scale*. The patient has had a right frontal craniotomy with a frontal resection. The *red reference lines* show the cross registration of the same voxel on the aligned image and maps

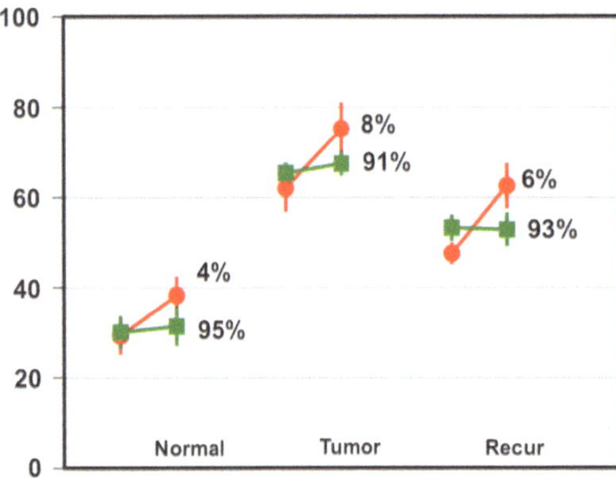

Fig. 13.9 Case #2 TSC responses to radiation from weeks 0–2 to 4–6 for different brain regions and in the region of recurrence found at within 12 weeks post radiation. Responses for voxels in regions not treated with high-dose radiation are labeled "Normal," those for voxels in the surgical bed and radiation portal are labeled "Tumor," and those responses for voxels within the region of recurrence are labeled "Recur." The TSC responses are measured in mM units. The percentage of voxels are shown for increases in TSC (*red lines with circles*) or no change in TSC (*green lines with squares*). Only a small percentage of voxels show increased TSC during radiation indicating lack of significant response

Future Developments at 9.4 Tesla

Although the TSC and IVF bioscales can be obtained at 3.0 T with an SNR that provides a linear calibration of the arbitrary MR signal into sodium concentration, the spatial resolution achieved in an acquisition time just above 8 min is limited to about a nominal isotropic voxel dimension of 5 mm which corresponds to a point spread function with an isotropic resolution of approximately 8.7 mm. As a 10-min acquisition time reflects an approximate upper limit of the tolerance of most patients to remain stationary, further improvements in resolution must improve SNR without further signal averaging. As the SNR increases with increasing magnetic field, this step has been taken with the construction of a 9.4 T magnet and scanner that performs sodium MR imaging in an almost identical fashion as the 3.0 T clinical scanner [18]. Although the power deposition from RF pulses also increases with field strength, quantitative sodium imaging uses long TR periods compared to the longitudinal relaxation times, thereby eliminating this concern. The SNR improvement also allows the B0 shimming and mapping to be performed directly with the sodium signal. There does not appear to be any significant variation in relaxation characteristics with field strength, probably reflecting the quadrupolar properties of the sodium nucleus.

The current FDA guideline for MRI as an insignificant risk for human subjects imposes an upper limit on the static magnetic field of 8.0 T.

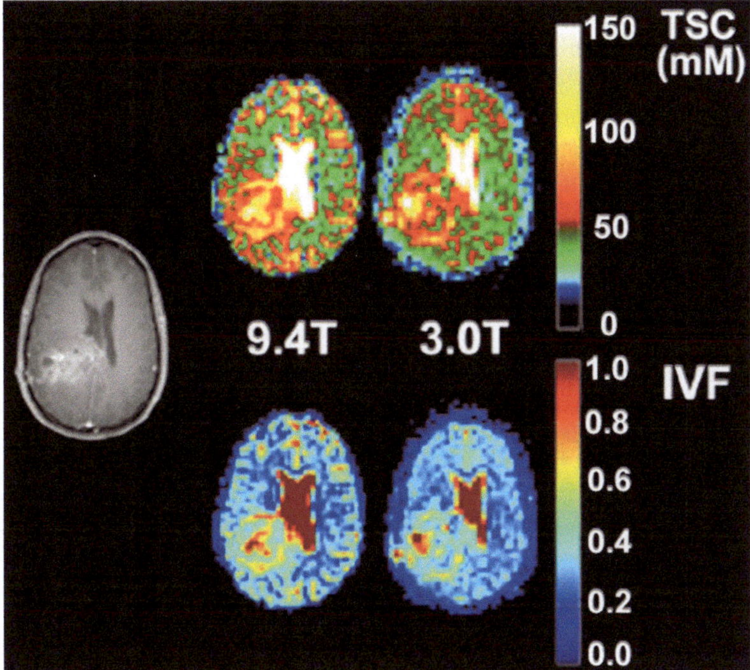

Fig. 13.10 Comparison of axial partitions of tissue sodium concentration (TSC, *upper row*) and interstitial volume fraction (IVF, *lower row*) bioscales from 9.4 and 3.0 T for Case #3 which is from a young woman with a grade III glioneuroma in the right parietal lobe treated with radiation and chemotherapy without surgical resection. The 3.0 T bioscales were obtained after radiation therapy. The 9.4 T bioscale was obtained 6 months after the 3.0 T imaging. The color scales are shown on *right*. The proton image on *left* is an intravenous contrast-enhanced axial T1-weighted image from 3.0 T. The higher resolution possible at 9.4 T reduces partial volume averaging, thereby improving accuracy of the bioscales

This limit was based on safety testing performed on a now decommissioned 8.0 T scanner at Ohio State University [19]. Safety testing using humans at 9.4 T over the last 6 years has also demonstrated no significant irreversible adverse effects on vital signs or cognitive function [20, 21]. Although the clinical scanner vendors are providing commercial research 7.0 T scanners for human imaging, there are now at least four 9.4 T MR scanners suitable for human imaging available in the world today. Such advances suggest that such ultrahigh-field scanners are likely to see clinical applications in the near future. The sodium-based bioscales shown in Fig. 13.10 allow comparison of current 9.4 and 3.0 T images for the same subject, albeit at different times separated by 6 months. This case #3 is of a 29-year-old woman with a grade III glioneuroma who did not undergo surgery but was treated with radiation and chemotherapy. This tumor also responded to radiation treatment, although incompletely, but the patient remains well 3 years later.

Summary

Quantitative sodium MR imaging produces TSC and IVF bioscales and can be performed efficiently at both 3.0 and 9.4 T. Weekly MR imaging of patients undergoing fractionated radiation treatment of brain tumors is well tolerated. The bioscales are sensitive to changes within the tumor on this time scale and indicate the desired tumor response when TSC and IVF increase. The elimination of edema gives a decrease in TSC. The isotropic spatial resolution of these bioscales is limited to about 8–9 mm at 3.0 T, but this can be improved to 5–6 mm at 9.4 T without extending the acquisition time. The hypothesis that a lack of a TSC response in tumors undergoing radiation treatment has prognostic significant for local early recurrence still requires testing in a larger number of patients. A lack of response detected by imaging during radiation may provide an indication that follow-up surveillance imaging should be performed at a shorter interval than the usual 3–4-month follow-up if other treatment options are to be considered.

Acknowledgments The authors acknowledge financial support from PHS RO1 CA1295531A1. This work was supported in part by a SPARK award from the Chicago Biomedical Consortium with support from The Searle Funds at The Chicago Community Trust. We thank Dr. Peter Johnstone from the Indiana University Health Proton Therapy Center, Bloomington, Indiana, for the proton beam radiation treatment plan for case #1.

References

1. Gilbert MR, Armstrong TS. Management of patients with newly diagnosed malignant primary brain tumors with a focus on the evolving role of temozolomide. Ther Clin Risk Manag. 2007;3(6):1027–33.
2. Lacroix M, Abi-Said D, Fourney DR, et al. A multivariate analysis of 416 patients with glioblastoma multiforme: prognosis, extent of resection, and survival. J Neurosurg. 2001;95(2):190–8.
3. Hall WA, Kowalik K, Liu H, Truwit CL, Kucharezyk J. Costs and benefits of intraoperative MR-guided brain tumor resection. Acta Neurochir Suppl. 2003;85:137–42.
4. Dolecek TA, Propp JM, Stroup NE, Kruchko C. CBTRUS Statistical Report: Primary brain and central nervous system tumors diagnosed in the United States in 2005–2009. Neuro-oncology 2012;14(suppl 5): v1–v49.
5. Tofts PS, Kermode AG. Measurement of the blood-brain barrier permeability and leakage space using dynamic MR imaging. 1. Fundamental concepts. Magn Reson Med. 1991;17(2):357–67.
6. Roberts HC, Roberts TPL, Brasch RC, Dillon WP. Quantitative measurement of microvascular permeability in human brain tumors achieved using dynamic contrast-enhanced MR imaging: correlation with histologic grade. Am J Neuroradiol. 2000; 21(5):891–9.
7. Thulborn KR, Lu A, Atkinson IC, Damen F, Villano JL. Quantitative sodium MR imaging and sodium bioscales for the management of brain tumors. Neuroimaging Clin N Am. 2009;19(4):615–24.
8. Lu A, Atkinson IC, Claiborne T, Damen F, Thulborn KR. Quantitative sodium imaging with a flexible twisted projection pulse sequence. Magn Reson Med. 2010;63(6):1583–93.
9. Hamstra DA, Galban CJ, Meyer CR, Johnson TD, Sundgren PC, Tsien C, Lawrence TS, Junck L, Ross DJ, Rehemtulla A, Ross BD, Chenevert TL. Functional diffusion map as an early imaging biomarker for high-grade glioma: correlation with conventional radiologic response and overall survival. J Clin Oncol. 2008;26:3387–94.
10. Somjen GG. Ions of the brain, normal function, seizures and stroke. New York, NY: Oxford University Press; 2004.
11. Nicholson C, Sykova E. Extracellular space structure revealed by diffusion analysis. Trends Neurosci. 1998;21(5):207–15.
12. Neeb H, Ermer V, Stocker T, Shah NJ. Fast quantitative mapping of absolute water content with full brain coverage. Neuroimage. 2008;42:1094–109.
13. Atkinson IC, Lu A, Thulborn KR. Clinically constrained optimization of flexTPI acquisition parameters for the tissue sodium concentration bioscale. Magn Reson Med. 2011;66(4):1089–99.
14. Johnson LA, Pearlman JD, Miller CA, Young TI, Thulborn KR. MR quantification of cerebral ventricular volume using a semi-automated algorithm. Am J Neuroradiol. 1993;14:1373–8.
15. Hilal SK, Maudsley AA, Ra JB, Simon HE, Roschmann P, Wittekoek S, Cho ZH, Mun SK. In vivo NMR imaging of sodium-23 in the human head. J Comput Assist Tomogr. 1985;9(1):1–7.
16. Ouwerkerk R, Bleich KB, Gillen JS, Pomper MG, Bottomley PA. Tissue sodium concentration in human brain tumors as measured with 23Na MR imaging. Radiology. 2003;227:529–37.
17. Thulborn KR, Davis D, Adams H, Gindin T, Zhou J. Quantitative tissue sodium concentration mapping of the growth of focal cerebral tumors with sodium magnetic resonance imaging. Magn Reson Med. 1999;41:351–9.
18. Thulborn KR. Chapter 5. The challenges of integrating a 9.4T MR scanner for human brain imaging. In: Ultra high field magnetic resonance imaging. Volume 26, Robitaille P-M, Berliner LJ, editors. New York, Springer; 2006. pp105–126.
19. Robitaille PM, Warner R, Jagadeesh J, Abduljalil AM, Kangarlu A, Burgess RE, Yu Y, Yang L, Zhu H, Jiang Z, Bailey RE, Chung W, Somawiharja Y, Feynan P, Rayner DL. Design and assembly of an 8 tesla whole-body MR scanner. J Comput Assist Tomogr. 1999;23(6):808.
20. Atkinson IC, Sonstegaard R, Pliskin NH, Thulborn KR. Vital signs and cognitive function are not affected by 23-sodium and 17-oxygen MR imaging of the human brain at 9.4 tesla. J Magn Reson Imaging. 2010;32:82–7.
21. Atkinson IC, Renteria L, Burd H, Pliskin NH, Thulborn KR. Safety of human MRI at static fields above the FDA 8T guideline: sodium imaging at 9.4T does not affect vital signs or cognitive ability. J Magn Reson Imaging. 2007;26:1227–52.

Future Clinical Applications of Molecular Imaging: Nanoparticles, Cellular Probes, and Imaging of Gene Expression

14

Arnav Mehta, Ketan B. Ghaghada, and Srinivasan Mukundan Jr.

Anatomical imaging has been the conventional paradigm for diagnosis since the advent of radiography a century ago. Computed tomography (CT), magnetic resonance (MR), and ultrasound (US) imaging have been at the forefront of anatomical imaging modalities. Under this conventional paradigm, pathology is identified by alteration of the typical anatomy, thus characterizing location and burden of disease. Changes in the morphological appearance have been used to assess response to treatments [1]. However, this convention provides little information of the physiological, molecular, and biochemical basis of disease.

The developments of CT perfusion and MR diffusion and perfusion methods have unlocked the door to a new paradigm—one of physiologic imaging. Rather than demonstrating anatomy only, these new techniques have been used to determine physiological parameters such as cerebral blood flow (CBF), cerebral blood volume (CBV), and mean transit time (MTT). These in turn provide the physician with new insight into underlying pathological processes, for example, a decrease in apparent diffusion coefficient (ADC) demonstrates the onset of an acute infarction. Similarly, changes in CBV are associated with response to tumor therapy. Despite the great utility of these techniques, they are unable to document fundamental changes at the molecular level [2].

Major advances in cell and molecular biology, in addition to the development of small-animal imaging instrumentation, have paved the way for noninvasive visualization of molecular events within living organisms. Molecular imaging (MI), the imaging paradigm of the future, seeks to describe processes at the subcellular and molecular level. MI techniques directly or indirectly monitor and record the spatiotemporal distribution of molecular and cellular processes for biochemical, biological, diagnostic, or therapeutic applications. Therefore, processes such as angiogenesis, receptor expression, tumor growth, and premalignancy can be directly interrogated.

To accomplish this goal, a constantly expanding set of molecular, biological, and chemical tools have allowed for imaging forays into biochemical pathways in vivo. Such biochemical tools include molecular cloning, chip array, microfabrication, X-ray crystallography and mass spectrometry (Fig. 14.1). These methods have been used to study pathways related to metabolism, cell proliferation, apoptosis, gene expression, mutation, and receptor occupancy. MI techniques have allowed for the transition from imaging gross anatomical changes to the molecular interactions that are beneath the spatial resolution of conventional imaging that are the basis for disease [3].

A. Mehta
Division of Biology, California Institute of Technology, Pasadena, CA, USA

K.B. Ghaghada
School of Biomedical Informatics, University of Texas Health Science Center, Houston, TX, USA

S. Mukundan Jr. (✉)
Brigham and Women's Hospital, 75 Francis St, Boston, MA 02115, USA
e-mail: smukundan@partners.org

J.J. Pillai (ed.), *Functional Brain Tumor Imaging*, DOI 10.1007/978-1-4419-5858-7_14,

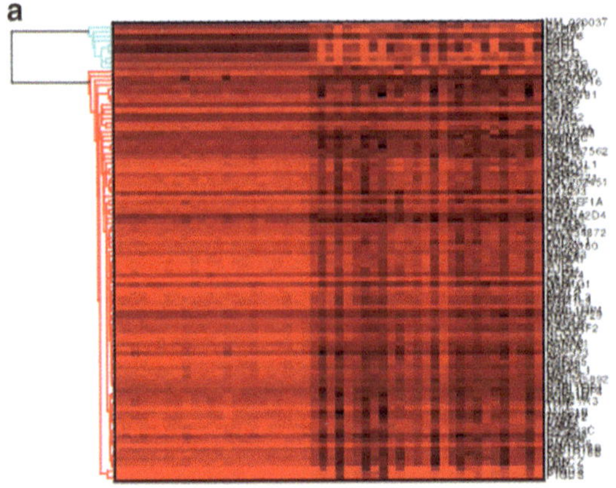

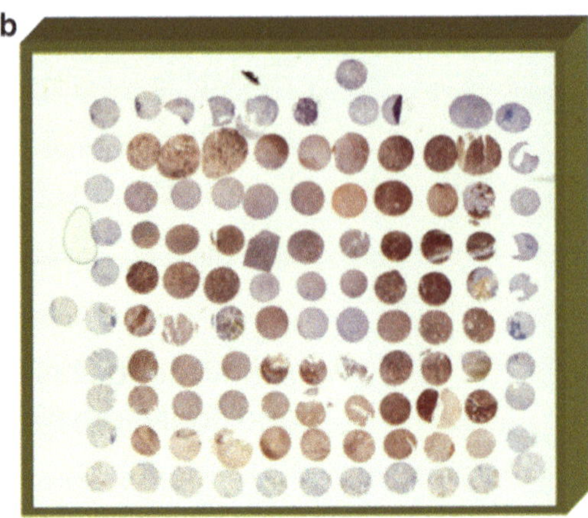

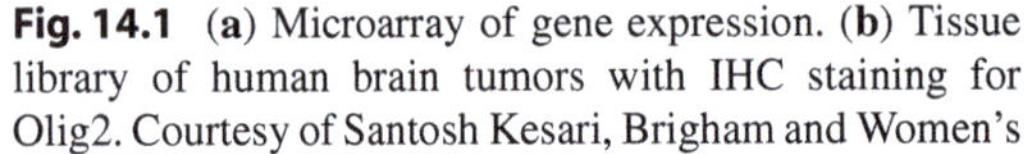

Fig. 14.1 (**a**) Microarray of gene expression. (**b**) Tissue library of human brain tumors with IHC staining for Olig2. Courtesy of Santosh Kesari, Brigham and Women's Hospital. Current address is University of California San Diego School of Medicine

Some of the key prerequisites for imaging biochemical processes in living systems include adequate substrate (mRNA, proteins, surface receptors, etc.) to serve as molecular targets, the development of high affinity probes to bind to the targets, and the availability of sensitive and high resolution imaging modalities. Typically, for a successful imaging system, all of these prerequisites are met.

This chapter explores recent advances that have been made in molecular imaging with discussion of their potential diagnostic and therapeutic applications in the clinic. We begin by discussing key targets and the limitations of current modalities in molecular imaging studies. We then highlight the versatility of nanoparticles and cellular probes and how this has significantly advanced our ability to study molecular events in vivo.

Molecular Targets

The question of identifying where to begin interrogating cellular processes using molecular imaging starts with the central dogma of molecular biology. The dogma provides a framework for understanding the flow of sequence information beginning with deoxyribonucleic acid (DNA) and ending with protein products that affect cellular physiology (Fig. 14.2). DNA is first transcribed to form messenger ribonucleic acid (mRNA) in the cell nucleus. The mRNA is then processed and transported into the cytoplasm where it is translated using the cell ribosome machinery to form proteins, which undergo further posttranslational modification to their fully functioning form.

The regulation points of each of these processes are key targets for molecular imaging techniques. The number of genetic targets increases exponentially down the transcription pathway, beginning with two genes of DNA, to 50–1,000 mRNA and 100–10^6 protein polypeptides, whose function further amplifies the number of targets several fold [4]. The Human Genome Project has opened an exciting array of new opportunities by uncovering the entire collection of over 20,000 human genes, and therefore the entire spectrum of possible molecular targets.

The search and design of potential high-affinity probes has been complemented by a number of rapidly evolving technologies and discoveries such as the development of combinatorial techniques, rational design studies, high-throughput testing, robotics, and identification of molecular targets [4]. The important challenges to successful probe design include delivery barriers for intracellular targets, since high molecular weight macromolecules do not diffuse well within the cytosol, nor do they enter the cell easily. DNA

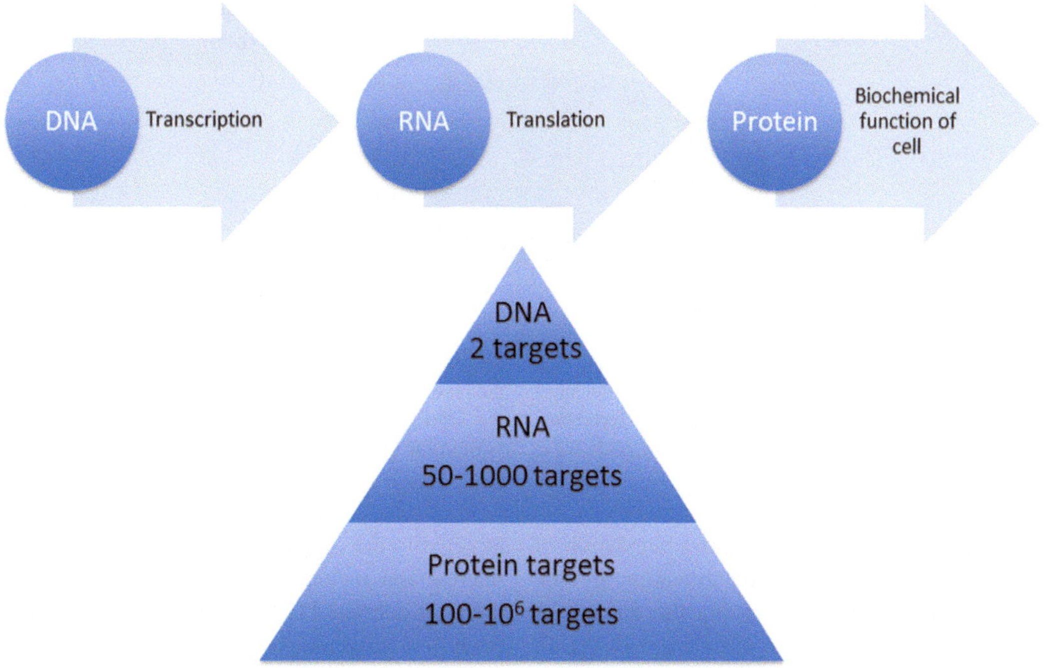

Fig. 14.2 Central dogma of molecular biology: DNA is transcribed into RNA, which is then translated to proteins. The number of targets increases several fold at each step, with any given cell containing two genes of DNA, between 50 and 1,000 mRNA molecules, and up to 10^6 protein molecules for each target

is replicated, transcribed, and stored in the cell nucleus, thus making it a particularly difficult target. To reach a DNA target, a molecular probe must traverse the cell membrane (to enter the cytoplasm) and then traverse the nuclear envelope, also a lipid bilayer. Intracellular proteins and mRNA are more accessible as they are stored and processed in the cytoplasm, therefore requiring traversal of only one membrane barrier. Cell-surface proteins are the most accessible targets to molecular probes, as binding does not require the probe to cross cell membranes (Fig. 14.3). Molecular probes may utilize a diversity of available membrane transporters and channels to transverse biological membranes. These proteins may be influenced by ligand binding, voltage sensitivity or second messenger systems. They include channels that allow for the passive diffusion of specific molecules, uniporters that facilitate the transport of large molecules down their concentration gradient, and symporters and antiporters. Symporters couple transport of one molecule with another molecule present in the cell environment, down its concentration gradient, and antiporters transport molecules actively, against their gradient, along with a molecule that has a favorable gradient. Other challenges include ensuring a sufficient concentration of probe is bound to its molecular target for enough time to be detectable in vivo. Conversely, unbound probe should not be present in appreciable quantities as this would result in a nonspecific "background" signal.

While significant effort has been made to design more efficient methods for the identification and delivery of probes, a number of procedures have been used in drug delivery to bypass the physiological barriers that exist to prevent foreign substances from circulating within the body. Such procedures include the use of drugs that circulate for longer periods of time to obtain a more homogeneous distribution, thus allowing the probe to distribute to all accessible regions of the cell. Other procedures include the local delivery of probes in conjunction with pharmacological

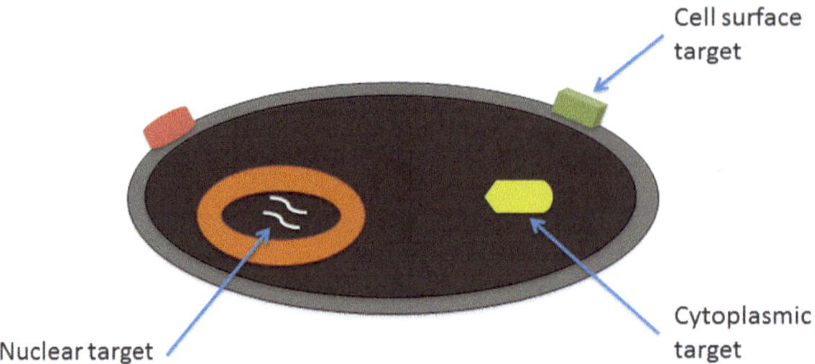

Fig. 14.3 Accessibility of molecular targets in a cell. Cell surface targets, such as surface proteins, are the most accessible since probes do not have to cross membrane barriers. Cytoplasmic targets, which include most intracellular proteins and mRNA, require a probe to traverse the plasma membrane. Nuclear targets, such as DNA, are the least accessible since probes must traverse both plasma and nuclear membranes

methods to improve targeting and pegylation of the drug to decrease its identification by the immune system, thus increasing the amount of time the probe remains in circulation [4, 5]. In addition, the use of signals, derived from peptides, which stimulate shuttling of the drug across cellular membranes has also been used [6]. This method directly uses the ability of the cell to shuttle molecules into the intracellular space using ligand activated transporters on the surface of the cell membrane.

DNA and mRNA are present at relatively low concentrations in cells and therefore would require levels of signal amplification when used as targets in MI that are difficult to achieve in clinical imaging [4]. In contrast, imaging of protein targets is efficient and practical, and a number of biochemical strategies have been developed for amplification of protein signals. These strategies have utilized the alteration of the physical and chemical behavior of probes after target interactions, capitalizing on unique cellular functions to trap probes, and pre-targeting and enhanced probe kinetics to increase target concentrations [4, 7–10].

Three classifications of molecular probes are generally discussed and utilized in MI modalities [11]. Compartmental probes are generally used to assess physiological parameters such as flow and perfusion (Fig. 14.4). Strictly speaking, it is not the molecular process being studied but a related biochemical interaction. Targeted probes are designed to complement a specific moiety targeted to the molecule, enzyme, or receptor of interest and include a component that provides physical contrast [11] (Fig. 14.5). The enhancement of angiogenic vessels in rats has been demonstrated in the magnetic resonance modality using antibodies against $\alpha_v\beta_3$ integrin, a transmembrane protein characteristic of angiogenic endothelium. These antibodies are bound to liposomes containing several Gd(III) moieties, which significantly increased relaxivity of the probe [12]. Finally, smart probes activate exclusively in the presence of a specific molecular agent [11]. These probes hold an advantage over targeted probes due to the absence of significant background signal. Perhaps the best known example of a smart probe is EgadMe, which consists of a Gd(III) chelating agent bound at eight coordination sites and a galactopyranose residue that blocks the remaining site. In the presences of β-galactosidase, the galactopyranose is cleaved therefore allowing water to access the blocked Gd(III) coordination site [13]. Other examples of smart probes include zinc and calcium activated gadolinium magnetic resonance contrast agents, which have demonstrated potential use in signal transduction and catalytic activity studies [14, 15]. Recent advances in probe technology have included the development of nanosensors that are able to detect specific DNA and RNA nucleotide pairings, in addition to hybridization chain reaction (HCR) and RNA fluorescence in-situ hybridization (FISH) technologies for detecting individual RNA molecules [16–18].

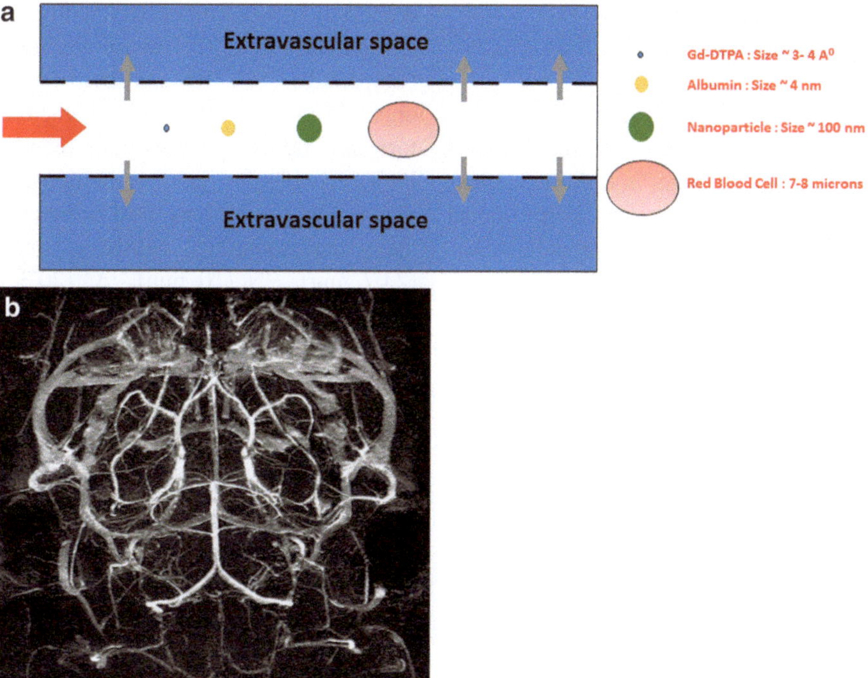

Fig. 14.4 (**a**) Illustration of a compartmental probe. Conventional contrast agents are sub-nm in size and can leak into the extravascular space. Nanoparticles, being typically 20–50-fold larger than traditional contrast agents, remain in the intravascular space. (**b**) MR Angiography demonstrating the mouse Circle of Willis obtained using a surface-conjugated liposomal gadolinium contrast agent, a vascular compartmental probe

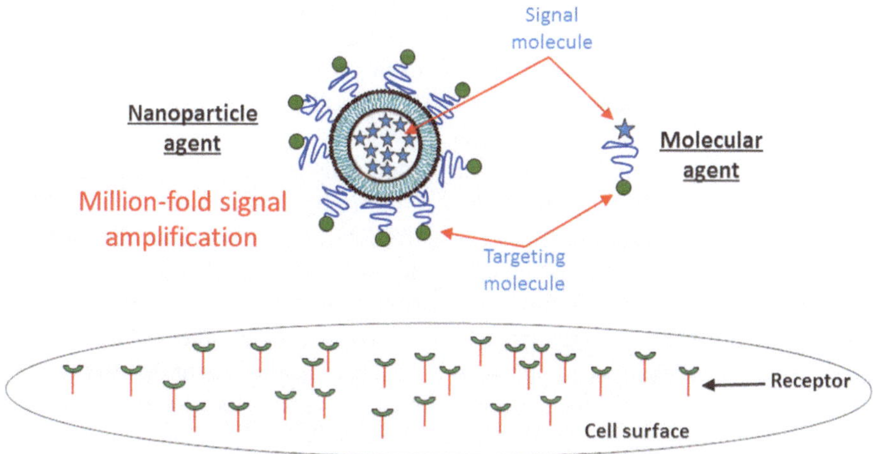

Fig. 14.5 Illustration of nanoparticle and conventional molecular targeted agents. A nanoparticle agent can enable a million-fold signal amplification by encapsulating millions of signaling molecules

Imaging Modalities

Prior to approaching any biological question, it is also essential to consider the most suitable imaging modality for the problem, in addition to identifying a suitable target. The conventional wisdom for molecular imaging modalities has been limited to nanosensor, optical, nuclear, and, to a lesser extent, MR imaging, with limited applications of the commonly used CT and ultra sound (US) modalities [4]. Recent advances in imaging technologies have seen broader molecular imaging applications of all of these and have resulted in variations such as photoacoustic ultrasound, fluorescence or luminescence imaging, and MR microscopy [11, 19]. Current MI modalities available include CT, MR, positron emission tomography (PET), single photon emission CT (SPECT), optical imaging techniques, and US [19]. These modalities differ in their sensitivity, spatial and temporal resolution, and complexity of use; however, they are applied with a shared goal of higher specificity. The important properties of several common MI modalities will be discussed in the following paragraphs.

Nuclear Imaging

Nuclear imaging has been used extensively for molecular imaging at the organ level, with recent extensions to the tissue, cellular, and genetic level. The fundamental concept underlying this imaging modality is that proteins in the cell can be probed with specific radiopharmaceuticals. The two classes of marker genes that have been largely investigated are those that encode cell-surface proteins and those that encode intracellular enzymes [4]. The two prominent nuclear imaging techniques currently in use are PET and SPECT.

PET has been used for molecular, physiologic and, to a lesser degree, anatomic imaging, and more specifically, has been used extensively for metabolism and in the preclinical realm, gene expression studies. It remains the paradigm for sensitivity to molecular events with nanomolar to femtomolar (10^{-9}–10^{-15}) sensitivity for biological compounds [11]. Its sensitivity provides the opportunity to quantitatively characterize receptors and ligands at molecular concentrations. PET technologies have resolutions of around 3 mm. Some commonly used radionuclides, with their corresponding half-lives, include ^{15}O (2.07 min), ^{13}N (10 min), ^{11}C (20.3 min), ^{18}F (1.83 h), ^{124}I (4.2 days), and ^{94}T^{m} (53 min) [11]. The disadvantages of this modality include the cost and accessibility of hardware, and availability of radionuclides. Gene expression studies using this modality have been conducted by incorporating a PET reporter gene, such as that for the intracellular enzyme herpes simplex virus thymidine kinase, into an adenovirus vector that is able to penetrate the cell nucleus. The final intracellular protein product of the reporter gene after transcription and translation can be detected by treatment of the cells with 8-[F-18]fluoroganciclovir, which penetrates the cell membrane and binds to the protein. Analogous studies have been conducted by utilizing reporter genes that produce cell surface receptor targets, such as the dopamine receptor, which are bound by [F-18] flurorethylspiperone [20].

SPECT is another powerful nuclear imaging technique that has been used largely for gene expression and structure studies. It provides a cheaper alternative to PET at the cost of much lower resolution, often around 1–2 cm. Some commonly used radionuclides for SPECT include ^{99}Tc^{m} (6 h), ^{111}In (2.8 days), ^{123}I (13.2 h) and ^{125}I (59.5 days) [11]. Disadvantages of this technique are the limited availability of radionuclides and complicated probe chemistry, since, unlike PET, it does not use physiological tracers and therefore requires chelating agents to incorporate the radionuclide within the tracer [19]. Radiolabeled Annexin V, which binds phosphatidylserine, a cell surface protein expressed during programmed cell death, has demonstrated the use of SPECT in detection of apoptosis and protein targets [19, 21]. Furthermore, radiolabeling of DNA oligonucleotides with ^{99}Tc^{m} has made mRNA and DNA targets accessible to SPECT studies [22, 23].

Optical and Bioluminescence Imaging

In recent years, optical imaging technologies have had a significant impact on the landscape of molecular imaging. These technologies have advanced from a better understanding of fluorescence, which is the absorption of one wavelength of light and its subsequent emission, and luminescence, which arises from the conversion of chemical energy into light [11]. While optical imaging technologies do not have any current clinical applications, they are much cheaper compared to the hardware requirements of other modalities and have been used for noninvasive anatomical localization. General optical imaging techniques have resolutions that range from 3 to 5 mm and possess nanomolar sensitivity. Some of the major disadvantages of general optical imaging techniques include low resolution and low depth penetration.

Fluorescence in the near infrared region is best of the optical imaging techniques and may be used to obtain greatest depth since the lowest coefficient of absorbance occurs in the 650–900 nm range, which coincides with minimal inherent fluorescence of body tissue [4, 11, 19]. This mode of optical imaging requires a light source of a defined bandwidth, which upon contact with an optical contrast agent, or fluorescent molecule, emits a signal with different spectral characteristics. This signal can then be resolved with an emission filter and captured with high sensitivity [3, 4]. Optical contrast agents that are detectable in the near infrared range have been designed by conjugating analogs of somatostatin, which bind to somatostatin cell surface receptors overexpressed in tumors, to cyanine dye [24]. In addition, near infrared labeled probes have been used to image protease activity of intracellular enzymes such as cathepsin B [10].

Bioluminescent imaging involves the administration of a substrate, luciferin, which emits light at specific wavelengths upon reaction with an enzyme, luciferase. Since most animals have no endogenous luciferase enzyme, there is very little background noise from this technique. This modality has low resolution, on the range of 3–5 mm, and is used largely for anatomical localization, gene expression and functional studies, and high-throughput screening [11, 19, 25]. Reporter genes encoding the firefly photoprotein luciferase, which utilizes energy from ATP to emit photons, have been used to image the distribution and clearance kinetics of tumor cells [26].

Magnetic Resonance Imaging

Magnetic Resonance (MR) Imaging has been used extensively in the clinic and is capable of extracting anatomical and physiological information concurrently. It is used primarily for anatomical evaluation and exhibits a resolution on the range of 1–2 mm. MR techniques are not naturally sensitive to label detection, and thus have low signal yield. As a result, they require robust signal amplification strategies such as cellular internalization of paramagnetic probes, contrast agents coupled with biological amplification strategies, such as trapping of probes within a cell, or secondary reporter systems, such as the use of an enzyme to catalyze the formation of detectable molecules in cells [27]. Signal amplification using targeted agents carrying several gadolinium moieties have been commonly used in addition to “smart” agents, whose cleavage allows water access to gadolinium [12, 13]. The major disadvantages of the MR modality include low-sensitivity, long scan times, and high-cost.

MR models for imaging transgene expression have been developed. MRI has been used for In vivo detection of tumor cells expressing transferrin receptors on their surface. In this system, transferrin is conjugated to monocrystalline iron oxides, which serves as an MR imaging probe [28, 29]. Magnetic nanosensors that can detect certain mRNA and DNA sequences have also been developed. These nanosensors may be used with MRI to detect the phenotype of tumors in vivo [30].

Functional Magnetic Resonance Imaging has seen remarkable growth in recent years and has been used for functional evaluation studies.

It demonstrates a resolution in the range of 0.5–2 mm. The major disadvantages of this technology include the availability of contrast agents and cost.

Computerized Tomography

Computerized tomography is not as prevalent in molecular imaging as in the clinic. However, it is much cheaper than MR and PET techniques previously described and has unlimited depth penetration and a fast scanning time. It is used primarily for structural imaging, especially of soft tissue, bones and lungs [11, 19]. CT resolution is usually around 0.5 mm. The major disadvantages of this modality are low contrast sensitivity and radiation exposure.

Nanoparticles

Nanoparticles have proven to be immensely useful in diagnostic imaging and in the delivery of therapeutics. For imaging, nanoparticle contrast agents have allowed for the visualization of drug delivery to tumors and other cellular and molecular events in vivo [31]. These contrast agents have further been used to guide surgical removal of solid tumors [32]. Nanoparticles can also be designed to enhance delivery of drugs poorly soluble in water, to prevent degradation of therapeutic molecules, and to increase the specificity and the efficacy of drugs [33]. This chapter focuses on nanoparticles used as contrast agents, which may be categorized into four groups: iron oxide, metal-based, lipid-based, and polymeric nanoparticles.

Iron Oxide Nanoparticles

Iron oxide nanoparticles have been studied for over 20 years as an MRI contrast agent and are the only nanoparticle contrast agent that has been approved by the FDA for use in humans [34, 35]. They consist of an iron-oxide core that is surrounded by an outer coat of hydrophilic polymers for stability of the particle [36]. The most commonly used polymers are dextran, polyethylene glycol (PEG), or polyvinyl alcohol (PVA) because of their biocompatibility [34].

Two varieties of iron oxide nanoparticles are commonly used: ultrasmall super-paramagnetic iron oxide particles (USPIOs) and supermagnetic iron oxide particles (SPIOs). USPIOs have diameters between 10 and 40 nm, and may be subcategorized into moncrystaline iron oxide particles with or without dextran coating. These particles have low T2 relaxivity compared to SPIOs and are generally used as blood pool contrast agents or for imaging macrophages [34]. Furthermore, targeting of inflammatory lesions using USPIOs has also been performed by grafting a sialyl-Lewisx mimetic, a ligand for E-selectin, onto the dextran coating of the particle [37].

SPIOs tend to be between 60 and 150 nm in size. They have high T2 relativities (R2) and are used primarily in T2-weighted imaging. Amino-PVA-SPIOs are actively taken up by brain-derived microglia and endothelial cells without any active inflammatory response. This has been confirmed with SPIO nanoparticles derivatized with a fluorescent reporter molecule. Thus, SPIOs represent a potentially important vehicle for drug delivery and the detection of neurodegenerative diseases [38].

Iron oxide nanoparticles coated with dextran, or various protein fragments, are also taken up by lymphocytes. In this way these particles may be used to image immune cells with almost single cell resolution [39]. Magnetic pre-labeling of cells may also be used to track the cell location and migration post-transplantation or transfusion [40]. Since these nanoparticles have half-lives in blood of over 18 h, they are particularly valuable for studying inflammatory diseases, lymph-node staging, and tumor imaging [41, 42]. Importantly, iron oxide nanoparticles have been used in dynamic contrast enhanced MRI to image brain tumors and tumor microvasculature, as well as the response to antiangiogenic therapies [43–45].

Metal-Based Nanoparticles

Over the past decade, metal nanoparticles have proven extremely useful as contrast agents and for dynamic imaging in many biological systems.

The most common nanoparticles currently used are metal nanoshells and quantum dots, both of which have tunable optical properties. Metal nanoshells are composed of a dielectric core nanoparticle, usually silica, surrounded by a thin metal shell [46]. These particles can be produced to either absorb or scatter light over most of the visible and infrared spectrum, depending on the dimensions and composition of the core and outer shell. For biomedical applications and optical imaging, gold nanoshells are most often used [47, 48]. These particles can be fabricated to absorb light in the near-infrared range, in which there is maximum penetration of light through tissue. This has made them particularly adept for photothermal therapy; in fact, gold nanoshells have been used for thermal ablation in canine brain tumors [49, 50].

Metal nanoshells can be effectively used as contrast agents in optical imaging when designed to scatter rather than absorb light [46]. The low levels of contrast between normal and diseased tissues limit the utility of optical imaging in the clinic. However, targeted optical contrast agents have recently been developed as in the case of a gold colloid conjugated to epidermal growth factor receptor (EGFR) antibodies [51].

Quantum dots are semi-conductor crystals whose size and shape can be controlled accurately by the duration, temperature and ligands used in their synthesis [52]. These nanoparticles usually have a cadmium-based core with a surrounding inert metallic sheet. As for metal nanoshells, the absorption and emission of quantum dots is dependent on their composition and size. Single quantum dots can be tracked over long periods of time with confocal microscopes, making them excellent candidates for single-molecule studies. Several techniques have been used to solubilize and stabilize quantum dots for live-animal imaging. Examples include ligand exchange with molecules containing thiol groups [53], and encapsulation in phospholipid micelles or polymer shells [54, 55]. For most targets, three steps are sufficient for labeling: (1) an antibody against a specific target, (2) a biotinylated antibody against the first antibody, and (3) a streptavidin-coated quantum dot [52]. Furthermore, these particles can be equipped with other properties, such as functional groups for better membrane permeability or enzymatic activity.

The long lifetimes of quantum dots make them adept for In vivo imaging. Intravenous injection of quantum dots with two-photon confocal microscopy has been used to image vasculature in live mice [56]. Additionally, quantum dots coated with PEG can be visualized in mouse bone marrow and lymph nodes several months after administration, with reduced accumulation in the liver [57]. Recently, these nanoparticles have been utilized for cellular and molecular imaging of numerous tumors and in surgical resection of brain tumors [58–60]. This is possible because quantum dots are phagocytosed by macrophages in the immune system, which go on to incorporate into brain tumors therefore labeling them. It should be noted that studies to date have not involved humans as the toxicity of the cadmium core raises significant challenges for their use clinically.

Lipid-Based Nanoparticles

Lipid-based nanoparticles have been extensively studied for development of contrast agents. The nanoparticles are primarily composed of amphiphilic lipid molecules that contain a hydrophobic and hydrophilic component. Depending on the structure and assembly, lipid nanoparticles can be divided into three categories: micelles, liposomes, and lipid-coated perfluorocarbon (PFC) nanoparticles.

Micelles are self-assembled lipid nanoconstructs, typically 10–50 nm in size, consisting of a hydrophobic core surrounded by a hydrophilic shell. Micellar contrast agents have been developed by conjugating imaging moieties, such as gadolinium chelates, to amphiphilic lipid molecules. Gadolinium micelles have been preclinically used as molecular MRI agents for detection of macrophages in atherosclerotic plaques [61].

PFC nanoparticles have been extensively studied as molecular MRI contrast agents and multifunctional nanoparticles in cardiovascular and cancer applications [62]. The nanoparticles consist of a hydrophobic liquid perfluorocarbon core surrounded by a lipid monolayer [63]. The lipid monolayer can be used for incorporating gadolinium chelates for use in MRI, optical probes, targeting ligands and therapeutic molecules, thus enabling the development of multifunctional nanocarriers. Large-sized PFC nanoparticles have also been investigated as ultrasound contrast agents [64].

Liposomes, one of the most extensively studied nanoparticle platforms, have been utilized as contrast agents for a variety of imaging modalities. Liposomes are spherical lipid bilayer vesicles with diameters ranging between 50 and 400 nm. The lipid bilayer separates the internal aqueous core of the liposome from the external medium. Liposomal contrast agents incorporating imaging moieties in the internal aqueous core and lipid bilayer have been synthesized and investigated.

Liposomal contrast agents have primarily been developed for CT and MRI applications. PEGylated liposomes encapsulating conventional small molecule iodinated agents within the core interior have been developed and investigated as blood-pool CT agents [65]. The iodinated liposomal contrast agents have also been used to image and probe the functional status of tumor vasculature [66, 67] in preclinical small animal models. Gadolinium-containing liposomal MR contrast agents have also been used as blood pool and molecular imaging agents [68–70]. High T1 relaxivity surface-conjugated gadolinium liposomes have also been used for MR neuro-angiography in a mouse model. Liposomal MRI agents have enabled ultra-high resolution imaging of the mouse Circle of Willis as well as other perforating vessels within the brain at ~50 μm in-plane resolution [71].

Liposomes also provide a high degree of flexibility in tailoring their in vivo chemical properties for specific imaging applications. For instance, the in vivo blood half-life of liposomes can be altered by modifying their outer surface. Long circulating liposomes containing a hydrophilic polymer, polyethylene glycol (PEG), have been developed and used as blood-pool contrast agents for both MRI and CT applications [65, 69]. Unlike conventional contrast agents, long circulating liposomal contrast agents provides uniform signal intensity and stable enhancement over an extended period of imaging. Similarly, the aqueous core of liposomes can be used to co-encapsulate a therapeutic and an imaging moiety, thus enabling image-guided drug delivery. This has been exemplified by use of liposomal gadolinium MRI contrast agents co-encapsulating a chemotherapeutic agent for monitoring convection-enhanced delivery in brain tumors [72]. The outer surface of liposomes can also be modified to present ligands at the distal end of polymer chains for targeting liposomal nanoparticles to specific cell-surface receptors. Ligand-targeted liposomes have been investigated as molecular imaging contrast agents in MRI applications [73].

Polymeric Nanoparticles

A wide variety of biocompatible and biodegradable polymers are available for synthesis of polymeric nanoparticles. Some of the most commonly used polymers for nanoparticle synthesis are polylactic acid (PLA), poly (lactic-co-glycolic acid) (PLGA), poly (lysine), and polyethylene glycol (PEG)-based co-polymers. The ability to control nanoparticle structure and functionality at the molecular level enables synthesis of a wide variety of polymeric nanoparticles for development of nanotherapeutics [74, 75] and imaging agents [76, 77] in a variety of cancers including brain tumors [78, 79]. Nanoparticles ranging from 10 to 1,000 nm in size can be fabricated by varying the polymeric backbone and synthesis process.

Dendrimers, one of the most extensively studied polymeric nanoparticles, are highly branched, multi-generational structures that can be functionalized with imaging moieties [32, 80–83], therapeutic molecules [33, 84], and affinity moieties [85, 86] for tumor targeting. Non-targeted and antibody-targeted dendrimers have been used for delivery of therapeutics to brain tumors [87–89]. MRI and CT compatible dendrimer contrast agents have also been used for monitoring convection-enhanced delivery of macromolecular therapeutics in brain tumors [90].

Conclusion

The range of problems open to the molecular imaging techniques described above is vast and continually expanding. Molecular imaging is an exciting new field that will continue to grow with the interdisciplinary efforts of engineers, physicists, chemists, biologists, and computer scientists. The constantly evolving technologies, along with the identification of new targets and the design of novel probes, will continue to help scientists uncover new problems and solutions in the fields of molecular biology and medical science.

References

1. Davis KR, Taveras JM, New PFJ, et al. Cerebral infarction diagnosis by computerized tomography. Am J Roentgenol. 1975;124:643–61.
2. Eastwood JD, Lev MH, Wintermark M, et al. Correlation of early dynamic CT perfusion imaging with whole-brain MR diffusion and perfusion imaging in acute hemispheric stroke. AJNR Am J Neruoradiol. 2003;24:1869–75.
3. Chen X, Conti PS, Moats RA. *In vivo* near-infrared fluorescence imaging of integrin $\alpha_v\beta_3$ in brain tumor xenografts. Cancer Res. 2004;64:8009–14.
4. Weissleder R, Mahmood U. Molecular imaging. Radiology. 2001;219:316–33.
5. Lewin M, Carlesso N, Tung CH, et al. Tat peptide-derivated magnetic nanoparticles allow in vivo tracking and recovery of progenitor cells. Nat Biotechnol. 2000;18:410–4.
6. Neuwelt EA, Weissleder R, Nilaver G, et al. Delivery of virus-sized iron oxide particles to rodent CNS neurons. Neuroscience. 1994;34:777–84.
7. Gambhir SS, Barrio JR, Phelps ME, et al. Imaging adenoviral-directed reporter gene expression in living animals with positron emission tomography. Proc Natl Acad Sci U S A. 1999;96:2333–8.
8. Barbet J, Peltier P, Bardet S, et al. Radioimmunodetection of medullary thyroid carcinoma using indium-111 bivalent hapten and anti-CEA x anti-DPTA-indium bispecific antibody. J Nucl Med. 1998;39:1172–8.
9. Hu S, Shively L, Raubitschek A, et al. Minibody: a novel engineered anti-carcinoembryonic antigen antibody fragment (single-chain Fv-CH3) which exhibits rapid, high-level targeting of xenografts. Cancer Res. 1996;56:3055–61.
10. Weissleder R, Moore A, Mahmood U, Bogdanov Jr A. In vivo imaging of tumors with protease-activated near-infrared fluorescent probes. Nat Biotechnol. 1999;17:375–8.
11. Dzik-Jurasz ASK. Molecular imaging *in vivo*: an introduction. Br J Radiol. 2003;76:S98–109. Special issue.
12. Anderson SA, Rader RK, Westlin WF, et al. Magnetic resonance contrast enhancement of neovasculature with $\alpha_v\beta_3$-targeted nanoparticles. Magn Reson Med. 2000;44:433–9.
13. Louie AY, Huber MM, Ahrens ET, et al. In vivo visualization of gene expression using magnetic resonance imaging. Nat Biotechnol. 2000;18:321–5.
14. Major JL, Parigi G, Luchinat C, Meade TJ. The synthesis and *in vitro* testing of zinc-activated MRI contrast agents. Proc Natl Acad Sci U S A. 2007;104(35):13881–6.
15. Li W, Parigi G, Fragai M, Luchinat C, Meade TJ. Mechanistic studies of a calcium-dependent MRI contrast agent. Inorg Chem. 2002;41:4018–24.
16. Perez JM, O'Loughin T, Simeone FJ, Weissleder R, Josephson L. DNA-based magnetic nanoparticle assemble acts as a magnetic relaxation nanoswitch allowing screening of DNA-cleaving agents. J Am Chem Soc. 2002;124:2856–7.
17. Choi HM, Chang JY, Trinh LA, et al. Programmable in situ amplification for multiplexed imaging of mRNA expression. Nat Biotechnol. 2010;28(11):1208–12.
18. Raj A, van den Bogaard P, Rifkin SA, van Oudenaarden A, Tyagi S. Imaging individual mRNA molecules using multiple singly labeled probes. Nat Methods. 2008;5(10):877–9.
19. Pomper MG. Molecular imaging: an overview. Acad Radiol. 2001;8:1141–53.
20. Phelps ME. Positron emission tomography provides molecular imaging of biological processes. Proc Natl Acad Sci U S A. 2000;97(16):9226–33.
21. Blakenberg FG, Katsikis PD, Tait JF, et al. *In vivo* detection and imaging of phosphatidylserine expression during programmed cell death. Proc Natl Acad Sci U S A. 1998;95:6349–54.
22. Shields AF, Lim K, Grierson J, Link J, Krohn KA. Utilization of labeled thymidine in DNA synthesis: studies for PET. J Nucl Med. 1990;31(3):337–42.
23. Hnatowich DJ, Winnard Jr P, Virzi F, et al. Technetium-99m labeling of DNA Oligonucleotides. J Nucl Med. 1995;36(12):2306–14.
24. Becker A, Hessenius C, Licha K, et al. Receptor-targeted optical imaging of tumors with near-infrared fluorescent ligands. Nat Biotechnol. 2001;19:327–31.
25. Contag CH, Ross BD. It's not just about anatomy: in vivo bioluminescence imaging of gene expression. J Magn Reson Imaging. 2002;16:378–87.
26. Sweeney TJ, Mailander V, Tucker AA, et al. Visualizing the kinetics of tumor-cell clearance in living animlas. Proc Natl Acad Sci U S A. 1999;96:12044–9.
27. Weissleder R, Simonova M, Bogdanova A, et al. MR imaging and scintigraphy of gene expression through melanin induction. Radiology. 1997;204(2):425–9.
28. Moore A, Joesephson L, Bhorade RM, Basilion JP, Weissleder R. Human transferrin receptor gene as

marker gene for MR imaging. Radiology. 2001;221:244–50.
29. Weissleder R, Moore A, Mahmood U, et al. *In vivo* magnetic resonance imaging of transgene expression. Nat Med. 2000;6(3):351–4.
30. Josephson L, Perez JM, Weissleder R. Magnetic nanosensors for the detection of oligonucleotide sequences. Angew Chem. 2001;113(17):3304–6.
31. Cheng Z, Thorek DL, Tsourkas A. Gadolinium-conjugated dendrimer nanoclusters as a tumor-targeted T1 magnetic resonance imaging contrast agent. Angew Chem Int Ed Engl. 2010;49(2):346–50.
32. Longmire M, Choyke PL, Kobayashi H. Dendrimer-based contrast agents for molecular imaging. Curr Top Med Chem. 2008;8(14):1180–6.
33. Medina SH, El-Sayed ME. Dendrimers as carriers for delivery of chemotherapeutic agents. Chem Rev. 2009;109(7):3141–57.
34. Ros PR, Freeny PC, Harms SE, et al. Hepatic MR imaging with ferumoxides: a multicenter clinical trial of the safety and efficacy in the detection of focal hepatic lesions. Radiology. 1995;196:481–8.
35. Weissleder R, Elizondo G, Wittenberg J, et al. Ultrasmall superparamagnetic iron oxide: characterization of a new class of contrast agents for MR imaging. Radiology. 1990;175:489–93.
36. Laurent S, Forge D, Port M, et al. Magnetic iron oxide nanoparticles: synthesis, stabilization, vectorization, physiochemical characterizations, and biological applications. Chem Rev. 2008;108:2064–110.
37. Boutry S, Laurent S, Elst LV, Muller RN. Specific E-selectin targeting with a superparamagnetic MRI contrast agent. Contrast Media Mol Imaging. 2006;1(1):15–22.
38. Petri-Fink A, Chastellain M, Jullierat-Jeanneret L, Ferrari A, Hofmann H. Development of functionalized superparamagnetic iron oxide particles for interaction with human cancer cells. Biomaterials. 2005;25(15):2685–94.
39. Modo M, Hoehn M, Bulte JW. Cellular MR imaging. Mol Imaging. 2005;4(3):143–64.
40. Bulte JW. Intracellular endosomal magnetic labeling of cells. Methods Mol Med. 2006;124:419–39.
41. Lahaye MJ, Engelen SM, Kessels AG, et al. USPIO-enhanced MR imaging of nodal staging in patients with primary rectal cancer: predictive criteria. Radiology. 2008;246(3):804–11.
42. Harisinghani MG, Barentsz J, Hahn PF, et al. Noninvasive detection of clinically occult lymph-node metastases in prostate cancer. N Engl J Med. 2003;348(25):2491–9.
43. Neuwelt EA, Varallyay CG, Manninger S, et al. The potential of ferumoxytol nanoparticle magnetic resonance imaging, perfusion, and angiography in central nervous system malignancy: a pilot study. Neurosurgery. 2007;60(4):601–11.
44. Christoforidis GA, Yang M, Kontzialis MS, et al. High resolution ultra high field magnetic resonance imaging of glioma microvascularity and hypoxia using ultra-small particles of iron oxide. Invest Radiol. 2009;44(7):375–83.
45. Gambarota G, Leenders W, Maass C, et al. Characterization of tumor vasculature in mouse brain by USPIO contrast-enhanced MRI. Br J Cancer. 2008;98(11):1784–9.
46. Hirsch LR, Gobin AM, Lowery AR, et al. Metal nanoshells. Ann Biomed Eng. 2006;34(1):15–22.
47. Lin AW, Lewinski NA, West JL, et al. Optically tunable nanoparticle contrast agents for early cancer deletion: model-based analysis of gold nanoshells. J Biomed Opt. 2005;10(6):064035.
48. Talley CE, Jackson JB, Oubre C, et al. Surface-enhanced Raman scattering from individual au nanoparticles and nanoparticle dimer substrates. Nano Lett. 2005;5(8):1569–74.
49. O'Neal DP, Hirsch LR, Halas NJ, et al. Photothermal tumor ablation in mice using near infrared-absorbing nanoparticles. Cancer Lett. 2004;209(2):171–6.
50. Schwartz JA, Shetty AM, Pierce RE, et al. Feasibility study of particle-assisted laser ablation of brain tumors in orthotopic canine model. Cancer Res. 2009;69(4):1659–67.
51. Sershen SR, Westcott SL, Halas NJ, West JL. Temperature-sensitive polymer-nanoshell composites for photothermally modulated drug delivery. J Biomed Mater Res. 2000;51(3):293–8.
52. Michalet X, Pinaud FF, Bentolila LA, et al. Quantum dots for live cells, in vivo imaging, and diagnostics. Science. 2005;307:538–44.
53. Chan WCW, Nie S. Quantum dot bioconjugates for ultrasensitive nonisotopic detection. Science. 1998;281:2016–8.
54. Dubertret B, Skourides P, Norris DJ, et al. In vivo imaging of quantum dots encapsulated in phospholipids micelles. Science. 2002;298:1759–62.
55. Pellegrino T, Manna L, Kudera S, et al. Hydrophobic nanocrystals coated with an amphiphilic polymer shell: a general route to water soluble nanocrystals. Nano Lett. 2004;4(4):703–7.
56. Larson DR, Zipfel WR, Williams RM, et al. Water-soluble quantum dots for multiphoton fluorescence imaging in vivo. Science. 2003;300:1434–6.
57. Ballou B, Lagerholm BC, Ernst LA, et al. Noninvasive imaging of quantum dots in mice. Bioconjug Chem. 2004;15:79–86.
58. Smith AM, Duan H, Mohs AM, et al. Bioconjugated quantum dots for in vivo molecular and cellular imaging. Adv Drug Deliv Rev. 2008;60(10):1226–40.
59. Jackson H, Muhammad O, Daneshvar H, et al. Quantum dots are phagocytized by macrophages and colocalize with experimental gliomas. Neurosurgery. 2007;60(3):524–9.
60. Popsescu MA, Toms SA. In vivo optical imaging using quantum dots for the management of brain tumors. Expert Rev Mol Diagn. 2006;6(6):879–90.
61. Mulder WJ, Strijkers GJ, Briley-Saboe KC, et al. Molecular imaging of macrophages in atherosclerotic plaques using bimodal PEG-micelles. Magn Reson Med. 2007;58(6):1164–70.

62. Tran TD, Caruthers SD, Hughes M, et al. Clinical applications of perfluorocarbon nanoparticles for molecular imaging and targeted therapeutics. Int J Nanomedicine. 2007;2(4):515–26.
63. Kaneda MM, Caruthers S, Lanza GM, et al. Perfluorocarbon nanoemulsions for quantitative molecular imaging and targeted therapeutics. Ann Biomed Eng. 2009;37(10):1922–33.
64. Marsh JN, Partlow KC, Abendschein DR, et al. Molecular imaging with targeted perfluorocarbon nanoparticles: quantification of the concentration dependence of contrast enhancement for binding to sparse cellular epitopes. Ultrasound Med Biol. 2007;33(6):950–8.
65. Mukundan S, Ghaghada KB, Badea CT, et al. A liposomal nanoscale contrast agent for preclinical CT in mice. AJR Am J Roentgenol. 2006;186(2):300–7.
66. Ghaghada KB, Badea CT, Karumbaiah L, et al. Evaluation of tumor microenvironment in an animal model using a nanoparticle contrast agent in computed tomography imaging. Acad Radiol. 2011;18(1):20–30.
67. Karathanasis E, Chan L, Karumbaiah L, et al. Tumor vascular permeability to a nanoprobe correlates to tumor-specific expression levels of angiogenic markers. PLoS One. 2009;4(6):e5843.
68. Mulder WJ, Strijkers GJ, Griffioen AW, et al. A liposomal system for contrast-enhanced magnetic resonance imaging of molecular targets. Bioconjug Chem. 2004;15(4):799–806.
69. Ghaghada KB, Bockhorst KHJ, Mukundan S, et al. High resolution vascular imaging of the rat spine using liposomal blood pool MR agent. AJNR Am J Neuroradiol. 2007;28(1):48–53.
70. Ghaghada KB, Ravoori M, Gnanasabapathy D, et al. New dual mode gadolinium nanoparticle contrast agent for magnetic resonance imaging. PLoS One. 2009;4(10):e7628.
71. Howles GP, Ghaghada KB, Qi Y, et al. High-resolution magnetic resonance angiography in the mouse using a nanoparticle blood-pool contrast agent. Magn Reson Med. 2009;62(6):1447–56.
72. Grahn AY, Bankiewicz KS, Dugich-Djordjevic M, et al. Non-PEGylated liposomes for convection-enhanced delivery of topotecan and gadodiamide in malignant glioma: initial experience. J Neurooncol. 2009;95(2):185–97.
73. Mulder WJ, Strijkers GJ, Habets JW, et al. MR molecular imaging and fluorescence microscopy for identification of activated tumor endothelium using a bimodal lipidic nanoparticle. FASEB J. 2005;19(14): 2008–10.
74. Blanco E, Kessinger CW, Sumer BD, et al. Multifunctional micellar nanomedicine for cancer therapy. Exp Biol Med. 2009;234(2):123–31.
75. Danson S, Ferry D, Alakhov V, et al. Phase I dose escalation and pharmacokinetic study of pluronic polymer-bound doxorubicin (SP1049C) in patients with advanced cancer. Br J Cancer. 2004;90:2085–91.
76. Torchilin VP. Polymeric contrast agents for medical imaging. Curr Pharm Biotechnol. 2000;1(2):183–215.
77. Torchilin VP. PEG-based micelles as carriers of contrast agents for different imaging modalities. Adv Drug Deliv Rev. 2002;54:235–52.
78. Kuroda J, Kuratsu J, Yasunaga M, et al. Antitumor effect of NK012, a 7-ethyl-10-hydroxycamptothecin-incorporating polymeric micelle, on U87MG orthotopic glioblastoma in mice compared with irinotecan hydrochloride in combination with bevacizumab. Clin Cancer Res. 2010;16(2):521–9.
79. Inoue T, Yamashita Y, Nishihara M, et al. Therapeutic efficacy of a polymeric micellar doxorubicin infused by convection-enhanced delivery against intracranial 9L brain tumor models. Neuro Oncol. 2009;11(2):151–7.
80. Tomalia DA, Naylor AM, Goddard WA. Starburst dendrimers: molecular-level control of size, shape, surface chemistry, topology, and flexibility from atoms to macroscopic matter. Angew Chem Int Ed Engl. 1990;29:138–75.
81. Wiener EC, Magnin RL, Gansow OA, et al. Dendrimer-based metal chelates: a new class of magnetic resonance imaging contrast agents. Magn Reson Med. 1994;31(1):1–8.
82. Tan M, Wu X, Jeong EK, et al. Peptide-targeted Nanoglobular Gd-DOTA monoamide conjugates for magnetic resonance cancer molecular imaging. Biomacromolecules. 2010;11(3):754–61.
83. Cheng Z, Thorek DL, Tsourkas A. Gadolinium-conjugated dendrimer nanoclusters as a tumor-targeted T1 magnetic resonance imaging contrast agent. Angew Chem Int Ed Engl. 2010;49(2):346–50.
84. Choi YS, Thomas T, Kotlyar A, et al. Synthesis and functional evaluation of DNA-assembled polyamidoamine dendrimer clusters for cancer cell-specific targeting. Chem Biol. 2005;12:35–43.
85. Singh P, Gupta U, Asthana A, et al. Folate and folate-PEG-PAMAM dendrimers: synthesis, characterization, and targeted anticancer drug delivery potential in tumor bearing mice. Bioconjug Chem. 2008;19(11): 2239–52.
86. Boswell CA, Eck PK, Regino CA, et al. Synthesis, characterization, and biological evaluation of integrin alphavbeta3-targeted PAMAM dendrimers. Mol Pharm. 2008;5(4):527–39.
87. Yang W, Wu G, Barth RF, et al. Molecular targeting and treatment of composite EGFR and EGFRvIII-positive gliomas using boronated monoclonal antibodies. Clin Cancer Res. 2008;14(3):883–91.
88. Sarin H, Kanevsky AS, Wu H, et al. Effective transvascular delivery of nanoparticles across the blood-brain tumor barrier into malignant glioma cells. J Transl Med. 2008;6:80.
89. Han L, Zhang A, Wang H, et al. Tat-BMPs-PAMAM conjugates enhance therapeutic effect of small interference RNA on U251 glioma cells in vitro and in vivo. Hum Gene Ther. 2010;21(4):417–26.
90. Regino CA, Walbridge S, Bernardo M, et al. A dual CT-MR dendrimer contrast agent as a surrogate marker for convection-enhanced delivery of intracerebral macromolecular therapeutic agents. Contrast Media Mol Imaging. 2008;3(1):2–8.

Editor's Biography

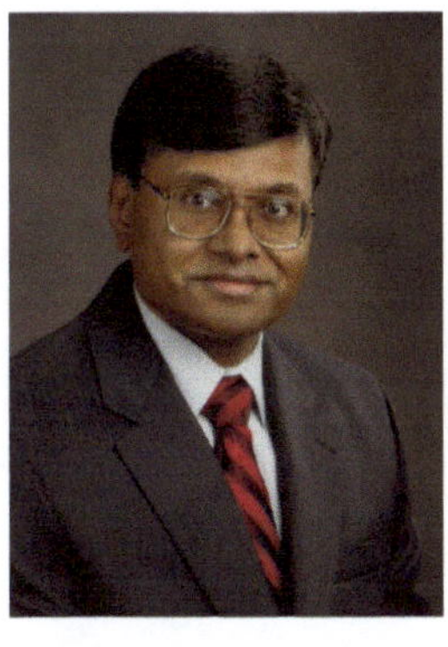

Dr. Pillai graduated *cum laude* from Yale University with a major in chemistry and obtained his medical degree from Jefferson Medical College in Philadelphia. After completion of an internship in internal medicine and residency in diagnostic radiology, he completed a 2-year fellowship in neuroradiology at Case Western Reserve University/University Hospitals of Cleveland. After 7 years on the faculty at the Medical College of Georgia, where he was Associate Professor of Radiology and Director of Neuro-Magnetic Resonance Imaging as well as President of the School of Medicine Faculty Senate in 2006–2007, he joined the faculty of Johns Hopkins University School of Medicine in 2007. He is currently Associate Professor of Radiology and Radiological Science as well as Director of Functional MRI within the Neuroradiology Division of the Russell H. Morgan Department of Radiology and Radiological Science at the Johns Hopkins Univ. School of Medicine. He has also been the director of the clinical fMRI service at the Johns Hopkins Hospital since 2008.

Dr. Pillai is currently on the Editorial Boards of the American Journal of Neuroradiology, Public Library of Science (PLoS-ONE) and the World Journal of Clinical Oncology and has served as reviewer for many other professional journals. He has received research grant funding from the Radiological Society of North America (RSNA), Siemens Medical Solutions, the National Institutes of Health (NIH) and the Johns Hopkins Brain Science Institute during his academic career for work in functional MRI as applied to the study of brain tumors, brain plasticity and the phenomenon of neurovascular uncoupling. He has published extensively in scientific journals, mostly in the field of functional MRI, and has authored multiple book chapters as well as lectured at numerous national and international meetings. Dr. Pillai served as the President of the American Society of Functional Neuroradiology in 2008–2009. He has been very active in both the American Society of Neuroradiology and RSNA over the last decade including membership on the Scientific Program Committees of both organizations over the last decade. He is currently a member of the Annual Meeting Program Committee of the International Society for Magnetic Resonance in Medicine (ISMRM).

J.J. Pillai (ed.), *Functional Brain Tumor Imaging*, DOI 10.1007/978-1-4419-5858-7,

Index

A
AAs. *See* Amino acids (AAs)
ACC. *See* Anterior cingulate cortex (ACC)
N-acetylaspartate, 40
Adenosine triphosphate (ATP), 213
Adiabatic fast passage (AFP), 204, 205
AFP. *See* Adiabatic fast passage (AFP)
American Society of Functional Neuroradiology (ASFNR), 62
Amide proton transfer (APT)-MRI
  assessment, brain cancer treatment response, 177–178
  and CEST, 172–173
  description, 171
  gadolinium, 171
  Gd-induced renal toxicity, 171
  gliomas (*see* Gliomas)
  limitation, 178–179
  optimal neurosurgery and radiotherapy, 173
  pseudopalisading necrosis, 173–174
  and radiation necrosis, 177, 178
  rat model, 173
Amino acids (AAs)
  and FET, 133
  and FLT, 134
  methionine, 130
  non-metabolizable analogues, 130
Anisotropy, 28, 30
Anterior cingulate cortex (ACC), 196, 199
Antiangiogenic therapy, 15–16
Apparent diffusion coefficient (ADC), 225
APT-MRI. *See* Amide proton transfer (APT)-MRI
Arterial spin labeling (ASL)
  magnetization transfer, 9
  MR perfusion technique, 8
  radio-frequency, 8
  specific absorption rate, 9
ASFNR. *See* American Society of Functional Neuroradiology (ASFNR)
ASL. *See* Arterial spin labeling (ASL)
ATP. *See* Adenosine triphosphate (ATP)
Axonal bundles
  description, 183
  fiber tractography, 186
  interdigitate and cross, 184
  voxel, 184

B
BBB. *See* Blood-brain barrier (BBB)
Bioluminescence imaging, 231
Bisdas, S., 14
Blood-brain barrier (BBB), 5, 143, 150
Blood oxygenation level-dependent (BOLD) signals, 111
Blood oxygen level dependent functional magnetic resonance imaging (BOLD fMRI)
  activation maps, 60, 61
  ASFNR, 62
  block design silent word generation paradigm, 59–60
  breath-hold task, 63–64
  CBF and oxygen consumption, 59
  clinical validation, 68–69
  coronal composite BOLD language, 75
  CPT, 61
  CVR, 63
  EPI, 60
  expressive paradigms, 64–66
  fMRI protocol, 63
  functional imaging, 72
  GLM, 60
  imaging technique, 61
  inferior temporal gyrus, 76
  language fMRI, 72–76
  language mapping, 64, 65
  motor deficits, 71–72
  neurovascular uncoupling, 73
  presurgical planning, 74
  receptive paradigms, 66–68
  semantic paradigms, 68
  stereotactic biopsy, 69–71
  susceptibility artifacts, 63
BOLD signals. *See* Blood oxygenation level-dependent (BOLD) signals
Brainlab neuronavigation system, 90
Brain pathology, MRS
  demyelinating diseases, 206
  field strengths, 195
  glutamate, 206
  HD, 206
  PCC, 206
  sagittal MRI, 199, 202
  spectra, 196, 197

J.J. Pillai (ed.), *Functional Brain Tumor Imaging*, DOI 10.1007/978-1-4419-5858-7,

Brain tract. *See* Diffusion tensor imaging (DTI)
Brain tumors
ASL, 12, 18
channel head coil, 45
characterization
diffusion anisotropy, 30
diffusion metrics, 30–34
DTI, 29
mean diffusivity and tumor cellularity, 29–30
water diffusion, 28–29
chemical shift imaging, 44
DCE MRI acquisition, 6
2D-PRESS-MRSI, 44
EPSI, 45
GABA and GSH, 46
metabolic imaging and molecular functions, PET (*see* Positron emission tomography (PET))
metabolites, 39–42
MRI data, 10
MRS, 39
MRSI, 42
neoplastic *vs.* non-neoplastic lesions, 48–49
PRESS voxel, 44
prognosis, 49
pulse sequences, spatial localization, 42–43
single-voxel MRS localization sequences, 43
treatment planning and monitoring, 50–51
tumor grading and diagnosis, 47–48
Brown, T.R, 44
Bucci, M., 186

C

Caseiras, G.B., 10
CBF. *See* Cerebral blood flow (CBF)
CBV. *See* Cerebral blood volume (CBV)
Central nervous system, 131, 137, 138
Cerebral blood flow (CBF), 12–13, 59
Cerebral blood volume (CBV), 8
Cerebrospinal fluid (CSF), 215
Cerebrovascular reactivity (CVR), 63
CEST, 172–173
Chan, A., 153
Chao, S.T., 136
Cha, S., 4
Chemical shift displacement (CSD)
artifact, 201
RF pulses, 198
slice selection, 195
Chemical shift imaging (CSI), 42, 44
Chen, W., 137
Cher, L.M., 134
Choline, 39
Chung, J.K., 133
Clinical translation, DTI, 95–96
Computed tomography (CT)
meningioma, 139
molecular imaging, 139
molecular modalities, 232
somatostatin analogue, 131
Contrast agent
lipid-based nanoparticles, 233
metal-based nanoparticles, 232
nanoparticle, 228, 229
CPT. *See* Current procedural terminology (CPT)
Cranial and paraspinal nerves, 139
CSD. *See* Chemical shift displacement (CSD)
CSF. *See* Cerebrospinal fluid (CSF)
CSI. *See* Chemical shift imaging (CSI)
CT. *See* Computed tomography (CT)
Current procedural terminology (CPT), 61
CVR. *See* Cerebrovascular reactivity (CVR)

D

Data visualization, DTI
color-coded FA maps, 101
echoplanar imaging, 102, 103
ellipsoid, 101
fiber tracking/tractography, 101–102
HARDI, 102
limitations, 102–103
NPV and PPV, 103
Diffusion metrics
anisotropy, 30–31
brain metastases, 30, 34
cerebral diffuse, cell lymphoma, 30, 33
glioblastomas, 31
metastatic lung adenocarcinoma, 30, 32
Diffusion MR tractography, surgical planning
acquisition and reconstruction
component, 185
diffusion-weighted images, 185–186
DSI, 186
fiber crossing techniques, 185
HARDI, 186–187
capabilities and limitations, 183
DTI (*see* Diffusion tensor imaging (DTI))
framework, 192
functional mapping, 189–190
HARDI (*see* High angular resolution diffusion imaging (HARDI) tracrography)
motivation and translation
complex white matter architecture, 184
3D Gaussian pattern, 184, 185
DTI and HARDI, 184–185
measures, water diffusion, 183
white matter tract, neurosurgery, 183
Diffusion spectrum imaging (DSI), 186
Diffusion tensor imaging (DTI)
biopsy samples, 27
brain tumor characterization (*see* Brain tumors, characterization)
data visualization (*see* Data visualization, DTI)
definition, 183
description, 95
ellipsoid, 28–29
fiber tracking, 188–189
and HARDI
acquisition requirements, 186, 187

callosal tracts, 184
detection, anisotropic diffusion, 184
identification, single fiber population, 185
histogram analysis, 34–35
interpretation
anaplastic astrocytoma, 105–106
description, 104
FLAIR and post-contrast SPGR images, 104, 105
fMRI (*see* Functional magnetic resonance imaging (fMRI), and DTI)
high-grade gliomas, 104
immediate and relative proximity, 104
localization sources
clinical presentation, 97–98
functional anatomy standard imaging, 98, 99
intraoperative electrocortical mapping, 100
intraoperative functional white matter testing, 99–100
techniques, presurgical mapping anatomy, 98–99
MD and FA, 28
metrics, classification, 35
neurosurgery, brain tumors (*see* Neurosurgery, brain tumors)
planar anisotropy, 28
presurgical mapping process, 95, 97
protocols and acquisition, 100–101
quantification, 107
software data, 106–107
standard of care, 107
translation, 95–96
and tumor infiltration, 32–33
water molecules, 28
white matter architecture, 184, 195
Diffusivity, 28, 30
Dowling, C., 149, 152
DSC. *See* Dynamic susceptibility contrast (DSC)
DSI. *See* Diffusion spectrum imaging (DSI)
DTI. *See* Diffusion tensor imaging (DTI)
Dynamic susceptibility contrast (DSC), 4

E

Echo planar imaging (EPI), 60
Echo-planar imaging and signal targeting with alternating radio frequency (EPISTAR)
HGGs, 12
LGGs and lymphomas, 12
Echo-planar spectroscopic imaging (EPSI), 45, 204
Echo times (TE)
bandwidth refocusing pulses, 205
centrum semiovale, 196, 197
scan parameters, 199, 205
spectra, 196
spin-echo experiment, 205
ECM. *See* Extracellular matrix (ECM)
EEG. *See* Electroencephalography (EEG)
Electroencephalography (EEG), 89–90, 111–112
EPI. *See* Echo planar imaging (EPI)
Epidermal growth factor receptor (EGFR), 233
Epilepsy surgery
adaptive spatial filtering method, 118, 119
cortical resection, 118
epileptogenic zone, 118
MSI, 119–120
non-lesions and lesions, MEG, 118
secondary bilateral synchrony, 118–119
spikes, 118
tuberous sclerosis, 119
EPISTAR. *See* Echo-planar imaging and signal targeting with alternating radio frequency (EPISTAR)
EPSI. *See* Echo-planar spectroscopic imaging (EPSI)
Ewelt, C., 135
Expressive paradigms
hemispheric language lateralization, 65
rhyming task, 66
silent word generation task, 64
stimuli, phonological, 66
supplementary motor area, 65
Extracellular matrix (ECM), 157–158

F

FDG. *See* 2-[^{18}F]-fluoro-2-deoxy-D-glucose (FDG)
FET. *See* O-(2-^{18}Ffluoroethyl)-L-tyrosine (FET)
2-[^{18}F]-fluoro-2-deoxy-D-glucose (FDG)
cerebral cortex, 131
glioblastoma multiforme, 136
gliomas, 131
glucose metabolism and malignancy, 130
and PCNSL, 137
RT and RS, 135
^{18}F-fluoromisonidazole (FMISO), 131, 134, 136
Fiber tractography, 186, 188, 191
FLAIR. *See* Fluid attenuated inversion recovery (FLAIR)
Flexible twisted projection imaging (flexTPI), 216, 217
flexTPI. *See* Flexible twisted projection imaging (flexTPI)
Floeth, F.W., 133
Fluid attenuated inversion recovery (FLAIR), 143, 151
Fluorescence in-situ hybridization (FISH) technologies, 228
FMISO. *See* ^{18}F-fluoromisonidazole (FMISO)
fMRI. *See* Functional magnetic resonance imaging (fMRI)
Forsen, S., 172
Fractional anisotropy (FA)
metastasis, 32
and tumor cellularity, 30
Functional connectivity, preoperative neurosurgery
abnormalities, 122
definition, 122
disconnection grade, 122, 125
ECS mapping, 122–123
fronto-temporo-insular low-grade glioma, 122–123, 125
MEG imaging, 122, 124
time-frequency space, 122

Functional imaging
  CPT, 61
  deoxyhemoglobin and oxyhemoglobin concentrations, 79
  neuronavigation, 106
Functional magnetic resonance imaging (fMRI)
  advantages, 85, 86
  artifacts, 87, 88
  block design, 86
  confidentiality, 91
  deoxyhemoglobin and oxyhemoglobin concentrations, 79
  description, 79–80
  diffusion tractography, 90
  digit mapping, 91–92
  and DTI
    speech and language, 104, 105
    visual field difficulties, 104, 105
    white matter, 104
  early 1990s, 79
  effects, tumor
    abnormal neovasculature, 87–88
    bilateral finger-tapping, 88
    decoupling, 89
  finger tapping, 85, 86
  inspection, 92
  integration, 91
  intraoperative mapping (*see* Intraoperative mapping, fMRI)
  MEG, EEG and PET, 89–90
  paresis/weakness, 86–87
  sensory motor system (*see* Sensory motor system, fMRI imaging)
  tongue and foot motion, 85
  7T scanner, 91–92

G

Gaa, J., 12
Gaggl, W., 99
Ganslandt, O., 156
General linear model (GLM), 60
Glioma grading, 9–10
Gliomas
  advantages, APT, 174
  fMRI, 83, 88
  hematoxylin and eosin, 173
  human glioblastoma xenografts, 173
  MTR images
    glioblastoma, 174–176
    9L gliosarcoma, 173, 174
    low-grade glioma, 176–177
  protocols, 179
GLM. *See* General linear model (GLM)
Grosu, A.L., 135
Grummich, P., 122

H

HARDI. *See* High angular resolution diffusion imaging (HARDI) tracrography
HCR. *See* Hybridization chain reaction (HCR)
HD. *See* Huntington's disease (HD)
Hematopoietic neoplasms, 137
Henry, R., 186
Herholz, K., 135
HGG. *See* High-grade glioma (HGG)
High angular resolution diffusion imaging (HARDI) tracrography
  diffusion-weighted signal, 187
  and DTI (*see* Diffusion tensor imaging (DTI))
  fiber tracking
    motor system and DTI, 188–189
    performance, 189, 190
    white matter tracts, 188
  fiber tractography, 186
  and HYDI, 187
  motivation and translation, 184–185
  and ODF, 186, 187
  presurgical imaging and tractography protocol
    acquisitions, 190–191
    clinical tool, 190
    fiber tractography, 191
    interactive data language, 191
    q-ball reconstruction, 191
    registered binary mask, 191–192
    surgical navigation system, 192
    work flow and communication, 190, 191
  q-ball reconstruction, 186–187
  requirements, 186
  spherical convolution, 187
High-grade glioma (HGG)
  EPISTAR tumor, 12
  LGG, 10
  and meningiomas, 12
  necrosis, 155
  neurosurgical resection, 150
  radiotherapeutic and neuro-navigational surgical techniques, 151
  temozolomide, 154
  therapeutic response, 14
High magnetic field
  pulse sequences, 200–202
  safety and physiological effects, 207
Hoffman, R.A., 172
Holodny, A.I., 88, 89
Huntington's disease (HD), 206
Hybrid diffusion imaging (HYDI), 187
Hybridization chain reaction (HCR), 228
HYDI. *See* Hybrid diffusion imaging (HYDI)

I

Image alignment, 219
Inoue, T., 30
Interstitial volume fraction (IVF)
  axial partitions, 223
  bioscales, 222, 223
  human brain, 214
  quantitative sodium MRI, 212
  tumor response, 213
  voxel volume, 213

Intraoperative mapping, fMRI
bilateral finger-tapping, 90, 91
Brainlab neuronavigation system, 90
direct cortical stimulation, 90
procedure, 90
real-time (rtfMRI), 90–91
surgical units, 90
visualizing fiber tracks, 90
Iron oxide nanoparticles, 232
IVF. *See* Interstitial volume fraction (IVF)

J
Jacobs, A.H., 134
Jakab, A., 34
Jones, C.K., 179

K
Karantanis, D., 137
Kesari, S., 226
Keupp, J., 179
Kober, H., 89, 122
Koga, T., 135
Korvenoja, A., 89
Kracht, L.W., 133
Krings, T., 88
Kumar, M., 31
Kuo, L., 186
Kwee, S.A., 134
Kwock, L., 145, 149

L
Lactate, 47–49
Language cortex, 82, 83
Language lateralization, 120–123
Lee, M.C., 15
Lipid-based nanoparticles
contrast agents, 233
liposomes, 234
micelles, 233
PFC, 233–234
structure, 233
Lipids, 46, 48
Low-grade glioma (LGG)
and HGG, 10
therapeutic response, 14
Lu, S., 32

M
Magalhaes, A., 145, 149
Magnetic resonance imaging (MRI)
Cho/Cr peak intensity ratios, 145
and FDOPA, 133–134
and FET, 133
frameless stereotactic neuro-navigation system, 158, 159
Gd-contrast enhancement, 143
intracranial lesions, 144
MET uptake, 134
molecular modalities, 231–232
pediatric tumors, 139
and RTOG, 151
Magnetic resonance spectroscopic imaging (MRSI)
brain pathology, 206–207
and CSD effects, 195
field dependence
ACC, 196, 199
glutamate (Glu), 196, 198
glutamine (Gln), 196, 198
human brain, 195
metabolite, 196
sagittal MRI, 196, 199
SNR, 195–196
spectra, 196, 197
strengths, field, 196
TE, 196, 197
7 T spectrum, 196
high magnetic fields, 207
magnetic field strengths (B_0), 195
pulse sequences (*see* Pulse sequences, MRS)
and SNR, 195
Magnetic resonance spectroscopy (MRS)
application, 145
3D MRS technique, 152
and FLAIR, 151
and HGG, 150
hypoxic/psuedopalisading tumor population
Cho and NAA levels, 155
Lip/Lac peak, 156, 157, 162
metstatic lesion, post-radiosurgery, 155, 161
infiltrative glioma population
Cho/Cr and Cho/NAA ratios, 158, 159
Cho/NAA levels, 157
ECM, 157
metabolic maps, 156
neurosurgical intervention, 159–160
tissue samples, 156
infiltrative Grade 4 Glioma, 152, 153
proliferative glioma population, 155
proton MRSI, 152
and RTOG, 151
Magnetic resonance spectroscopy imaging (MRSI)
anaplastic astrocytoma, 160
Cho and Cr, 163–164
Cho/Cr and Cho/NAA ratios, 158
Lip/Lac peak, 162
metastatic lesion, 161
noninvasive technique, 144
radiation necrosis, 160, 163
tumor infiltration, 156
Magnetic source imaging (MSI), 119–120
Magnetoencephalography (MEG)
applications, preoperative neurosurgery (*see* Preoperative neurosurgery)
BOLD signals, 111
brain sensing, 112
cortical functional measures and temporal changes, 111
diffusion MR tractography, 189

Magnetoencephalography (MEG) (*cont.*)
 and EEG, 111–112
 and fMRI activation, motor task, 89
 high resolution spatial and temporal cortical activity, 124, 126
 modalities, fMRI, 111
 primary motor gyrus, 89
 sensor data analysis (*see* Sensor data analysis, MEG)
 spatial resolution, 89
 temporal and spatial resolution, 117–118
Mandelli, M.L., 186
Mapping, 63, 64
Martin, A.J., 155
McKnight, T.R., 149, 155
Mean diffusivity (MD)
 FA and tumor cellularity, 30
 histogram analysis, 34
Measuring cell density
 ATP, 213
 brain tissue, 213
 CSF, 215
 ion homeostasis, 213
 ionic environment, brain, 213
 IVF (*see* Interstitial volume fraction (IVF))
 quantitative sodium imaging, 215
 spatial resolution, 214
 TD, 214
 TSC (*see* Tissue sodium concentration (TSC))
 in vivo and in vitro, 214
MEG. *See* Magnetoencephalography (MEG)
Meningioma
 FDG PET, 138
 MET uptake, 138
 SSTR2, 138–139
Metabolites
 choline, 39
 cyclic sugar alcohol, 41
 glutamate and glutamine, 41
 human brain, 39, 40
 2-hydroxyglutarate, 42
 NAA, 39
 post-radiation therapy, 42
 tumor necrosis, 41
Metal-based nanoparticles
 cellular and molecular imaging, 233
 contrast agents, 232
 EGFR, 233
 nanoshells, 233
 quantum dots, 233
Metastases, 12, 30–32, 35
L-[methyl-^{11}C]-methionine (MET)
 astrocytomas, 132–133
 and FDG, 134
 necrosis, 136
 radiation treatment planning, 135
MI. *See* Molecular imaging (MI)
Mil, S.J., 11
Miwa, K., 134
MNS. *See* Multinuclear spectroscopy package (MNS)
Molecular imaging (MI)
 and ADC, 225
 apparent diffusion coefficient (ADC), 225
 biochemical processes, living systems, 226
 central dogma, molecular biology, 226, 227
 diagnostic and therapeutic applications, 225, 226
 innovation, 226–227
 modalities
  CT and ultra sound, 232
  description, 230
  MRI, 231–232
  nuclear, 230
  optical and bioluminescence, 231
 nanoparticles (*see* Nanoparticles)
 regulation, 226
 targets
  antibodies, 228
  cell surface, 227–228
  compartmental probe, 228, 229
  DNA, 227
  drug delivery, 227
  genetic, 227
  identification and delivery, probes, 227–228
  mRNA and DNA, 228
  nanoparticle agent, 228, 229
  protein
 techniques, 225
 tools, 225, 226
Molecular probes
 cell-surface proteins, 227
 classifications, 228
 identification and delivery, 227–228
Moller-Hartmann, W., 145, 149
Monitoring treatment response, neoplasms
 antiangiogenic therapy, 15–16
 BBB disruption, 15
 delayed radiation necrosis, 14
 metastatic brain tumors, 14
 progression, 15
 pseudoprogression, 14–15
 pseudoresponse, 16
 radiation effects, 15
Motor cortex. *See* Sensory motor system, fMRI imaging
MRI. *See* Magnetic resonance imaging (MRI)
MR perfusion imaging
 adiabatic tissue homogeneity model, 7
 ASL, 8
 BBB, 5
 CBV, 8
 contrast agent leakage, 4–5
 DCE MRI acquisition time, 6
 DSC, 4
 GBCA, 6–7
 neoplasms, 13
 PKMs, 6
 primary glial neoplasms, 9–12
 signal intensity changes, 6
 tumor biology, 3
 T1W DCE sequence, 5

MRS. *See* Magnetic resonance spectroscopy (MRS)
MRSI. *See* Magnetic resonance spectroscopic imaging (MRSI)
MRS metabolic tumor population profiles, 155–156
MRS monitoring of tumor therapies, 160
MSI. *See* Magnetic source imaging (MSI)
Multinuclear spectroscopy package (MNS), 216
Murdoch, J.B., 197, 201

N
NAA. *See* *N*-acetyl aspartate (NAA)
Nabavi, A., 179
N-acetyl aspartate (NAA), 39
Nanoparticles
  agents, 232
  diagnostics and therapeutics imaging, 232
  iron oxide, 232
  lipid-based, 233–234
  metal-based, 232–233
  polymeric, 234
Narang, J., 14
Neoplasms
  biopsy guidance, 13
  lymphoma *vs.* glioma, 13
  meningioma, 13
  monitoring treatment response, 14–16
  solitary metastasis *vs.* glioma, 13
Neoplastic *vs.* non-neoplastic lesions
  diagnosis, 48
  diffusion and perfusion MRI, 49
  NAA, 48
Neurosurgery
  brain tumors
    diagnosis, 96
    maximal cyto-reduction, 96
    risk-benefit analysis, 96
    speech and motor deficits, 97
  magnetoencephalography (*see* Magnetoencephalography)
Nguyen, T.B., 10
Nuclear imaging, 230

O
ODF. *See* Orientation distribution function (ODF)
O-(2-^{18}Ffluoroethyl)-L-tyrosine (FET)
  and MRI, 133
  radiation and chemotherapy, 137
  stereotatic biopsies, 135
Ogawa, T., 132
Optical imaging, MI, 231
Orientation distribution function (ODF), 186, 187
Outer-volume suppression (OVS), 204
OVS. *See* Outer-volume suppression (OVS)
Ozsunar, Y., 14

P
Padma, M.V., 131
Patronas, N.J., 131
PCC. *See* Posterior cingulate cortex (PCC)
PCNSL. *See* Primary central nervous system lymphoma (PCNSL)
Peck, K.K., 83
Pediatric tumors, 139
Perfluorocarbon (PFC) nanoparticles, 233–234
Perfusion. *See* MR perfusion imaging
Permeability
  BBB, 15
  DRN, 14
  MR imaging, 6
PET/CT. *See* Positron emission tomography (PET)
Petrella, J.R., 85
PFC nanoparticles. *See* Perfluorocarbon (PFC) nanoparticles
Pharmacokinetic models (PKMs), 6
Piroth, M.D., 137
Pirotte, B.J., 134, 139
Pirzkall, A., 152
PKMs. *See* Pharmacokinetic models (PKMs)
Polymeric nanoparticles, 234
Positron emission tomography (PET)
  AAs, 130
  angiogenesis and hypoxia, 131
  cell surface receptor, 131
  cerebral cortex, 131
  choline, 130, 134
  cranial and paraspinal nerves, 139
  FDG, 130–132
  FDOPA, 133–134
  FMISO, 131
  glial tumors, 135
  hypoxia, 134
  intensive irradiation/chemotherapy, 136
  malignant tumors, 131
  measure tumor cell proliferation, 130
  meningioma, 137–139
  metastatic brain tumors, 139
  methionine, 130
  MET uptake, 134
  molecular imaging, 129
  neuroepithelial tumors, 131
  PCNSL and hematopoietic neoplasms, 137, 138
  pediatric tumors, 139
  PET/CT aim, 139
  photon energy, 129
  positron-emitting radionuclides, 129–130
  presurgical planning, 89–90
  quantitative imaging method, 129
  RT and RS, 135, 136
Posterior cingulate cortex (PCC), 206
Preoperative neurosurgery
  assessment, functional connectivity (*see* Functional connectivity, preoperative neurosurgery)
  epilepsy (*see* Epilepsy surgery)
  functional mapping, tumors, 120
  language laterality, 120–123
Presurgical (brain) mapping, 95, 97
Presurgical planning. *See* Blood oxygen level dependent functional magnetic resonance imaging (BOLD fMRI)

Price, S.J., 151
Primary Brain Tumors, 1H-MRSI. *See* Proton magnetic resonance spectroscopy imaging (1H-MRSI)
Primary central nervous system lymphoma (PCNSL), 137
Primary glial neoplasms
- CBF, 12–13
- cellularity and grade, 11
- DCE MR, 12
- EPISTAR, 12
- LGG and HGG, 10
- MR perfusion, glioma grading, 9–10
- rCBV, 9
- tumor grade, 9

Proton magnetic resonance spectroscopy imaging (1H-MRSI)
- astrocytoma and oligodendroglioma, 149, 150
- BBB, 143
- capability, MRI, 143
- Cho/Cr
  - and Myo/Cr, 145, 148
  - peak intensity ratios, 145, 149
- description, 143
- Gd-contrast enhancement, 143
- gliomas, 144–145
- 1H MRSI, 145
- MI/Cr ratio, 145
- MRS (*see* Magnetic resonance spectroscopy (MRS))
- MRSI (*see* Magnetic resonance spectroscopy imaging (MRSI))
- neurosurgical and radiotherapy treatment approaches, 144
- noninvasive technique, 144
- proton MRS spectral patterns, 148
- reduction, NAA and Cr, 145
- single voxel MRS technique, 145
- spectral profiles, 148
- surgical and radiotherapy (RT) tumor treatment plans, 144

Pruel, M.C., 148
Pseudoprogression (PsP), 14–15
Pseudoresponse, 16
Pujol, J., 85
Pulse sequences, MRS
- AFP pulses, 204, 205
- automated shimming routines, 197
- coupled spin systems, 205–206
- EPSI, 204
- high bandwidth slice, 203
- lipid suppression, 204
- mesial temporal lobe epilepsy, 204
- OVS, 204
- 3D-PRESS, 203
- RF coil design, 197
- single slice, 204, 205
- slice-selective, 204
- spatial dimensions, 202
- spectral resolution, 197
- 2D-STEAM, 203
- SVMRS (*see* Single voxel (SV))
- 7 T 2D-MRSI scan, 203
- transmit B_1 inhomogeneity, 197–198

Q

Quantitative sodium MRI
- applications
  - axial partitions, TSC, 221, 223
  - contrast-enhancing mass, 220
  - CT images, 220
  - frontal craniotomy, 221, 222
  - high-grade tumors, 221
  - oligoastrocytoma, 220
  - proton beam radiation treatment, 220, 221
  - TSC bioscales, 219–222
  - voxels, 220–222
- B0 homogeneity, 216
- brain imaging, 215
- CT images, 219
- developments, 9.4 Tesla
  - SNR, 222
  - spatial resolution, 222
  - TSC and IVF bioscales, 222
- flexTPI, 216, 217
- image blurring, 219
- k-space trajectory, 216, 217
- metabolic parameters, 215
- MNS, 216
- nuclear relaxation properties, 215
- phantoms, 217
- protons, 215
- RF coils, 216, 217
- SNR, 217–219
- spatial resolution, 217, 219
- transformations, 219
- TSC bioscale, 218, 219
- tumor response over time, 219

R

Radiation response
- IVF, 221
- surgical resection, 212
- TSC (*see* Tissue sodium concentration (TSC))
- voxels, 219, 221, 222

Radiation therapy (RT), 135–136
Radiation therapy oncology group (RTOG), 151
Radio-frequency (RF), 197, 216, 217
Radiosurgery (RS), 135–136
rCBV. *See* Regional cerebral blood volume (rCBV)
Real-time (rtfMRI), 90–91
Receptive paradigms
- hemispheric language, 67
- semantic encoding decision paradigm, 68
- word listening, 67–68

Regional cerebral blood volume (rCBV), 9
Reiche, W., 30
RF. *See* Radio-frequency (RF)
Ribom, D., 133
RS. *See* Radiosurgery (RS)
RT. *See* Radiation therapy (RT)
RTOG. *See* Radiation therapy oncology group (RTOG)

S

Sanchez-Panchuelo, R.M., 91
SAR. *See* Specific absorption rate (SAR)
Saur, D., 69
Semantic paradigms, 68
Sensor data analysis, MEG
  adaptive beamformers, 115
  auditory responses, 115–116
  Bayesian inference procedure, 115
  brain activity, 112
  Cartesian coordinate system, 113
  coregistration, 113
  description, forward-field matrix, 113
  Gaussian thermal and electrical noise, 117
  measurement system, 113
  outside head, source model, 112–113
  parametric dipole fitting, 113–114
  source localization, 117
  spontaneous brain activity, sensory/cognitive events, 116
  time-frequency analysis, adaptive spatial filters, 115, 116
  tomographic imaging, 114–115
  volume conductor, 113
Sensory motor system, fMRI imaging
  primary motor cortex
    extra-axial lesions, motor gyrus, 80, 82
    foot motor and SMA, 80, 84
    hand and tongue movements, 80, 83
    precentral gyrus, 80, 81
    reverse-omega sign, 80, 81
  secondary motor areas, 82
  SMA (*see* Supplementary motor area (SMA))
Signal-to-noise ratios (SNR)
  field strengths, 195, 196, 198
  MRS, 195, 196
  7 T spectrum, 196
Single voxel (SV)
  and ACC, 199, 202
  adiabatic RF pulses, 199–202
  bandwidth amplitude and frequency, 198, 201
  conventional pulse sequences, 198, 200
  and CSD effects, 198, 200, 201
  metabolite concentrations, 202
  and OVS, 202
  phase-cycling, 202
  pulse sequences, 199
  sagittal MRI, 199, 202
  and SAR, 198, 199
  short TE, 198, 199
  slice selective pulses, 198, 200
SNR. *See* Signal-to-noise ratios (SNR)
Sodium magnetic resonance imaging (Sodium MRI)
  anatomical imaging, 212
  interstitial volume fraction, 213
  intraoperative imaging, 211
  IVF (*see* Interstitial volume fraction (IVF))
  local tumor recurrence, 211, 212
  measuring cell density, 213–215
  prognosis, 211
  quantitative sodium (*see* Quantitative sodium MRI)
  surgical resection, 212
  treatment, brain tumors, 211
  TSC (*see* Tissue sodium concentration (TSC))
Sodium MRI. *See* Sodium magnetic resonance imaging (Sodium MRI)
Somatostatin receptor subtype 2 (SSTR2), 138–139
Source localization, MEG, 117
Specific absorption rate (SAR), 198, 199
SPIOs. *See* Supermagnetic iron oxide particles (SPIOs)
SQUIDs. *See* Superconducting quantum interference devices (SQUIDs)
SSTR2. *See* Somatostatin receptor subtype 2 (SSTR2)
Stadlbauer, A., 30, 135, 149, 158
Stall, B., 151
Superconducting quantum interference devices (SQUIDs), 112
Supermagnetic iron oxide particles (SPIOs), 232
Supplementary motor area (SMA)
  cortical compensation, 83
  and foot motor, 80, 84
  high-grade gliomas, 83–85
  language cortex, 82
  localization, 82, 84
  lower animals, 82
  planning and activation, 83
  pre-SMA, 82
Surgical planning. *See* Diffusion MR tractography, surgical planning
SV. *See* Single voxel (SV)

T

Tanaka, Y., 135
Taylor, J.S., 164
TD. *See* Tissue density (TD)
TE. *See* Echo times (TE)
7 Tesla
  ACC, 196
  brain pathology, 206–207
  MRSI, 203, 204
  pathological conditions, 195
  reproducibility, 202
  SNR, 196, 197
Tissue density (TD), 214
Tissue sodium concentration (TSC)
  axial partitions, 223
  bioscales, 219, 220, 222, 223
  human brain tissue, 214
  ion homeostasis, 213
  MR measurement, 214
  quantitative sodium MRI, 212
  voxels, 221, 222
Tozer, D.J., 34
Treatment planning and monitoring, brain tumors
  high-grade gliomas, 51
  proton MRSI measurements, Cho, 51
  pseudo-response, 51

TSC. *See* Tissue sodium concentration (TSC)
Tsien, R.D., 145
Tumor biology
  angiogenesis, 3
  glioblastomas, 3
Tumor cell density, 213–215
Tumor grading and diagnosis
  Cho values, 48
  high-grade brain tumors, 47
  metastatic lesions and glioblastomas, 48
Tumor infiltration
  FA and CP, 33
  glioblastomas and metastases, 32
  peritumoral region, 32
Tumors. *See* Brain tumors
Tzika, A.A., 163

U
Ultrasmall super-paramagnetic iron oxide particles (USPIOs), 232
USPIOs. *See* Ultrasmall super-paramagnetic iron oxide particles (USPIOs)

V
Van Laere, K., 136
van Westen, D., 12, 32

W
Wang, S., 30, 31, 172
Wang, W., 30, 33–35
Ward, K.M., 172
Warmuth, C., 12
Weber, D.C., 135
Weber, M.A., 14
Westin, C.F., 28
Wetzel, S.G., 16
White matter tract, 104, 183
Wilkinson, I.D., 85

Z
Zhang, K., 158
Zhang, S., 31
Zhou, J., 173, 177, 178
Zhu, H., 179

MIX
Papier aus verantwortungsvollen Quellen
Paper from responsible sources
FSC® C105338

If you have any concerns about our products,
you can contact us on
ProductSafety@springernature.com

In case Publisher is established outside the EU,
the EU authorized representative is:
Springer Nature Customer Service Center GmbH
Europaplatz 3, 69115 Heidelberg, Germany

Printed by Libri Plureos GmbH
in Hamburg, Germany